Praise for

THE PROTEIN BOOST DIET

"Clear, comprehensive, and incredibly useful . . . the best thyroid resource I have ever read."

—Kathleen DesMaisons, PhD, author of *Potatoes Not Prozac*

THE PROTEIN BOOST DIET

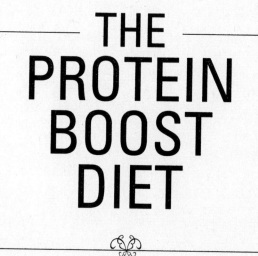

Improve Your Hormone Efficiency for a
Fast Metabolism and Weight Loss

RIDHA AREM, MD

Previously published as *The Thyroid Solution Diet*

ATRIA PAPERBACK

New York   London   Toronto   Sydney   New Delhi

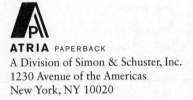

ATRIA PAPERBACK
A Division of Simon & Schuster, Inc.
1230 Avenue of the Americas
New York, NY 10020

First Atria Paperback edition January 2014
Previously published as *The Thyroid Solution Diet*

ATRIA PAPERBACK and colophon are trademarks of Simon & Schuster, Inc.

For information about special discounts for bulk purchases,
please contact Simon & Schuster Special Sales at
1-866-506-1949 or business@simonandschuster.com.

The Simon & Schuster Speakers Bureau can bring authors to your live event.
For more information or to book an event contact the Simon & Schuster Speakers
Bureau at 1-866-248-3049 or visit our website at www.simonspeakers.com.

Designed by Mspace/Maura Fadden Rosenthal

Manufactured in the United States of America

10 9 8 7 6 5 4 3 2 1

Library of Congress Cataloging-in-Publication Data is available.

ISBN 978-1-4516-9951-7
ISBN 978-1-4516-9952-4 (pbk)
ISBN 978-1-4516-9954-8 (ebook)

NOTE TO READERS

This publication contains the opinions and ideas of its author. It is intended to provide helpful and informative material on the subjects addressed in the publication. It is sold with the understanding that the author and publisher are not engaged in rendering medical, health, or any other kind of personal professional services in the book. The reader should consult his or her medical, health, or other competent professional before adopting any of the suggestions in this book or drawing inferences from it.

The case histories included in this book are based on the author's experience with his patients. Names and certain personal information have been changed.

The author and publisher specifically disclaim all responsibility for any liability, loss, or risk, personal or otherwise, that is incurred as a consequence, directly or indirectly, of the use and application of any of the contents of this book.

To all those who cherish and respect life,
a precious gift from God.
It is my hope that this book will inspire millions
of people to embrace the path of mind-body
balance for a healthy and happy life.

ACKNOWLEDGMENTS

Writing this book and putting my innovative weight-loss program in print would not have been possible without the help and support of so many wonderful people. First, I would like to thank the thousands of patients who taught me so much about challenges with weight loss and who gave me the opportunity to help. These patients have allowed me to refine my program over the years. Special thanks go to the patients who permitted me to share their struggles with weight in this book. Without the support and understanding of my wife, Noura, and my two sons, I would not have been able to write this book. Noura was instrumental in the design of the wonderful recipes, which are in line with the unique guidelines of my diet. The outcome of this tremendous work has been a compilation of delicious and healthy recipes that will help millions of people adhere to this diet. Special thanks also go to Paul Diedrich, an exercise expert, for helping me design, structure, and illustrate the resistance exercise portion of the 20/10 exercise program.

My deepest gratitude goes to Leslie Meredith, my editor at Atria, for her vision, her conviction that this book, like my first book, will benefit millions of people in the United States and throughout the world. I also thank her for the help, guidance, and thoroughness in editing and restructuring the manuscript. It was a joy and an enriching experience working with Heidi Hough, who did an outstanding job refining and editing the manuscript. Thank you to Jenn Garbee for her superb contribution editing and refining the recipes provided in this book. I also thank the team at Atria, in particular Donna Loffredo for her assistance and guidance and Suzanne Fass for her thorough copyediting. I thank my agent, Angela Rinaldi, for her help and guidance throughout the process of delivering the final version of the book. A special thanks also goes to Dr. Elizabeth Lee Vliet, sex hormone expert and author of *Screaming to Be Heard*, for reviewing the manuscript and giving me insightful advice. Finally, I want to thank Anne Marie Nguyen, Sara Jones-Burns, Melinda Huang, and Kimberly Garland for assisting me at various phases of this project and helping me with the preparation of the manuscript.

CONTENTS

CONTENTS

References are online at www.aremwellness.com.

THE
PROTEIN
BOOST
DIET

INTRODUCTION

Do You Have a Sluggish Metabolism? Revive It by Resetting Metabolism-Regulating Hormones

Do you want to lose weight? Have you tried diet after diet and yet the stubborn pounds remain? Regardless of why you gained weight, once you're wearing those extra pounds, your metabolism shifts gears, triggering multiple hormonal changes that perpetuate weight gain by making your body resistant to losing weight. The only way to lose weight is to rebalance your hormone systems, and the Protein Boost Diet is meticulously crafted to do just that.

As an endocrinologist with extensive experience in treating thyroid disorders, as well as other hormone and metabolic disorders, I've spent nearly thirty years caring for patients seeking to lose weight. Thyroid and weight issues go hand in hand, and my primary interest in thyroid disorders grew into a passion for designing the best weight-loss program for anyone with a weight challenge. The truth is, regardless of what made you start gaining weight, my program is effective because I designed it to speed up metabolism on a molecular level by reversing the multiple hormone problems that underlie any weight gain.

Several hormonal systems work in concert to regulate your eating behavior, energy balance, and body fat. But thyroid hormone is one of the most important key players. It is one of the master controllers of weight and the touchstone of metabolism. In fact, the other primary hormones that regulate your metabolism and weight—leptin and ghrelin—work *through* thyroid hormone. The Protein Boost Diet has been meticulously designed to make thyroid hormone and leptin more efficient at burning off fat. Over the years, the Protein Boost

Diet has helped hundreds of my thyroid patients boost their stubborn metabolisms. Because if your metabolism is low, you *will* have trouble losing weight.

The Protein Boost Diet has shown equally impressive results for people with normal thyroids who haven't been able to lose weight on other popular diets. For overweight people without thyroid problems, my diet rebalances the hormones that regulate metabolism and makes them more successful at burning off fat.

In other words, this book can help anyone trying to lose weight.

ARE YOUR HORMONES MAKING YOU FAT?

Ask yourself these questions: Are you always tired? Do you have dry skin and dry hair? Is your hair thinning? Are your hands and feet always cold? Do you have a lack of motivation or are you moody, anxious, irritable, or depressed? A thyroid imbalance could be causing any of these symptoms . . . and your weight gain, too. For decades, researchers knew that the thyroid, a butterfly-shaped gland at the front of the neck, governed metabolism, mood, body fat, brain function, and even hearing and vision. But the details on how thyroid hormone controls appetite, energy, and weight weren't clear until recently. Even if you haven't been diagnosed with a thyroid condition, or your doctor has told you your blood tests are normal, you might have a subclinical thyroid imbalance, meaning your blood tests are minimally abnormal or borderline. Many doctors ignore these small abnormalities, but losing weight with a borderline low thyroid condition is extremely difficult.

Other, different hormone imbalances, including growth hormone deficiency, can lower your energy and mood, decrease muscle, and increase fat. Does extra fat go right to your belly? Did your metabolism slow significantly as you transitioned into menopause or after you became menopausal? Do you have polycystic ovary syndrome (PCOS)? If you have any of these conditions, you no doubt have a sluggish metabolism and can find help in this book. Balancing hormone levels with hormone medications will give you the ingredients to succeed in losing weight, but that's not enough. You also need to follow a diet that will improve your hormone efficiency.

The Protein Boost Diet helps you rebalance hormone efficiency. It will help boost metabolism, tame cravings, energize your body, and improve mood naturally. You can lose weight and keep it off. You can outsmart aging, thyroid issues, menopause, and other hormone conditions that make you gain weight by embracing the Protein Boost Diet, the complete program for a happy mind and vigorous metabolism.

THE PROTEIN BOOST DIET WILL IMPROVE YOUR HORMONE EFFICIENCY FOR A SPEEDIER METABOLISM

When I started my career as a hormone and metabolism specialist, I quickly realized that one of the most challenging issues facing my patients was their struggle with weight gain and their inability to lose weight. Even those who lost weight by dieting often had a hard time keeping it off. Yet back then, I took a very narrow view of how to lose weight and I would give a generic response to my frustrated patients: "Eat less food; eat less fat and carbs; exercise more." My thinking, like that of many other physicians at the time, was that weight control was a matter of simple math—eat less and you'll lose weight; increase activity and you'll lose even more. In recent years, though, with new discoveries about the process of storing fat and how metabolism is regulated, it's become clear this advice was not the full answer.

Metabolism has to do with your body's complex system for processing and distributing the nutrients in food for use by your organs. Nutrients are converted—metabolized—into energy molecules that are dispersed throughout the body for three purposes: for energy so you can move and function, for generating heat by burning calories, or for storage as fat. When your body can efficiently convert energy molecules into heat, you burn calories instead of holding on to them and converting them to fat. If your system loses its efficiency, the distribution of energy then shifts toward fat storage, indicating a slow metabolism. Conversely, you can achieve heightened calorie burn—a speedy metabolism—by making your body produce more heat.

My program is based on the science that underlies the hormonal interactions that slow down metabolism and contribute to increasing weight gain. These hormone interactions can keep you from reaching your ideal weight and keeping the weight off. Most diet books don't even acknowledge the very real issues of metabolic slowdowns and the challenges people have in resetting their sluggish metabolisms. Nor do they guide you to eat foods that can energize your metabolism and abate food cravings, which I will do. I've perfected the Protein Boost Diet program over the past decade.

For years throughout my career I have been convinced that, besides balancing your hormones, addressing stress and accelerating metabolism are also crucial for successful weight loss. Extensive new research on metabolism and body fat, coupled with my experience in this field, prompted me to write this book. I've examined the effectiveness of the many diets available and found that the Mediterranean diet is the one that offers the most health and weight-loss benefits. But the generic Mediterranean diet, while effective, is not structured enough to completely reverse the multiple hormone imbalances that all overweight people have. So I've adapted the Mediterranean diet for the Protein Boost Diet eating plan so that it's low-glycemic (meaning it doesn't have a lot of carbohydrates that cause jumps in your blood sugar when digested), high-fiber, higher-protein, and low saturated fat. These properties make my unique diet the most efficient program for weight loss and optimal health.

The Protein Boost Diet is more than a simple meal plan to help you lose weight. It's a comprehensive program designed to restore your sluggish metabolism to its proper pace and allow it to respond normally to what you eat and don't eat. Following my plan can effectively break the vicious cycle of multiple hormone imbalances that are perpetuating your weight gain and weight-loss resistance. I'll also help you appreciate why your body behaves as it does—in other words, your physiology (which endocrinologists like me find fascinating)—and give you a prescription for reversing all this weight gain. My goal is for you to understand that treating your weight problem is as serious as treating a life-threatening medical condition.

ACTIVATING WEIGHT-LOSS HORMONES

Our biological clocks have a real say in when we get hungry and how fast our metabolism functions. So I use this information as the basis for the eating schedule I lay out for you as well as the food I advise you to eat—and not to eat—at each meal. Adjusting your diet and eating schedule are important for increasing your metabolism, yes, but so are sleep, reducing stress, finding out your food sensitivities, and identifying any toxic environmental factors that are triggering your weight gain. Once you discover and correct these and begin the meal plans and workouts I've devised, your weight will drop and the pounds that creep back on after most diets will not return.

THE PROTEIN BOOST DIET: AN INNOVATIVE, HIGH-PROTEIN DIET

An important pillar of The Protein Boost Diet is eating specific combinations of protein-rich foods throughout the day to deliver a complete spectrum of the amino acids—the building blocks of proteins—that boost energy-burning in your cells. These foods also enhance the action of the weight-loss hormones leptin and thyroid hormone in your body. We now know from scientific research that certain amino acids have the ability to activate the fat-burning process. For this reason, I designed the Protein Boost Diet to include at least two different protein sources at each meal to provide you with the most complete and well-balanced amino acid profile. The selection of specific proteins at each meal also aims at providing you with the amino acids that improve hunger, cravings, anxiety, and mood. The Protein Boost Diet is more than just a high-protein diet. I structured it so that it fulfills other important fundamentals such as eating an optimal amount of fiber and eating good fats rather than bad. Another pillar of my diet is reducing the sugar in your system, especially at certain times of the day, so you regain control over insulin, another hormone that affects weight. That's part of why I ask you to synchronize mealtimes with certain times of the day. For your weight-related hormones to function effectively, you must eat when your internal clock can best regulate your hormone levels and how you metabolize nutrients. No other diet program that I know of takes this meal timing seriously or helps you understand how you can do this.

Part of the Protein Boost Diet is an exercise program designed to supercharge the performance of thyroid hormone, growth hormone, insulin, and leptin, all of which help with weight loss. The exercise program, called "20/10," is a combination of twenty minutes of aerobic activity, including high-intensity intermittent sprints, and ten minutes of daily resistance exercises for toning your whole body and maximizing your weight loss. You will be amazed at the powerful effects that just half an hour of daily exercise has on your waistline. Here's a sneak preview. On the Protein Boost Diet, you'll . . .

- *Enjoy satisfying multiprotein combinations for each of your meals and daily menus.* These proteins contain exactly the right amino acid combinations for optimal efficiency of two powerhouse weight-loss hormones—leptin and thyroid hormone. Eating these selected proteins will also strengthen your production of growth hormone, a fat-burning, muscle-building all-star that gets recharged during dream sleep. When you increase leptin sensitivity, you lift thyroid activity—and your entire metabolism as a consequence.

- *Enjoy whole fruits and higher-glycemic carbs earlier in the day,* when you most need them to fuel activity. This timing also aligns with your body's natural ability to use up carbs with the help of insulin.

- *Clear your system of destructive sugar loads by eating fiber in every meal and snack,* to improve insulin efficiency and make you feel fuller.

- *Eat delicious, healthful fats (monounsaturated and polyunsaturated) and acquire the ability to burn fat.* Forget "fat-free." These fats can improve every aspect of your health from appetite, mood, and metabolism to cardiovascular vigor.

- *Eat very-low-glycemic foods at dinner* to keep insulin levels down while you sleep, so you aren't storing fat while dreaming of a trim body.

- *Reduce inflammation and oxidative stress* with the abundant antioxidants in recommended fruits, vegetables, herbs, spices, and supplements.

- *Detox* by sidestepping foods to which you're sensitive and by drinking my do-it-yourself Sensational Detox Smoothie (in Chapter 8).

My comprehensive plan should leave you looking better physically and feeling energetic. Let's get started by getting your hormones into balance.

PART ONE

HOW HORMONES MAKE US FAT

Unraveling the Mystery of Hormone Imbalance and Sluggish Metabolism

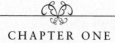

CHAPTER ONE

THE ROLE OF METABOLISM IN WEIGHT GAIN

Fat-Busting and Fat-Boosting Hormones

Getting your hormones into balance is the only way to lose weight in the long term.

Here's a common scenario: you're having dinner at a restaurant and you're served a basket of bread and butter. Before starting your meal, you eat fresh bread with a thin spread of butter. Most likely the bread isn't whole grain and is loaded with the carbohydrates that quickly turn to glucose (sugar) in your body. Immediately, your brain feels a surge of glucose that makes you want to eat more bread. As your stomach digests the butter, your body senses the saturated fat and makes you crave more animal fats. Restaurants probably know they're manipulating your hormones to make you hungrier with their complimentary bread and butter. By the time you order, chemicals in your brain cause you to crave even more quickly digested carbs and fat, and you probably end up ordering and eating more than you need or intend to eat. If you do this too often, your body learns to crave the foods that make you fatter, and loses its sensitivity to leptin, the hormone or chemical signaler that tells you that you've eaten enough. Along with your appetite, your waist size gradually grows as well.

For many years, experts thought losing weight was about eating less and exercising more. And yet the latest evidence shows it's not simply how much you eat but *the very foods you eat* that have an extraordinary impact on slowing your calorie-burning metabolism. A slow metabolism makes you pack on the pounds. Eating high-glycemic, processed foods like sugar, refined wheat bread, and other junk foods turns you into an insulin-generator. And the more insulin you have, the bigger your waistline, period. By the same token, foods like the ones in my meal plans can reverse weight gain and energize your metabolism so it burns more calories.

Hormone imbalances cause weight gain, and weight gain itself triggers abnormal levels and action of nearly every hormone involved in metabolism. This cascade of metabolic dysfunction and weight problems starts with a downgrade in the efficiency of the hormones involved in weight control, and in this chapter we'll review the major players.

Hormones are chemicals produced in your body by your tissues and endocrine glands that regulate the biological functions of many organs and tissues. If you're overweight, it's a virtual certainty that the most crucial hormones that regulate calorie burning—leptin and thyroid hormone—aren't functioning efficiently, meaning you become resistant to these master controllers of weight. "Resistant" means your body no longer hears or reacts to the beneficial signal of the hormone. My diet helps reverse this resistance. You need these helpful hormones to function properly so they offset the action of the hormones that make you fatter—cortisol and ghrelin. Once your body becomes resistant to the helpful weight-loss hormones, these unhelpful hormones escalate weight gain. Another beneficial and powerful player in revving up your calorie-burning metabolism is growth hormone (GH), which you want to maintain at high levels in order to stay youthful and lean.

YOUR METABOLISM'S DEFAULT STRESS RESPONSE: ADD FAT NOW

Think of your metabolism as a computer equipped with a complex and synchronized software system (your hormones) that reacts to anything that disturbs your mental or physical well-being. This system takes in a wealth of signals from the environment (your emotions, stress level, nutrition, and sleep quality), interprets them, and responds by *making your body accumulate fat*—essentially storing all those data. That's because your body is programmed to do one thing: survive when it senses a threat. When functioning properly, your hormone system maintains your weight in a near-constant range, responding as it should to the amount of calories you take in. It's a balanced design to prevent you from losing weight—the body's vital energy stores—during lean times and from accumulating too much fat when you overeat.

Under normal circumstances, our metabolic machinery adjusts itself constantly according to what we eat. In overweight and obese people, however, the body "misreads" its own energy balance, starting when fat-burning/fat-storing hormones get out of whack and make you hungry for the wrong foods, which cause blood sugar levels to skyrocket. That's the start of a real weight-gain trend, when appetite increases and you begin to store more fat. With fat-burning and fat-storing hormones out of balance, your brain soon stops relaying hormone signals to the power plants in your cells—the mitochondria—to generate energy to get rid of the unwanted weight. Once you start losing the activity of mitochondria, you burn fewer calories and your entire metabolism shifts into low gear, slowing everything down.

A perpetual cycle of these slowdowns leads to accumulating extra fat over time and not being able to lose it. Even if you weren't born with an underactive metabolism or with powerful overeating impulses designed to make you store more fat, your metabolism can become slower, sluggish, and underreactive in response to being "trained" by what, when, and how you eat. Metabolism can also decelerate in response to a wide range of environmental factors perceived by your system as threats to its very survival. We're constantly bombarded by internal and external hormone disruptors that seem to shape us into people with extra fat ready to survive.

TOO MUCH BODY FAT

Being overweight is a fast-spreading epidemic in our world, a shift toward obesity that's occurred in less than a single generation. Faced with centuries of threats of undernutrition—of *not enough* to eat— the human body's regulating mechanisms are biased toward fat preservation rather than fat elimination. Obesity in adults and children alike is directly responsible for devastating health problems and early death. In the United States, one-third of the adult population is obese and more than half of all Americans are overweight or obese. The trends are alarming: In 1994, seventeen states reported 15 to 19 percent of their population as obese, while all other states had a 10 to 14 percent obesity rate. In 2009, twelve states reported more than 30 percent of their population as obese, and in a majority of other states, 25 to 29 percent are obese. If this trend continues, fully half of the US population will be obese by 2020.

And yet you can't say that we're unwilling to try to lose weight—American adults spend more than $50 billion a year on weight-loss efforts (many of dubious quality, however). But the abundance of readily available government-supported, cheap, nonnutritious food—much of it processed and high in calories—and our sedentary lifestyle keep us fat.

ARE YOU OVERWEIGHT OR OBESE?

Many people are overweight and not even aware of it. This issue of skewed self-perception becomes clearer if you look at movies and TV shows from thirty years ago. The "fat kid" appears average compared with children today and many of the adults seem very skinny. In fact, most overweight people view their body weight as "about right," "appropriate," or "acceptable," with 82 percent underestimating their actual weight. If you're overweight and you don't perceive it, you're more likely to smoke, eat an unhealthy diet, and be physically inactive. Clearly if you don't consider yourself to be overweight or obese, you're less likely to make the changes necessary to improve your weight and overall health. So get out a tape measure and let's get started.

There are several ways to evaluate body fat. My favorite methods are waist circumference, waist-to-hip ratio, and waist-to-height ratio. Body mass index (BMI), based on weight and height, has some drawbacks as you'll see below, but it's helpful in giving you a rough idea of body fat. It's also a good indicator of the health risks related to how overweight you are.

- *Waist Circumference:* Wrap a tape measure around the narrowest part of your waist, just above your navel. This is waist circumference. Measurements greater than 35 inches in women and 40 inches in men are directly linked to a high risk of metabolic disorders such as diabetes. Waist circumference is related to visceral fat, which collects at your belly and around vital internal organs. It's an indicator of internal inflammation that damages your metabolism's ability to process fats and sugars. Having a waist circumference in the high zone points to insulin resistance, cholesterol problems, high blood pressure, and increased risk for diabetes, stroke, and heart disease.

- *Waist-to-Hip Ratio:* Standing with your feet together, wrap the tape measure around the widest part of your buttocks. This is your hip measurement. To obtain waist-to-hip ratio, take your waist circumference and divide it by your hip measurement. For example, one of my patients, Sarah, came to my office with a waist circumference of 45 inches and a hip measurement of 50 inches: 45 divided by 50 makes her ratio .90. A waist-to-hip ratio of more than 1.0 in men and more than .85 in women indicates abdominal fat accumulation. This visceral fat increases your risk for type 2 diabetes, stroke, and heart disease.

- *Waist-to-Height Ratio:* Calculating waist-to-height ratio involves the same math, except you divide your waist circumference by your height in inches. Returning to Sarah, who is five feet, six inches (66 inches), we divide her waist measurement of 45 inches by 66 to get a ratio of .68. A waist-to-height ratio over .50 indicates you are likely to be obese. A ratio more than .60 makes you very likely to be obese.

- *BMI:* Body mass index (BMI), based on your weight and height, estimates whether you have too much body fat. BMI charts place you in an underweight, normal weight, overweight, or obese category compared with other people in general. To calculate your BMI, Google "calculate BMI" and look for the National Heart, Lung, and Blood Institute (NHLBI) calculator, which will ask for your height and weight and then quickly do the math for you. A BMI between 18.5 and 24.9 is considered normal. You're overweight if your BMI is between 25 and 29, obese if your BMI is higher than 30. For example, a five-foot, nine-inch man weighing more than 169 pounds is considered overweight, and a five-foot, four-inch woman who weighs 145 pounds is also considered overweight. In "Weigh In and Measure" in Chapter 9, I show you how to use a BMI chart to identify your ideal weight and weight-loss goal.

BMI can be misleading because it measures weight instead of body fat and ignores where you carry fat on your body—such as the risky visceral fat around your waistline. It also doesn't distinguish between the weight of muscle and the weight of fat. If you're an athlete or bodybuilder, or if you don't have much muscle, BMI may not be the best way to tell whether you're carrying too much fat. People who have lots of nice lean muscle and very little body fat can seem to fall into the overweight or obese range while actually being in peak physical condition. Also, Asians are in general 3.5 percent leaner than Caucasians, so if you're Asian you may be overweight and have too much fat even though your BMI is apparently within a healthy range.

THE HORMONE TRIANGLE

Your weight is determined by the calories you eat and how much body fat you have—as well as the calories you burn when you're active and how many you burn when you're sitting (your resting metabolic rate). To keep your weight stable, a control center in your brain—the hypothalamus—acts as your body's main energy balance monitor. Other sites in your brain, stomach, and fat tissue contribute to the balancing act. Some hormones, such as leptin, ghrelin, and thyroid hormone, regulate long-term weight balance. Let's review them here so you know what you're dealing with.

LEPTIN: YOUR POWERFUL METABOLISM- AND HUNGER-CONTROLLING FRIEND

Leptin's job is to make you limit food intake and speed up metabolism to burn extra fat. It accomplishes this by telling your brain and body how much fat you're carrying. This hormone, produced by fat tissue itself, is one of the primary players in maintaining a stable body–fat balance. Women have two to three times the leptin of men because women tend to have more body fat generally, especially under the skin, and this subcutaneous fat produces much more leptin than visceral abdominal fat.

Leptin's paradox is plain to see. The more fat you have, the more leptin your body produces in an effort to reduce fat stores. This sounds like a good thing—more leptin to help burn fat—but there's a catch. Even though all that body fat is churning out leptin to make you get rid of fat, you don't lose weight because the fat you already have causes leptin to work less efficiently. This is leptin resistance. Put simply, when you're overweight or obese, leptin loses its ability to suppress your appetite and speed up metabolism. As you gain weight—or if you already have leptin resistance for other reasons such as thyroid imbalance or growth hormone deficiency—leptin levels become higher than normal, even though it's not doing its job. Chronically high levels of leptin make the hormone even less efficient, perpetuating a cycle of weight gain and slow metabolism. This is why it's so easy to start on a cycle of continuous weight gain once you start gaining weight. Leptin resistance leads to a higher level of leptin resistance, and the cycle continues.

Fasting or severely limiting calorie intake isn't the way to achieve weight loss, because when you eliminate food or drastically lower your intake, your leptin levels plummet. You won't lose fat at the same rate you're losing weight-loss-friendly leptin. A dramatic drop in leptin occurs during calorie restriction and will make you lose control over your appetite (remember, leptin decreases appetite) even as it slows your metabolism to make you burn far less fat.

Falling leptin levels as a result of calorie restriction also drive down levels of other metabolism-energizing hormones, including your sex hormones, thyroid hormone, and growth hormone. Calorie restriction is a virtually impossible means of losing weight in the long run because it throws all the other relevant hormonal reactions out of sync. For long-term success in losing weight and keeping it off, instead of severely restricting calories, you want to focus on eating foods that help leptin work at peak efficiency in your body. This is how the Protein Boost Diet helps reshape your hormone balance. You'll be reducing calorie intake, your body fat will start to drop, and your leptin levels will fall ... without making you hungrier. Leptin: your appetite-reducing, fat-burning friend.

When you're trying to lose weight, your goal is not to increase leptin but rather to make it work more effectively. (Interestingly, injecting overweight or obese people with leptin has proved ineffective for weight loss. However, once you've lost weight, leptin treatment may prevent you from regaining the fat you've lost.)

The key focus in losing weight and keeping it off is to counteract leptin resistance in the brain. As a result, your ferocious appetite will gradually subside and you'll burn more calories. High-fat diets encourage leptin resistance, and reducing bad dietary fat restores normal leptin efficiency in the brain. By eating a moderate amount of good fat, you'll cut calorie intake without becoming unnecessarily hungry, and you'll lose body fat as a result. Your leptin levels will gradually fall without making you hungrier. Eating protein also makes leptin more efficient, suppressing appetite and revving up your calorie-burning metabolism. Protein variety and reducing bad fats—both central to my program—will help your leptin work even better so you'll have even less hunger.

GHRELIN: YOUR WEIGHT ENEMY

Ghrelin is another powerful hormone, but this one stimulates appetite and slows your calorie-burning metabolism. It's produced primarily in your stomach, and also in small amounts in the pituitary gland, pancreas, brain, and testicles. Ghrelin levels automatically rise before a meal, signaling you to eat. Levels decline when you've eaten enough, and the decline prompts you to stop eating when ghrelin sends the "I'm full" signal, sixty to ninety minutes after eating. High amounts of ghrelin not only make you feel as though you're starving, they also slow metabolism and make your body hold on to fat. High ghrelin levels slow the activity of thyroid hormone, and—as you'll see in the next section—that's a recipe for weight gain. If you try to lose weight by just eating less, your ghrelin will stay high, making you constantly hungry and tempted to eat.

Ghrelin encourages the proliferation of fat cells, keeping them healthy and allowing them to hold on to all their fat. In fact, ghrelin discourages your body from burning fat. It's also partly responsible for fat storage, weight gain, and obesity. (Insulin, another hormone, has a role to play, too, as you'll soon see.) Injecting lab rats and humans with ghrelin rapidly stimulates hunger and food intake. When people lose weight as a result of an illness like cancer, ghrelin levels zoom upward in response to the body's call to preserve its remaining, life-sustaining body fat. Ghrelin is the hormone that makes it very difficult for you to keep off weight that you lose. Ghrelin makes you feel hungry and pushes you to select high-calorie foods over low-calorie choices.

In my view, the reason the procedure called roux-en-Y gastric bypass (RYGB) is the most long-term-effective bariatric surgery is that it removes the pouch in the lower stomach called the fundus, where ghrelin is produced. Without the fundus, you're far less hungry, and having less ghrelin in your system helps speed your metabolism. Obese people with non-insulin-dependent diabetes experience spectacular improvement in their blood sugar levels after this surgery, with many no longer requiring diabetes medication. Other remarkable benefits include lower cholesterol and triglyceride levels. However, there are ways to reduce ghrelin's effects on your body and behavior even without this surgery.

THYROID HORMONE: YOUR METABOLISM'S VIP

Your mind and body operate through the intricate thyroid hormone network to regulate most physiological functions, including weight. The two most powerful hormones regulating metabolism, leptin and ghrelin, are themselves regulated by thyroid hormone—and at the same time work through thyroid hormone. Clearly, your long-term weight loss depends on reestablishing harmony among these three hormone systems. Thyroid hormone is as essential and influential in regulating appetite and metabolism as leptin and ghrelin. Without an optimal balance of thyroid hormone in your body and brain, you simply cannot achieve or maintain a normal weight.

Here's how it works: Your brain's almond-sized hypothalamus— a powerful little gland that's also in charge of body temperature, feelings of fullness, mood, and emotions—prompts your thyroid gland to produce the right amounts of thyroid hormones T4 and T3 by sending signals to the thyroid via the pituitary, the master gland. T4 (thyroxine) moves throughout your body via your bloodstream.

T3 (triiodothyronine) is produced by the thyroid and other organs by converting T4 to T3 through the loss of an iodine atom. Throughout the book whenever I use the term "thyroid hormone," I am referring to both T4 and T3, the two biologically active forms of thyroid hormone. T3 is the most biologically active form of thyroid hormone and wields the power to help you lose weight by interacting with leptin and ghrelin, increasing energy burn and altering mood and appetite.

Thyroid hormone directly affects appetite centers of the hypothalamus, your food choices, and fat burn. It also affects leptin, ghrelin, growth hormone, and almost all chemicals involved in regulating metabolism.

The intimate relationship between leptin and thyroid hormones is amazing. First, leptin promotes thyroid growth and thyroid hormone production. Leptin signals the hypothalamus to send a message to the pituitary to tell your thyroid to produce the right amount of hormone needed for ideal metabolism. Without leptin, or when leptin is inefficient, the communication between your hypothalamus, pituitary, and thyroid gland fails to produce the right amount of hormones. Leptin also tells the cells in your body to convert enough T4 to T3. When leptin signaling isn't at its best, thyroid hormone becomes less efficient in your cells and your body burns even less energy and fat.

Essentially, leptin is the messenger that triggers your metabolism, while thyroid hormone kicks up metabolic activity by spurring thermogenesis (heat production) in cells, helping you burn more calories. Bottom line: you want a highly functional leptin signaling system so your body gets more T3, which energizes you and gives you that calorie-burning efficiency.

Just as leptin affects the thyroid, however, thyroid hormone itself affects leptin levels and leptin efficiency. Leptin requires thyroid hormone to carry out its healthy metabolizing, energy-producing, fat-burning benefits. If your T3 is low, leptin won't efficiently spark your metabolism. Low levels of thyroid hormones can be caused by a disorder of the hypothalamus or pituitary or a thyroid gland that isn't producing enough thyroid hormone (hypothyroidism, or low thyroid). Even low-grade hypothyroidism affects how well leptin works, and low thyroid always puts the brakes on metabolism and makes you gain weight.

Low thyroid hormone activity can also be caused by what's called "tissue hypothyroidism," the result of poor conversion of T4 to T3 in your body due to leptin resistance, a lack of essential micronutrients (such as selenium or zinc), too much of the stress hormone cortisol, or thyroid hormone resistance related to defective or reduced thyroid hormone receptor activity in the cells. Thyroid hormone resistance and thyroid hormone inefficiency will promote leptin resistance, resulting in a sluggish metabolism and weight gain.

As you can see, an imbalance of leptin–thyroid hormones is centrally involved in weight gain. Until balance is restored, you won't be able to boost your metabolism enough to lose the extra weight and keep it off. The Protein Boost Diet is designed to help you reestablish that balance.

The foods in my meal plans include a variety of specific protein combinations that provide the nutrients needed to help improve thyroid hormone levels and efficiency in the tissues. They're also effective in balancing sex hormones as well as the other weight-related hormones (cortisol, growth hormone, and ghrelin) and in improving leptin signaling.

Thyroid hormone also has a profound effect on hunger–hormone ghrelin levels. Low thyroid causes ghrelin to rise, making you hungrier and slowing metabolism even further. Happily, restoring thyroid hormone to correct levels causes ghrelin levels to drop.

Here's yet another factor that illustrates how thyroid hormone is the VIP of metabolism: well-balanced thyroid hormones have a significant effect on mitochondria—your cells' power plants—where molecules are converted into body heat. Thyroid hormone directly activates the heat burning of mitochondrial proteins that help regulate body temperature and metabolism. If you have low thyroid levels or leptin inefficiency, the energy-burning effect of these proteins slows down, and you'll end up with a sluggish calorie burn, and the extra calories are stored as fat tissue. Amazingly, thyroid hormone has the ability to convert fat cells into calorie-burning, heat-producing cells. Even leptin cannot produce this effect without thyroid hormone. *The Protein Boost Diet in its entirety aims to energize mitochondria so you'll burn more calories and store less unwanted fat.*

Thyroid hormones have a key regulating effect on abdominal obesity, insulin sensitivity, heart function, cholesterol levels, and blood pressure. Your mental well-being depends on healthy thyroid hor-

mone levels because thyroid hormones affect how much you have
of several key neurotransmitters (brain chemicals) involved in regulating appetite, feelings of fullness, cravings, food choices, and taste.
Abnormal thyroid hormone levels in your body and brain will drive
down levels of all of them. You simply cannot be successful in long-
term weight loss without balancing the hormone triangle of fat storage: leptin, ghrelin, and thyroid hormone.

Thyroid hormone is the touchstone of your metabolism regula-
tion: the ultimate energizer of metabolism through which the entire
hormonal system works to maintain optimal energy balance.

This diagram shows how your hormones and the food you eat
affect metabolism and appetite, and in turn how your metabolism
affects your hormones and the food you eat. The hypothalamus is
in charge of activating the autonomic nervous system and regulating
many of the hormones involved in metabolism. The hormones leptin,
ghrelin, and thyroid hormone work on the mitochondria to either
enhance calorie burning and heat production (leptin and thyroid
hormone) or slow heat production, which slows metabolism (ghrelin). Foods rich in certain amino acids also energize mitochondria
to produce more heat and burn more calories. The heat generated is

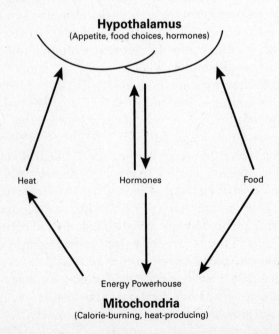

sensed by the hypothalamus, which prompts you to eat less. Specific foods (certain proteins, different fats) also affect the hypothalamus, either making you feel full or increasing appetite. The hypothalamus affects levels of thyroid hormone, growth hormone, and cortisol, and in turn leptin, ghrelin, cortisol, and thyroid hormone affect the hypothalamus, which has a say in appetite and food choices.

It's worth noting again that if you're trying to lose weight solely by cutting many calories, thyroid hormone will work against you, slamming the brakes on your metabolism. Starvation and calorie restriction lower both thyroid hormone and leptin, causing your mitochondria to burn fewer calories and generate less heat. After all, your body is trying to preserve your life—why would it burn up your energy stores?

Why the Protein Boost Diet Will Help Boost Your Metabolism

The Protein Boost Diet enhances thyroid hormone activity, lowers ghrelin levels and activity, and boosts leptin sensitivity to revive metabolism.

- Protein combinations nourish the body for optimal calorie-burning efficiency, so your body stores less fat and burns more energy.
- Specific food selections at each meal diversify protein consumption to enhance efficiency of leptin and thyroid hormone. The food also acts in your brain and gut to give you feelings of fullness rather than hunger.
- Fiber-rich foods eaten at every meal lower levels of the hunger hormone ghrelin to prevent hunger pangs.

TOO MUCH INSULIN = TOO MUCH FAT

Insulin is one of your body's most important regulators of sugar and fat. Here's how it works.

- After you eat, glucose (the by-product of all sugars) enters your bloodstream and signals your pancreas to release insulin.
- Your pancreas is animated by your cellular clock (see "Your Cellular Clock: *When* to Eat *What*" in Chapter 5) to most optimally respond to sugar at specific times of the day. If you eat a high load of sugar at the wrong time, the amount of

glucose in your blood is too much for the amount of insulin released to process it. Over time, this weakens insulin efficiency and your metabolism.

Insulin's role is to "unlock" cells so glucose can get into liver, muscle, and fat tissue and be used to power your body. If you eat too much sugar or refined carbohydrates (which act like sugar in your body), all the glucose not processed by your liver and muscles will be converted into fat. Insulin is key in storing away excess glucose—processing it into fat molecules and putting it into fat cells.

- With too much sugar in your system, your body loses sensitivity to insulin; your liver and muscles cannot recognize insulin and allow it into their cells to process glucose. As a result, glucose is stored as fat, mostly packed into your abdomen as dangerous visceral fat.

- When the liver and muscles can't process glucose, blood sugar levels rise, making your pancreas produce more insulin. The result: too much insulin floating in your system, working on fat cells to convert sugar into fat.

- All this extra fat generates damaging inflammation, which makes insulin resistance worse.

Insulin is nicknamed "the fat-storing hormone" for a reason. You need some sugar and insulin, but you don't need any extra.

DRIVING DOWN INSULIN LEVELS AND KEEPING THEM LOW ARE KEY OBJECTIVES IN LOSING WEIGHT

Your food choices have a dramatic impact on insulin levels. For example, the more refined carbohydrates you eat (most breads, all sweets and crackers, virtually all processed foods), the more insulin you'll have. Too much sugar and too much insulin in your system cause you to pack on the fat. As you gain weight, your liver and muscles become unable to respond appropriately to insulin, or resistant to it; and the more insulin-resistant you become, the more weight you gain.

Weight gain in turn causes you to become depleted of adiponectin, a hormone that tells your body to burn fat for fuel. The more fat you have, the lower your levels of adiponectin—not good, since adiponectin has multiple benefits: reducing inflammation, bolstering the immune system, protecting your heart and blood vessels, and making insulin work efficiently. This is one of the reasons why with weight gain you become more insulin-resistant and prone to cardiovascular disease. Low levels of adiponectin contribute to diabetes and cardiovascular disease.

The ultimate consequence of your blood sugar imbalance is not only weight gain from stored fat but also bodywide inflammation, which infiltrates your liver and muscles with fat and makes them resistant to insulin. The more your glucose levels rise, the more inflammation you'll have, pushing your metabolism into a downward spiral of inefficiency.

Inflammation also generates leptin resistance and affects the hypothalamus, your body's appetite control center and energy balance monitor.

FOODS LOADED WITH FAT AND SUGAR CAN INFLAME AND DAMAGE THE APPETITE-REGULATING AREAS OF THE HYPOTHALAMUS—THE ONES THAT SHAPE YOUR FOOD CHOICES

Significant weight gain and obesity are common symptoms in people suffering from hypothalamic disorders such as a tumor, inflammation, or a destructive condition such as surgery or radiation. When you lace your diet with too many simple sugars and bad fats, you make your body and brain respond less effectively to leptin. When you are leptin resistant, you burn off fewer calories even as you consume more. Adding to the melee, when you're leptin resistant your body begins to crave fatty foods.

Leptin resistance hinders your body's ability to recognize how much fat it has stored. Inflammation in the hypothalamus makes it unable to sense leptin, making you hungry so you eat more. In an experiment on rats eating a high-fat diet, inflammation in the crucial hypothalamic areas involved in regulating fullness occurred within twenty-four hours. After sixteen weeks on the high-fat diet, cell death in these areas increased—the cells that normally suppress appetite were working at just 80 percent of their normal effectiveness. Too much glucose and fat set off a vicious cycle of inflammation and resistance to both insulin and leptin. Insulin resistance and leptin resistance work together to escalate and perpetuate the weight-gain trend.

THE PROTEIN BOOST DIET HELPS DRIVE DOWN INSULIN

My meal plans are designed to limit glucose and insulin overload . . . and thus fat storage. You'll eat low-carb, low-glycemic meals rich in fiber and protein that minimize glucose surges and naturally lower insulin levels so you'll store less fat. Scheduling meals to coincide with peak insulin response to sugar is part of it. At night, you want the lowest blood sugar and insulin levels to shift metabolic activity from storing fat to burning calories while you sleep.

My diet also lowers inflammation by providing the antioxidants you need to improve insulin sensitivity and leptin and thyroid hormone efficiency.

INSULIN AND METABOLIC SYNDROME

With too much extra body fat, insulin loses its ability to work efficiently, and your insulin levels become higher than normal. This resistance to insulin also opens the door to a disorder called "metabolic syndrome." Indications that you may have metabolic syndrome include visible excessive fat around the abdomen and waist, high BMI, high blood pressure, abnormal blood sugar levels, high cholesterol, and high levels of triglyceride fats. If this describes you, you're also likely to have inflammation in your organs, fat accumulation in your liver (fatty liver), and a high level of oxidative stress (see "Antioxidants Protect Your Body from Oxidative Stress" in Chapter 8). Metabolic syndrome can ultimately lead to type 2 diabetes, cardiovascular disease, and stroke. High blood sugar from insulin resistance triggers your pancreas to release more insulin in an effort to return blood sugar to normal levels, but the pancreas can't continue this process indefinitely—it becomes exhausted. As insulin resistance worsens, the pancreas becomes inflamed and damaged and starts to fail from overuse. As the damage continues, the amount of glucose circulating in the blood continues to rise. This is diabetes, which has awful health consequences, including eye and nerve damage, infection and limb amputation, kidney damage, heart attack, and stroke.

In order to halt your weight gain trend and the further deterioration of your metabolism, you must stop the progression of insulin resistance. Following the Protein Boost Diet helps insulin work more efficiently, reduces inflammation, and reverses the toxic effects of glucose loading in your system. Addressing insulin resistance and losing your extra fat will help prevent the progression of metabolic syndrome to diabetes. In fact, this program can help you reverse both conditions.

Health Effects of Too Much Weight

Metabolic syndrome and diabetes aren't the only consequences of being overweight or obese. You're also more likely to have

- High blood pressure

- Decreased breathing capacity of the lungs caused by more pressure on the diaphragm from too much abdominal fat

- Sleep apnea (see Chapter 5)

- Pseudotumor cerebri, a condition related to a poorly understood increase of pressure inside the head that causes nausea, dizziness, and vision problems—symptoms similar to those of a brain tumor but without any tumor. It affects more women than men

- GERD (gastroesophageal reflux disorder), often related to increased pressure on the stomach caused by excessive abdominal fat

- Pregnancy complications: gestational diabetes, high blood pressure, congenital malformations of the newborn, increased risk of fetal death

- Urinary incontinence, often related to increased pressure on the bladder by abdominal contents

- Fatty liver, related to impaired fat clearance by the liver

- Depression (lowered self-esteem and serotonin levels)

- Cancers of the breast, ovaries, and prostate, related to excessive oxidative stress and genetic damage caused by free radicals

- Osteoarthritis in hips and knees, often related to damage of weight-bearing joints from excess weight

THE HYPOTHALAMUS AND BRAIN,
UNDER STRESS, ADD BODY FAT

As it regulates your metabolism, the hypothalamus constantly takes in signals from the environment and from your own behavior and state of mind. Stress, chronic illness, and infection are transmitted in a nanosecond to the hypothalamus, which triggers hormonal responses that cause you to store calories as fat, a form of energy ready to counterattack threats to your well-being when needed.

Chemicals and hormones produced in your gastrointestinal tract (such as ghrelin) and in fat tissue (such as leptin) also provide the hypothalamus with data about the food you eat (how it tastes, what food is available around you) and about how much body fat you have. Each distinct area of the hypothalamus actually "talks" to the others to make certain you're carrying enough calories for survival, and produces chemicals that directly affect your food choices and feelings of fullness. Your hypothalamus can also either speed up metabolism to burn calories or slow it down to conserve that fat. The willpower you need to break bad eating habits is no match for your hypothalamus's supremacy over appetite. Bottom line: unless you keep your hypothalamus healthy and stop sending it signs that it perceives as threats to your survival (stress, lack of sleep, hunger), you cannot stop your body from storing fat or stop your urges to eat fast and often.

WHY YOU BINGE WHEN YOU'RE FEELING STRESSED

Powerful signals from the hypothalamus can make you choose a candy bar because the sugar in it activates the pleasure center in the brain. Just like drugs, fattening foods can be addicting, and they affect the brain similarly via the pleasant yet potentially perilous hormone dopamine. You can see that, in order to lose weight and keep it off, you need to keep your hypothalamus healthy and to control the signals it receives. Once the areas in the hypothalamus that sense hunger-controlling leptin become inflamed or damaged, your feelings of fullness will be lessened and you'll end up eating more and choosing the bad fats that will make you fatter. Amazing.

By working with your hormones through the Protein Boost Diet and by working to reduce stress and boost your fat burning, you'll help keep your hypothalamus happy and in turn keep your hormones in balance so you can lose weight.

HOW TO ENHANCE THE POWER OF YOUR METABOLISM

Losing weight can be tough compared with how easily you gained it. When your metabolism slows down, your body stubbornly retains its weight regardless of your efforts to limit calories or change your lifestyle. Simply consuming fewer calories and burning off more won't help you lose weight and keep it off, because your extremely resilient hormone network is programmed to hold on to the fat.

Hormone imbalance initiates and perpetuates the vicious cycle of retaining weight. Eating foods high in sugar or fat causes your body to develop a resistance to the hormones that break them down and the result is a body with high levels of blood glucose (sugar) and the inability to metabolize it. Your system interprets glucose loading—eating high-glycemic foods such as sugar and most refined carbohydrates—as yet another signal that you're trying to accumulate fat to survive a threat of starvation. Your metabolism responds by burning fewer calories and conservation of fat. Eating these foods triggers a multihormone disorder that impels you to eat more of the same fattening foods and gain weight.

To halt this vicious cycle and regain your metabolism's momentum, you need to eat the foods that will support maximum metabolic efficiency. The key to losing weight and keeping it off is preventing/correcting hormonal resistance by eating a diet designed to maintain a healthy metabolism. An absolute necessity is to avoid quickly digested carbohydrates (including sugar, refined grains, high amounts of any carbohydrate, and virtually all processed foods) and bad animal fats (such as red meats, full-fat cheeses, and butter). A diet rich in fiber, a variety of proteins, good fats, and complex carbohydrates will free your body of these deleterious setbacks.

Most diets don't require you to eat foods in a specific order, but you can reshape your metabolism by eating certain foods first, such as protein- and fiber-rich sources, significantly reducing the early sugar load you get from eating foods like bread while taking in balanced blends of high-quality proteins to control your ferocious hunger and boost your metabolism. My diet will help reset your metabolism for the long term to reestablish a new energy balance and make your system feel at ease.

CHAPTER TWO

WHAT SLOWED YOUR METABOLISM AND CAUSED YOUR WEIGHT GAIN?

The Role of Your Genes, Your Parents, and Environmental Toxins

The human body can survive for several weeks without food, testament to its ability to store fat in the face of perceived emergency. But this same ability to hold on to fat also makes it difficult to lose weight. An abundance of junk food and a sedentary lifestyle upset your hormone balance, and apparently innocuous behaviors (which we'll discuss in this chapter) can alter hormonal balance too. Your body responds by storing more fat. There are also hidden chemicals in the environment in which we live that make us fat; our world is filled with obesogens, chemical hormone disruptors that boost fat cell production, slow metabolism, and change the way hormones manage appetite. Your genes and the environment in which you grew up also play a role in your weight gain. In a perfect world, the percentage of body fat we carry would be roughly the same for all people, with women having more body fat than men. But many factors are working against us.

HOW A WEIGHT-GAIN TREND BEGINS

You gain weight when your sensitive, complex metabolism registers a threat and responds by storing fat. Your metabolism responds to any threat—junk food, fatigue, illness, stress—by slowing way down to limit the calories it burns. It's kicking into defense mode, storing energy (as fat) for the future. This same sequence occurs when you severely restrict food intake. Your metabolism senses this powerful starvation signal and it becomes sluggish in order to conserve energy. "We might need that fat later," it's saying.

Overwhelming your cells with too much sugar and bad fats causes a snowball effect of both slowing metabolism and increasing cravings for the same bad foods. That's because, amazingly, hormone imbalances and survival-threatening conditions prompt your metabolic machinery to make you eat more of the very nutrients that are easily converted to the ultimate energy storage, fat.

WHAT OTHER FACTORS MIGHT HAVE SLOWED MY METABOLISM?

Common habits have powerful effects on hormones and weight. Everything we do is connected to hormones that increase our appetite for fattening foods and encourage our body's tendency to accumulate fat. Your uncontrollable eating behavior is likely to be the result of your sluggish metabolism. We who are trying to lose weight face an incredibly resilient metabolism.

Think about your life as you review the list below. The more of these factors you've been subjected to in the past, the more your metabolic machinery reacts by pushing you to select weight gain–promoting foods. Each and every one of these slows down your metabolism, causing it to burn fewer calories. And if you're not burning them off, you are gaining them as weight. Unless you address these issues, put a halt to them on every level, and reset your metabolism, you'll continue your weight gain and have a hard time reversing it. I discuss each of these in greater detail in the chapters indicated.

1. Eating meals rich in carbohydrates and animal fat at erratic times, nighttime eating, or skipping meals (Chapters 5 and 10)
2. Physical inactivity (Chapter 11)
3. Stress and anxiety (Chapter 4)
4. Depression (Chapter 4)
5. Insulin resistance (Chapter 1)

6. Sleep deprivation, sleep apnea, and poor-quality sleep (Chapter 5)

7. Polycystic ovary syndrome (PCOS; in this chapter and Chapter 6)

8. Menopause (Chapter 6)

9. Low testosterone (Chapter 6)

10. Thyroid hormone imbalance (Chapters 1 and 3)

11. Growth hormone deficiency (Chapter 3)

12. Toxic buildup, including obesogens (in this chapter and Chapter 8)

13. Food sensitivities (Chapter 9)

14. Medications (in this chapter)

15. GI bacterial imbalance (Chapters 4 and 8)

16. Antioxidant deficiency (Chapter 8)

As you can see, people who gain a lot of weight over a period of years don't necessarily gain it just because they started eating a crummy diet. It's more typical for life events such as the ones listed above to add to the struggle. For most of my patients, a constellation of factors causes the metabolic machinery to trigger fat storage. No matter which of these events occurred in your past or present, you can be sure of one thing: the appetite and satiety (fullness) centers in your hypothalamus are in charge of making you crave foods rich in sugar and fat.

My patient Meredith, a 25-year-old-librarian, is a good example of how multiple factors can cause a series of setbacks or slowdowns in metabolism. She came to me because of her slow but steady weight gain and other symptoms, including fatigue, low-grade depression, and irregular periods, having read on the Internet that her symptoms might point to low thyroid.

Meredith's weight history—from when she was young until now—amazed me. When she was six, she'd been diagnosed with a kidney condition that required treatment with prednisone, a glucocorticoid drug often prescribed for this condition. Glucocorticoids are a type of steroid and are derivatives of cortisol, the stress hormone produced by your adrenal glands. When you're stressed, your

glands release adrenaline and cortisol as a fight-or-flight response—
to get you out of trouble fast. But if you're stressed out constantly,
you have a lot of cortisol floating in your system, which increases
cravings for fattening foods and causes fat to be stored around
your waist. You can see why little 6-year-old Meredith gained fifteen pounds during her first year of treatment with this cortisol-like
drug. And her weight gain continued even after she stopped taking
the medication.

Since she went through puberty at age 10, Meredith's periods had
been irregular and hair had grown on her face and lower abdomen.
These are symptoms of polycystic ovarian syndrome (PCOS), caused
by an imbalance of female sex hormones and frequently accom-
panied by weight gain and insulin resistance. Tests confirmed her
PCOS, which, though unrelated to the medications she had taken at
age 6, had triggered her thirty-pound weight gain. Coinciding with
another jump in her weight five years ago, she began to have symptoms of low-grade hypothyroidism (low thyroid) including fatigue,
low-grade depression, dry skin, and constipation. Her weight gain
continued; she experienced yet another abrupt increase in weight
two years ago, coinciding with her sister telling her she'd started
snoring at night, the first sign of sleep apnea.

Meredith's weight reached 256 pounds. She cried a little as she
told me that over the last six months, "I don't want to get up and
exercise anymore, so I nap instead. I'm still tired, though, when I
wake up. Even if I spend ten hours lying in bed, I feel like I don't
sleep well. Plus, I'm depressed most of the time because I hate the
way I look and don't go out with my friends."

At least five life events triggered and perpetuated a slowdown of
Meredith's metabolism and her weight gain: the glucocorticoid medication when she was six; her PCOS; the low-grade hypothyroidism;
sleep apnea; and depression.

For Meredith and many others, the scenarios that slow metabolism and trigger subsequent weight gain can begin as early as childhood. Each of her triggers established a new weight set point that in
turn initiated a new trend of weight gain, which would continue for
years unless the contributing factors were reversed and her metabolism was reset.

We started with medication for Meredith's underactive thyroid, but she also needed help for the sleep apnea and PCOS. She began using a special breathing machine (see "Sleep Apnea" in Chapter 5) to prevent sleep apnea, giving her the first good night's sleep in months. For the PCOS, I prescribed metformin (see "Metformin and Birth Control Pills Can Also Help" in Chapter 6), antioxidant supplements, and the eating plan in this book, which is ideal for PCOS because its low-glycemic, higher-fiber, high-protein foods help reverse the insulin resistance and other hormone imbalances that occur with this condition. After she started all these remedies, Meredith began to exercise, too, and in two weeks started to lose weight, something she couldn't have done without a proper hormone balance. After about four weeks, her depression lifted, thanks to proper thyroid treatment, mood-enhancing nutrients, and weight loss.

Meredith's weight problem was more complicated than some because of her coexistent PCOS and thyroid condition, but her story illustrates the importance of addressing hormone imbalances in order to lose weight.

COULD IT BE YOUR GENES?

You can inherit a genetic tendency to be overweight or obese, but severe genetic obesity disorders are fortunately very rare and unlikely to be the root of your weight problem. Only about 5 percent of childhood obesity is caused by major genetic defects, and patients with these impairments typically have a ferocious appetite, slow metabolism, and thus severe obesity. If you're overweight as a result of hormonal imbalances or your calorie intake is out of control because of poor food choices, the genes that affect weight can become even more active, causing a further slowdown in metabolism.

HOW MUCH YOUR PARENTS WEIGH MATTERS

The household environment you grew up in can also influence your weight. Stronger than genes, parental weight has a powerful influence on childhood obesity and the risk of adult obesity. You may be obese owing to metabolic shifts that occurred during childhood, and your metabolic makeup as a child can date all the way back to how much both your parents weighed as well as to your mother's eating habits, her overall health, and how much stress she experienced while pregnant. Many studies show that overweight mothers are more likely to have overweight children than are mothers of normal weight. Children born to obese or overweight women have an increased risk for being overweight by age 4, showing how the uterine environment can modify the way a child's genes will be expressed, affecting both growth and the amount of fat children carry. In fact, two obese parents have an 80 percent chance of having obese children; this figure strongly supports the powerful effect of a genetic contribution to obesity. Also, your risk for being obese is five times greater if you have an obese first-degree relative (father, mother, brother, or sister).

Birth mothers with type 2 diabetes (caused by insulin resistance) place their offspring at greater risk for childhood metabolic dysfunction, leading to a vicious cycle of obesity and insulin resistance later in the child's life. Women with high cholesterol who eat unhealthy diets during pregnancy are also more likely to have obese children. Two-thirds of women in the United States are overweight or obese when they conceive. Likewise, women who don't eat enough during pregnancy have children with a distortion in their genes and an increased risk of cardiovascular disease, insulin resistance, metabolic syndrome, and obesity.

It's clear that a damaged metabolism in a pregnant woman—from eating too much or too little—passes to her children. Research also shows that a woman eating a high-fat diet during pregnancy can affect her child's development by damaging the brain's melanocortin pathway (appetite center) and serotoninergic system (satisfaction center). This results in her child having an increased appetite, anxiety-like behavior, and weight gain from birth.

STRESS, WEIGHT, AND GENES: VICTIM OF YOUR ENVIRONMENT

Your environment influences your genes. Weight-promoting genes are affected by what you eat and don't eat, and how much you exercise, as well as by smoking, infection, stress, and medications. As these life events occur, metabolism slows down and weight gain follows. During this process your genes actually change, and you're likely to pass on these altered genes to your children, who are more likely to become overweight or obese themselves.

Researchers call this "gene-environment interaction." Your genes respond to the environment in which you live and to your own behavior. Your environment during childhood, including any stress experienced, can affect your genes, causing mutations that lead to weight gain and obesity. Growing up in a stressful environment often leads to weight problems in children, with stressed children at risk of developing depression and being overweight later in life. Animals subjected to stress early in life have persistent alterations in their genes that make them susceptible to behavioral dysfunction and persistent high levels of the fat-inducing stress hormone corticosterone (similar to our human stress hormone cortisol).

Stress at a young age alters the hormone balance that leads to weight changes later. Gaining weight and becoming obese as a result of stress are caused by the adrenal glands producing too much cortisol, the stress hormone that increases abdominal fat along with cravings for fattening foods. Cortisol overload causes your body to break down muscle protein and produce high levels of glucose, sending blood sugar skyrocketing. This explains how stress can ultimately lead to insulin resistance and type 2 diabetes. In addition to suffering physically, obese children are more likely to be affected by emotional problems that worsen socialization later in adolescence. Overweight or obese young people are at greater risk of being overweight or obese adults.

Clarissa, a 35-year-old patient of mine, is a good example of how stress and an unhappy childhood can alter genes. Clarissa came from a family in which everyone was slim and trim. She herself was actually extremely skinny. "When I was a kid, I was so thin my ribs would show," she told me. But a stressful, unhappy childhood was enough to override Clarissa's "skinny" genes. "My father was abusive, and my mother was weak and didn't protect me. I was so unhappy growing up." To offset the stress, as a child and in her early teens, Clarissa sought refuge in junk food like chips and ice cream, which she took to her room to eat in peace.

"I started getting fat before age ten. Then when I was twelve or thirteen, I started gaining weight weirdly. It just got worse and worse." Clarissa's father repeatedly called her a fat pig and told her, "You'll never be successful. You're too big." As her depression deepened, Clarissa started eating even more junk food in high school. By the time she graduated, she'd gained 120 pounds.

After more than a decade of yo-yo dieting, Clarissa married and quickly became pregnant. During her pregnancy, Clarissa was depressed and ate enormous amounts. "For the first time I wasn't worried about what people thought about my weight because I had the excuse of being pregnant," she said. Now the mother of two young—and obese—children, she was struggling to keep her household healthy, and came to see if I could help her lose weight and keep it off.

I explained that she needed to stop bingeing on nutritionally empty snacks and to get them out of the house. This would also encourage her children to eat more healthfully. Clarissa put her entire family on the Protein Boost Diet. She lost the weight, and by using my exercise program faithfully, she has maintained herself at a well-balanced 145 pounds for several years now. Her children also quickly lost their extra fat and are now healthier. The entire family benefited and became more active. With her kids into soccer, Clarissa joined a women's league and she and the family kick the ball around after school almost every day.

Clarissa and her children will always be vulnerable to gaining their weight back fast if they deviate from eating right and exercising because of their own genetic propensity for gaining weight, caused by Clarissa's own childhood stress and unhappy childhood. This is the haunting effect of the slowdowns in metabolism established early in life. Stress at any period in life elicits adverse effects as powerful as inherited genes, but weight gain is itself detrimental to your genes, altering your genetic makeup during your lifetime and affecting your children.

Weight gain brought on by stress isn't the only way your weight genes are affected. Regardless of the stress that caused your weight gain, your weight genes can be altered by being exposed to too much oxidative stress (see "Antioxidants Protect Your Body from Oxidative Stress" in Chapter 8) caused by free radicals in your system. These are the by-products of biochemical reactions in cells that are overproduced when you become overweight. Oxidative stress then contributes to the perpetuating trend of weight gain.

It is possible to reshape your genetic makeup so it works for you instead of against you. When you follow the Protein Boost Diet and change the types of foods you eat, and also address the list of metabolism decelerators that may have prompted your weight-gain trend, you can turn around the deep-rooted effects of stress and readjust your metabolism so that you can lose weight and become healthy for the long term.

OUR HIDDEN TOXIC ENVIRONMENT: OBESOGENS AND WEIGHT GAIN

Day after day, just by living your life, you're exposed to numerous man-made chemical toxicants that are slowly destroying you from within. Known as "obesogens," these endocrine-disrupting (hormone-disrupting) compounds enter your body via high fructose corn syrup, pesticides, dyes, medicines, flavorings, personal care products, plastics, and contaminated water. Obesogens mimic or suppress the action of your own hormones, changing your body's weight-regulating system in myriad ways. One major effect they have is impairing leptin and thyroid hormone function. This impairment leads your body to store fat and limit the number of calories you burn. Obesogens also make your liver become resistant to insulin, causing your pancreas to churn out more fat-storing insulin. Your body reacts adversely to hormone disruptors, even in small amounts. In short, obesogens are a recipe for metabolic malfunction and weight gain. They also can alter your genes to make you even more susceptible to weight gain and obesity.

In addition to weight gain, endocrine-disrupting chemicals disturb hormones in other ways: triggering early puberty, reducing sperm quality, and increasing the risk of PCOS, ovulation dysfunction, testicular cancer, infertility, thyroid cancer, and congenital hypothyroidism.

Many hormone disruptors build up in fat tissue, but some circulate in your bloodstream, wrecking the function of hormones by attaching to cell membranes. Hormone-disrupting chemicals interfere with the biological activity of fat tissue and alter the calorie-burning efficiency of your cells' mitochondria—their power plants. The frightening reality is that hormone-disrupting chemicals are also transferred from a woman to her baby in pregnancy and via breast milk. When you are an adult, your metabolism may be sluggish simply because you were exposed to chemicals while you were developing in your mother's uterus; this means that metabolic syndrome may originate even before birth. Obesogens influence prenatal development, resulting in weight gain and other metabolic disruptions later in life.

Multiple obesogens are found in tap water, so get a water filter. Many filter types (carbon, resin, reverse osmosis, etc.) are available online, and while basic filters may not purify your tap water 100 percent, they can protect you from many of the chemicals discussed below. Because you'll be drinking plenty of water on the Protein Boost Diet, you'll want a water source with as little contamination as possible.

In addition to the following hormone-disrupting chemicals and sources, heavy metals and other toxins can also alter the fat-burning capabilities of mitochondria and contribute to weight gain (see Chapter 8).

FUNGICIDE: TRIBUTYLTIN (TBT)

You're exposed to this widespread hormone-disrupting fungicide through timber products, food, tap water, and plastics. TBT has been added to paint used on boats and in fish-farm cages to prevent parasite growth, so it has polluted marine life and food sources. This toxic chemical, even in small amounts, causes high cortisol levels and can cause metabolic setbacks and fat accumulation. TBT affects genes and makes you grow more fat cells. When a pregnant woman is exposed to TBT, her child is likely to have more fat mass and gain more weight throughout his or her life.

To avoid TBT: Filter your water and avoid eating farm-raised fish and shellfish.

PLASTIC BOTTLES: BISPHENOL A (BPA)

Bisphenol A (BPA), used to harden plastics, acts like a synthetic estrogen and affects your hormones, making you gain fat. BPA causes insulin resistance by inhibiting the release of adiponectin (which tells your body to burn fat). Even low doses of BPA (which most of us already have in our bodies) can harm thyroid receptors and promote insulin resistance, causing you to have a high body mass index, a large waist circumference, and high blood sugar levels.

To avoid BPA: Buy a reusable water bottle that's BPA-free and fill it yourself. Avoid plastics with numbers 3 or 7 on the bottom, as they can leach BPA. Because BPA is used to line metal cans (though some companies are introducing BPA-free cans), limit the number of canned goods you eat. Don't handle cash register receipts any more than needed—some contain a lot of BPA.

PESTICIDES

Both prenatal exposure and prolonged exposure to pesticides have unhealthy consequences on weight. Long-term exposure to pesticides provokes insulin resistance, chronically high insulin levels, and even diabetes.

To avoid pesticides: Soak conventionally grown vegetables (which contain pesticides) in a solution of one part vinegar to one part water before rinsing thoroughly to minimize risk. The best way to go is organic. If you eat organic produce for just five days, the body clears itself of most pesticide residue. Some pesticides, such as atrazine, leach into tap water sources—another reason to filter your drinking water.

DRY-CLEANING AND INDUSTRIAL CHEMICALS

Tetrachloroethylene is a man-made chemical commonly used in dry cleaning, in metal degreasing, and as an anesthetic. It pollutes the water in many countries and disrupts hormones, leading to weight gain. The negative outcome seems to be more from long-term exposure, so this is not as dangerous as some of the other obesogens, but with so many in our environment, you want to avoid all that you can.

To avoid tetrachloroethylene: Remove the plastic covering from dry-cleaned garments and let clothes air out before wearing.

PAINTS AND DYES: PCBs

Even though polychlorinated biphenyls (PCBs) are carcinogenic and were banned in 1979, a study in Dallas proved that there's little observation of the ban. Researchers measured food samples from supermarkets and found PCBs in foods, including meats, dairy prod-

ucts, canned foods, eggs, apples, cereal, and peanut butter. PCBs
have been used for fifty years in hydraulic equipment, electric insu-
lation, oil-based paint, rubber, pigments, and dyes. Improper dumping or burning can release the chemical into the environment. Fish
and crops can absorb small amounts. PCBs are routinely detected
in the environment and human tissues. This means you probably
consume detectable quantities. Effects of PCB include lowered IQ,
reduced visual recognition memory, attention and motor deficits,
reduced sperm count, and (in animals) low levels of the thyroid hormone T4.

To avoid PCBs: Don't eat farm-raised salmon, a major carrier of
PCBs, and other farm-raised fish.

PERCHLORATE AND LITHIUM

Ammonium perchlorate and lithium are soluble and easily contaminate water supplies. These contaminants encourage low thyroid
function and the slower metabolism that contribute to your weight
gain trend. Lower levels of thyroid hormones stymie your weight-
loss efforts.

To avoid perchlorate and lithium: Filtering drinking water provides the best protection.

NONSTICK COOKWARE

Perfluorooctanoic acids (PFOAs) are synthetic compounds found
in clothing, carpets, paints, adhesives and adhesive-backed contact
paper, coatings, food, food containers, and nonstick cookware. Being
resistant to water and oil, they persistently contaminate our environment because they resist breaking down. PFOAs alter fat metabolism, disrupt hormone balance, and have been linked to obesity and
metabolic changes in adulthood. Most people in the United States
have traces of PFOAs in their bodies, and given that PFOAs have a
half-life of several years, you won't rid yourself of them quickly.

To avoid PFOAs: The best and possibly only ways to avoid them
are to filter your tap water and not to use nonstick cookware.

PLASTIC WRAP, COSMETICS, SHAMPOOS

Phthalates are hormone-disrupting chemicals with effects similar to BPAs. They damage sex hormones and sex organ development and functions. As you'll learn in later chapters, thyroid and sex hormone imbalances cause weight gain. Sadly, phthalates are still often used to soften plastics and are found in many household items such as plastic food wrap/containers, cosmetics, shampoo, and even wallpaper. The toxic chemicals seep easily into your food or skin.

To avoid phthalates: Stay away from products made with DBP, MEHP, DEP, DEHP, DES, BzBP, or DMP. Fragrance added in any product can contain phthalates, too. Purchase plastic items with the numbers 1, 2, or 5 rather than 3 or 7 on the bottom. Safer products are easier to find at a health food store, and while they cost more, you're saving your family from many long-term health detriments.

CHECK YOUR MEDICATIONS

Many commonly prescribed drugs cause weight gain as a side effect, and the very medications used to treat diabetes, psychiatric conditions, autoimmune ailments, and neurological disorders cause weight gain. Some birth control pills promote weight gain, too. Make sure you're prescribed a newer-generation birth-control pill with less male hormone and fewer glucocorticoid and weight-promoting effects. Certain medications could make you end up with even more health problems because of the weight gain they have caused. I don't recommend that you stop taking medications linked to weight gain, but you should follow my carefully designed diet to reverse any metabolic issues your medicine causes. See "Protein and Its Aminos Help You Feel Full and Burn More Calories" in Chapter 7 for more on how specific foods can shore up fat-burning neurotransmitter activity.

The following lists include commonly used medications that can promote weight gain.

ANTIDIABETIC MEDICATIONS
Insulin
Sulfonylureas
Thiazolidinediones

GLUCOCORTICOIDS (USED FOR TREATMENT OF ASTHMA, ALLERGIC
    DISORDERS, AND AUTOIMMUNE DISORDERS)
Prednisone
Methylprednisolone
Other glucocorticoids

ANTIDEPRESSANTS, MOOD STABILIZERS, AND ATYPICAL ANTIPSYCHOTICS
Olanzapine (Zyprexa, Zydis)
Quetiapine (Seroquel)
Clozapine (Clozaril)
Divalproex (Depakote)
Risperidone (Risperdal)
Lithium (Eskalith, Lithobid)
Tranylcypromine (Parnate, Jatrosom)
Imipramine (Dynaprin, Desprinol, Antideprin, Deprimin)
Asenapine (Saphris, Sycrest)
Fluoxetine (Prozac)
Fluvoxamine (Effexor)
Paroxetine (Paxil)
Sertaline (Zoloft)
Mirtazapine (Remeron)
Phenelzine (Nardil)

The multiple potential slowdowns in metabolism I discuss in this
chapter, whether genetic, environmental, medication related, or hormonal, are some of the main contributors to the weight problems
people face around the world today. If you're affected by any of
these metabolism-crippling factors, try to address them before starting my diet.

In the next chapters I'll detail some of the common reasons for
a slowdown in metabolism that increasingly haunt many of us—
hormonal disorders, poor-quality or insufficient sleep, and stress.
You'll learn how to restore vivacious metabolism by eating the right
foods and rebalancing your hormones.

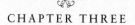

CHAPTER THREE

OVERCOMING THYROID AND GROWTH HORMONE PROBLEMS FOR OPTIMAL WEIGHT LOSS

More than thirty million people in the United States have a thyroid disorder—roughly 10 to 14 percent of the population. Another ten million to fifteen million people with thyroid imbalance are undiagnosed and may be suffering needlessly. Thyroid disorders generally affect ten women for every man. Hypothyroidism—low thyroid function—is roughly ten times more common than hyperthyroidism: too much thyroid hormone.

As a specialist in hormone disorders and metabolism, I think first of thyroid imbalance and growth hormone deficiency whenever I see a patient struggling with weight gain. Both thyroid and growth hormones have dramatic effects on your weight and mood. But with the right treatments and the Protein Boost Diet, you can rebalance these hormones.

Correcting thyroid imbalance with medication often provides the necessary ingredients for weight loss, but my patients do best at losing weight and keeping it off when they use thyroid medication in conjunction with the program in this book. Because I've seen so many patients gain weight as a result of incorrect thyroid hormone therapy, we'll take a close look at why that occurs, and I'll give you treatment advice that will help you and your doctor fix your imbalance without creating another problem.

Growth hormone (GH) is also a serious player in regulating metabolism, and a deficiency can cause significant weight gain, a fact that many people (doctors included) don't often consider. If you're not producing normal amounts of GH, you're likely to become over-weight or obese. In this chapter I'll explain why this happens and how to restore your GH.

Balancing your thyroid and growth hormones with the right foods and supplements is part of what makes the Protein Boost Diet so effective. The entire time you've been searching for why you can't lose weight, the problem may actually have been a hormonal imbal-ance. Unhealthy thyroid and growth hormone levels can block you from achieving your desired figure and health, but when you balance your hormones and follow the dietary prescriptions in my program, you can finally lose those stubborn pounds.

THYROID GLAND: METABOLISM ENERGIZER

In peak condition, your thyroid system is calibrated to provide the right amount of thyroid hormones needed to fulfill a wide range of bodily functions, including regulating metabolism, body tem-perature, heart rate, cholesterol levels, and blood pressure. Thy-roid hormones stimulate oxygen consumption by the cells in your body and are crucial for metabolizing fats, sugars, and proteins. This system is overseen by the pituitary, the master gland connected to your brain, which detects the amount of thyroid hormone in your bloodstream and organs and sends out signals to adjust levels as needed.

When your thyroid gland isn't functioning properly, the result can be either underproduction of thyroid hormones or overproduction. In *hypothyroidism (underactive thyroid),* also called "low thyroid," the amount of hormone produced by the thyroid gland isn't suffi-cient to maintain the metabolic balance of your body. This condition slows down your metabolism and you burn fewer calories. Low thy-roid can cause a wide array of symptoms including fatigue, mental fogginess, dry skin, hair loss, brittle nails, joint pains, muscle cramps, constipation, and sensitivity to cold, as well as mood swings, depres-sion, impaired memory, anxiety, decreased libido, and panic attacks. Women with low thyroid may also experience heavy menstrual peri-ods, discharge of the breasts, infertility, and miscarriages. Hypo-thyroidism changes your eating behavior and slows metabolism by making leptin inefficient. Weight-loss-friendly leptin tells your brain when you're full (signaling you to stop eating), boosts fat burning, and limits the amount of fat you store. Hypothyroidism will make you gain weight, make you burn less fat, raise your cholesterol, and put you at risk for cardiovascular disease. Even low-grade hypothyroidism (called "subclinical hypothyroidism"), in which you are missing just a very little amount of hormone, can cause symptoms and weight gain.

In *hyperthyroidism (overactive thyroid)*, your thyroid gland is churning out too much hormone. This has completely different effects on your metabolism, speeding it up and making you feel jittery and nervous. Hyperthyroidism also can cause multiple physical and mental symptoms, including weight loss, rapid heartbeat, shakiness, heat intolerance, abnormal menstrual periods, hair loss, anxiety, and mood changes. And just like hypothyroidism, hyperthyroidism changes your eating behavior and your metabolism. Excess thyroid hormone in your system will make you burn fat, but it also causes leptin levels to drop. Low leptin, coupled with an inefficiency of the leptin you do have, makes you hungry and produces cravings for the destructive foods you're trying to avoid, including sugar and bad fats.

It's important to know that once a slowdown in your metabolism has been triggered by thyroid problems, treatment with thyroid hormone won't necessarily make you lose all the weight you've already gained. A setback in metabolism induced by low thyroid cannot be overcome simply by normalizing your levels with thyroid hormone treatment. Losing the weight requires hormone treatment combined with a conscientious improvement in what, how, and when you eat and how active you are.

The Protein Boost Diet can help you reverse the multiple metabolic problems your body has been subjected to and help you successfully lose the extra weight. Alina is a good example of how it can work. A new patient in her mid-twenties from New York City, Alina saw me the week before she was to participate in a bicycle ride of more than 150 miles for the MS 150. I was stunned when she told me she had run a marathon or ridden in a bike race once or twice a month for several years, because this meant she was training consistently—yet she weighed 150 pounds, heavy for her average height. Alina came to see me for help understanding why she'd gained so much weight despite her extraordinarily active life. Here's what she told me.

"About two years ago I was in the best shape of my life. I'd just run the New York marathon and had never felt better. I probably weighed 118 or 120 pounds at the time. But starting in the winter of that year, I noticed a slow decline, a subtle change. I started feeling tired and gaining weight, and despite my exercise and healthy diet, I wasn't sleeping well. I was losing hair and my hands and feet were cold. I'd have to sleep with a heating pad on my feet every night and it was really frustrating because despite my good physical condition, I didn't feel that well.

"I continued to run and train and kept gaining weight. I thought maybe I was overexercising, so I laid off a little bit, altered my diet, and decided just to cross-train, ride my bike, swim, and run—preliminary training for a triathlon. Even with all this, I continued to gain weight, and I still wasn't sleeping well. I'm not old enough to feel how old I was feeling, and I continued to gain. Here I am two years later at 150. Last fall I ran a spring triathlon and I'm training to ride the MS 150 next weekend, and I'm thirty pounds heavier than I was two years ago. I eat well and not excessively. I feel really frustrated. I'm lethargic, kind of achy . . . I have a general lack of motivation, even though I push myself in all these sports. It's been a gradual decline over two years."

Several doctors told her that her thyroid was normal.

Our test results confirmed that the cause of Alina's weight gain and lack of wellness was low-grade hypothyroidism. Her thyroid test was in the borderline low–normal range, which is probably why the other physicians hadn't treated it. People who have low-grade hypothyroidism can experience rapid weight gain, just as Alina had, yet many doctors don't recognize low-grade hypothyroidism as having this effect.

To stop the weight gain and other symptoms, I started Alina on a well-balanced T4/T3 thyroid hormone therapy (a combination of the two thyroid hormones, mimicking what the thyroid gland normally produces). Her weight gain and other symptoms quickly stopped. Alina also started following my hormone-balancing eating plan as she restarted her training. Without the hormone imbalance urging her body to retain energy as fat, Alina lost her extra weight quickly. In four months she was back to 120 pounds and feeling great again. "I knew *something* was off with my hormones. I can't believe the other doctors didn't catch this. Your treatment turned my life around! Six months ago, I felt like I was aging. Now I'm back to being my 25-year-old self."

Quick Facts on Thyroid Disorders

- Nearly 2 percent of the population has moderate or severe hypothyroidism.
- Eight to 10 percent of the population has subclinical (low-grade) hypothyroidism, revealed as a mildly abnormal thyroid test result. Quite likely at least an additional 5 to 10 percent of the population has low-grade hypothyroidism with what is currently considered to be normal thyroid blood test results (I call this "covert hypothyroidism").
- Hashimoto's thyroiditis is an autoimmune thyroid disorder that inflames and destroys cells in the gland. It's the most common cause of hypothyroidism.
- Graves' disease is also an autoimmune thyroid condition, the most common cause of hyperthyroidism, affecting 1 to 2 percent of the population.

LOW THYROID AFFECTS METABOLISM AND WEIGHT

The number of calories you burn is determined by two things: how much energy (calories) you burn during physical activity and how much you burn at rest—sitting, sleeping, doing nothing. Thyroid hormones directly regulate the biochemical machinery in charge of burning calories at rest, called your "resting metabolic rate." If you have a deficiency of thyroid hormones, your resting metabolic rate will be lower and you'll burn fewer calories when you're not active than if your thyroid levels were perfectly normal. The calories you don't burn by having a slow resting metabolic rate can really add up, causing you to gain as many as ten to fifteen pounds a year. This partly explains how having hypothyroidism makes it so easy to gain weight, but there are other reasons, too.

As discussed in Chapter 1, thyroid hormone is essential for efficient functioning of leptin, which helps you limit your food intake and speed up metabolism. Low thyroid causes leptin to become inefficient at curbing appetite and making you burn calories at rest. The result is a gradual imbalance that makes you accumulate fat. Leptin inefficiency makes you want to eat more even as you're burning fewer calories doing nothing. The good news is that treating low thyroid will help restore leptin sensitivity unless you're obese, in which case the extra fat you've accumulated coupled with the insulin resistance will continue to impede leptin efficiency. Working with the Protein Boost Diet eating plan and exercise program will help restore leptin's effects.

Low thyroid also affects metabolism and appetite by making you produce more ghrelin, the hunger hormone. In people with hypothyroidism, ghrelin levels are about one-third higher than normal. Higher ghrelin exacerbates appetite and fat storage. Along with its effects on leptin and ghrelin, hypothyroidism also drives down levels of growth hormone (GH), slowing your metabolism even further. In "Growth Hormone Deficiency, a Cause of Relentless Weight Gain" in this chapter, I discuss in more detail the importance of GH on weight.

As a final blow, hypothyroidism also directly worsens insulin resistance. If you have low thyroid levels, insulin sensitivity is reduced by roughly a third of what it should be, but treatment to restore hormone balance improves insulin sensitivity, even in people with low-grade hypothyroidism. Insulin resistance causes you to convert more sugar to fat and to accumulate visceral fat (waistline fat and fat around vital internal organs). In fact, if you have any type of low thyroid condition (whether low-grade, moderate, or severe), you'll have more belly fat than someone whose hormone levels are normal. The only way to break this cycle of abdominal fat and worsening insulin resistance is to get your hypothyroidism treated, ideally while you follow an eating plan like mine to further balance all the other hormones involved in weight.

Having low thyroid distorts your hormonal harmony on so many levels that it actually can cause you to gain up to an extra one-third of your original weight. When you have hypothyroidism, the combination of higher visceral fat, increasing leptin resistance, worsening insulin resistance, and higher levels of the hunger hormone ghrelin exacerbate weight gain. This puts you on an escalating cycle of slow metabolism and added pounds, and raises your risk for many diseases. For people who stop taking needed thyroid hormone, metabolism predictably slows down. I cannot emphasize strongly enough the need for you to have your doctor monitor and regularly adjust your thyroid treatment so that you avoid falling back into the sluggish metabolism cycle that leads to extra weight.

Fortunately, if you have hypothyroidism, you can reverse your hormonal problems with proper treatment and a healthy lifestyle (including the program detailed in this book).

LOW THYROID OR WEIGHT GAIN: WHICH COMES FIRST?

The relationship between hypothyroidism and obesity is a two-way street. Low thyroid slows your metabolism and causes you to eat more, a situation that sets many of my patients on a downward spiral of repeated weight-gain cycles. But if you become overweight or obese for reasons other than low thyroid, the weight problem itself can cause low thyroid.

This means that weight gain and low thyroid feed off each other to escalate weight issues in many people. Being overweight, regardless of the reason, inevitably makes you hypothyroid at the cellular level, and this thyroid impairment in your tissues becomes part of the vicious weight-gain cycle. Obesity decreases the number of thyroid hormone receptors in your body and impairs the conversion of thyroid hormone T4 to T3. This makes you grow less responsive to metabolism-boosting thyroid hormones, as if your tissues were hypothyroid even though your gland is functioning normally. In other words, you become thyroid hormone resistant.

As discussed in Chapter 1, leptin inefficiency—a universal problem in most overweight and obese people—impairs the production of T3, the most metabolically active thyroid hormone in cells. This reduces thyroid hormone activity and promotes further slowing of metabolism. Being overweight puts a burden on your thyroid system and will make you more likely to develop problems with your thyroid gland. Impaired thyroid gland function is more common in overweight and obese people, and about one-fifth of obese people have hypothyroidism. Also, people who have higher BMIs have higher levels of the thyroid-stimulating hormone (TSH) made in the pituitary and released in an attempt to prompt the thyroid to produce more hormone. This could indicate that having a higher BMI makes the thyroid gland struggle and become more sluggish.

Being overweight or obese can also encourage your immune system to attack your thyroid, making it underactive. Again this has to do with leptin, which regulates immune function, and too much leptin in your system can promote an autoimmune attack on your thyroid—Hashimoto's thyroiditis, the most common cause of underactive thyroid. In essence, the more overweight you are, the more likely you are to have an underactive thyroid, leading to further weight gain.

If you have any symptoms of low thyroid (page 44) along with gradual weight gain, be proactive and have your thyroid tested promptly and treated if necessary to avoid escalation of symptoms and negative health effects. I'll give you specifics later in this chapter.

Complicating matters, not everyone with hypothyroidism necessarily has significant symptoms. So it's critical for you to be tested and treated because untreated hypothyroidism eventually causes major adverse health effects. Even low-grade hypothyroidism raises your cholesterol, blood pressure, triglyceride levels, and homocysteine levels. All of these increase your risk of coronary artery disease, the hardening of the blood vessels in your heart. Peripheral vascular disease is also a common complication of untreated low-grade hypothyroidism in older people.

TESTING FOR LOW THYROID

A high thyroid-stimulating hormone (TSH) level is the best indicator of an underactive thyroid. It's a sign your pituitary is churning out TSH, trying to get your sluggish thyroid to produce its hormones.

NORMAL TSH: CONVENTIONAL VIEW AND MY INTERPRETATION

The more impaired your thyroid gland, the greater the deficit of thyroid hormone in your system and the higher the TSH level in your blood. For this reason, TSH is used by doctors not only to diagnose low thyroid, but also to assess its severity. This chart shows the conventional normal range for TSH and what's considered by conventional medicine to be subclinical (low-grade) hypothyroidism, moderate hypothyroidism, or overt (severe) hypothyroidism.

TSH Level (mIU/L, milli-international units per liter of blood)	Diagnosis
0.4 to 4.5	Normal range
4.5 to 20	Subclinical (low-grade) hypothyroidism
20 to 40	Moderate hypothyroidism
Above 40	Overt (severe) hypothyroidism

I'd like to warn you about two important points often ignored by many doctors.

- The degree of your symptoms and weight issue has nothing to do with how severe your hypothyroidism is. In other words, you could be suffering from significant symptoms as a result of low-grade hypothyroidism while another person may have very few symptoms despite having much more severe hypothyroidism. The sensitivity to low thyroid is different from one person to the next, meaning the way you feel doesn't necessarily correlate with how abnormal your TSH level is.

- What's considered to be normal TSH as far as blood tests are concerned (0.4 to 4.5 mIU/L, as you can see in the chart) may not be normal for you, *meaning you may have low-grade hypothyroidism even with a test result that falls in the normal range.* Many people, especially those who have a TSH level between 2.0 and 4.5, are actually in the gray zone of normalcy. People with TSH in this range may actually have Hashimoto's thyroiditis or low-grade hypothyroidism with normal blood tests (covert hypothyroidism). Levels of T4 are typically in the normal range in low-grade hypothyroidism, even when TSH is clearly elevated (4.5 to 20 mIU/L).

Low thyroid can also be caused by central hypothyroidism (due to an impaired pituitary gland), in which case the TSH level is either normal or low. What indicates the pituitary as the source of low thyroid is a low level of free T4.

A HIDDEN CAUSE OF SLOW METABOLISM:
SUBCLINICAL (LOW-GRADE) HYPOTHYROIDISM

For decades, since TSH testing became widely available in the early 1970s, conventional medicine has questioned whether people with just slightly high TSH but normal thyroid hormone levels should be treated with thyroid hormone. For the most part, conventional medicine viewed these people as having a trivial biochemical abnormality not associated with symptoms and not having any bearing on their health. For this reason, this finding has been called "subclinical hypothyroidism," meaning with no clinical consequences. Before the 1999 publication of my first book, *The Thyroid Solution*, many doctors virtually ignored this biochemical abnormality and even refused to treat patients with "minor abnormal blood tests." Yet these patients were suffering from fatigue, depressive symptoms, and weight gain, along with other physical symptoms and health consequences such as heavy menstrual periods, infertility, hair loss, and lack of well-being.

I was treating patients for devastating symptoms that stemmed from this "trivial abnormality" because their concerns and symptoms had been dismissed by their doctors. Treating them made their symptoms abate or resolve, and this taught me that minor thyroid hormone deficit was not as trivial as most doctors believed. Minor thyroid hormone deficit shows up as just a slightly high TSH level. Even a normal TSH level doesn't necessarily mean that the function of the gland is perfectly normal. Millions of people actually have low-grade hypothyroidism as a result of a slightly impaired gland, even though their tests are viewed as normal. This is what I call "covert hypothyroidism." I'm happy to see there's been an increased awareness of this condition, and generally speaking, more doctors are taking it seriously. Sadly, however, even these days many patients who have thyroid tests in the borderline/gray zone of what's considered normal—along with many patients who clearly have Hashimoto's thyroiditis and/or slightly elevated TSH—are dismissed as having a biochemical abnormality that has no consequences. I can assure you that even covert hypothyroidism can sneakily, but surely, slow your metabolism and launch a trend of weight gain.

Low-grade hypothyroidism can cause low metabolism and weight gain especially when other weight-gain-promoting factors enter the picture. For example, a woman whose TSH levels are in the gray zone of normal, indicating she has low-grade hypothyroidism, but who might not have gained a lot of weight before menopause, will have a slower metabolism when she goes through menopause. The lowered estrogen, along with borderline-low thyroid hormone, can produce rapid, significant weight gain.

Even in cases where TSH levels are clearly elevated, some thyroid experts, physicians, and medical school professors claim—and teach new doctors—that low-grade hypothyroidism is not a cause of weight gain. These assertions reflect a poor understanding of how weight gain works. Low-grade hypothyroidism can definitely affect your metabolism and lead to insulin resistance and even metabolic syndrome. Research, in fact, found that people with metabolic syndrome have much higher TSH levels than healthy people and that having even slightly high TSH (indicating low-grade hypothyroidism) correlates with a bigger waist circumference. This points to one conclusion: low-grade hypothyroidism contributes to gaining body fat and can ignite a trend of weight gain over time.

HASHIMOTO'S THYROIDITIS AS A CAUSE OF LOW THYROID

Low thyroid can be triggered by a number of underlying thyroid conditions, but most commonly it's caused by an autoimmune disorder called "Hashimoto's thyroiditis." Hashimoto's is part of a spectrum of autoimmune disorders (including lupus, multiple sclerosis, and rheumatoid arthritis) in which the immune system mistakenly tries to destroy a healthy part of your body it views as an invader.

With Hashimoto's, antibodies and chemicals produced by your immune system attack your thyroid and the resulting inflammation causes thyroid cells to become impaired, no longer capable of producing a normal amount of hormones. This inflammation can even lead to gradual destruction of the thyroid gland, which causes severe hypothyroidism. Hashimoto's thyroiditis, to some extent, can indicate you have a genetic predisposition to all kinds of autoimmune conditions. Other members of your biological family might have Hashimoto's thyroiditis or Graves' disease, another type of autoimmune attack on the thyroid that causes overactive thyroid.

Other factors can contribute to the occurrence of Hashimoto's, including stress, depression, poor nutrition, and infection from bacteria and viruses. Being deficient in vitamins and antioxidants, including vitamins A, B$_6$, C, D, and E, copper, selenium, and folic acid can hamper your immune system and cause it to attack your thyroid. It's not uncommon to have Hashimoto's thyroiditis without having low thyroid, but you need to watch for the possibility of developing hypothyroidism in the future. You can be tested for Hashimoto's thyroiditis with a simple blood test called the "antithyroid antibody test." The most sensitive antithyroid antibody test is the antithyroperoxidase antibody (anti-TPO antibody). Unfortunately, nearly 30 to 40 percent of people with Hashimoto's thyroiditis have negative test results. Your doctor can use a thyroid ultrasound to diagnose this condition as well. Thyroid ultrasound is actually more sensitive for diagnosing even mild autoimmune thyroid conditions.

OTHER CAUSES OF HYPOTHYROIDISM

Your thyroid can produce too little hormone as a result of:

Treatment for an overactive thyroid
Surgery on your thyroid gland for lumps (nodules) or cancer
"Silent" thyroiditis, which is inflammation caused by a transient immune attack on the thyroid, a condition that causes hyperthyroidism for a few weeks followed by hypothyroidism that can either persist or resolve over time
Subacute thyroiditis (a viral infection of the thyroid that causes inflammation)
Radiation to the neck
Iodine deficiency
Taking medications that interfere with the thyroid, such as lithium (used to treat bipolar disorder) or amiodarone (used to treat abnormal heart rhythms)
Goitrogens (foods that interfere with thyroid function)

One of the patients whom I'd treated for low thyroid recommended her friend Maura come see me because Maura seemed to be having the same low thyroid symptoms. Maura was tired, couldn't focus, and had somehow gained weight without changing either her diet or her physical activity. Her test results revealed she had a low level of thyroid hormones, and her medical profile revealed that she was taking lithium for bipolar disorder. She'd started on the lithium about two months before her weight gain began and it was clearly interfering with her thyroid's production of hormone, making her body produce less than she needed. The resulting low thyroid and slowdown in metabolism had caused her weight gain. Since lithium was a necessary and effective medication for Maura, I prescribed thyroid hormone to balance her thyroid levels. With the right thyroid hormone treatment, and by following my diet, Maura lost all the weight she'd gained and her other thyroid-related symptoms dissipated over three months.

Up to 50 percent of people taking lithium have low-grade hypothyroidism. Lithium not only impairs the thyroid's ability to manufacture thyroid hormone, but can trigger an autoimmune reaction from your thyroid.

MEDICATIONS AND FOODS THAT INTERFERE
WITH THYROID FUNCTION

Many other medications can affect the function of the thyroid gland and cause either hypothyroidism or hyperthyroidism. For instance, excessive amounts of iodine can make your thyroid gland either underactive or overactive, resulting in significant thyroid imbalance. This can occur as a result of consuming supplements containing high amounts of iodine. Thyroid imbalance caused by too much iodine can also occur following CT or angiogram contrast imaging, for which you're injected with an iodine-containing contrast medium. Amiodarone, a medication used to treat heart irregularities, can also make the thyroid slow down or can make you hyperthyroid by causing inflammation and damage of the gland. Interferon α (Betaseron, Extavia), a medication used to treat chronic hepatitis C, and alemtuzumab (Campath, MabCampath), used to treat blood conditions, can cause an autoimmune attack on the thyroid gland that results in hypothyroidism. Sunitinib, a medication used to treat kidney cancer and gastrointestinal tumors, can also slow your thyroid.

Goitrogens, foods that interfere with the function of your thyroid, can also cause low thyroid when eaten in very large quantities on a routine basis. The list below shows foods that are goitrogens, but when they're cooked they have less effect on your thyroid. There's been much debate over the health benefits versus the thyroid risks of eating soy, given that it is a goitrogen. A study conducted a few years ago on rats showed soy consumption can produce low-grade hypothyroidism. Multiple studies recommend against feeding infants soy-based formula because it causes goiter—a swelling of the thyroid gland—in babies. You risk escalating low-grade hypothyroidism if you eat about 16 mg of soy phytoestrogens, the equivalent of one or two servings of soy per day, but other studies haven't seen a significant effect of soy on thyroid hormone in healthy people.

Soy does in fact have two proteins, genistein and daidzein, that impair the manufacture of thyroid hormone. After following much research, however, I continue to recommend eating soy and other foods with goitrogenic properties. Because soy has so many beneficial effects on your health and metabolism (as explained in Chapter 7), including reducing insulin resistance, inflammation, and blood pressure, I continue to view it as an excellent part of a healthy diet in which you eat other forms of protein as well. As long as you don't have untreated hypothyroidism or a sensitivity to soy, continue to enjoy it in reasonable amounts. Do not eat soy or soy products more than two or three times a week—whether your thyroid is normal or not.

FOODS THAT MAY LOWER THYROID FUNCTION*
Broccoli
Brussels sprouts
Cabbage
Cauliflower
Kale
Mustard greens
Peaches
Soy
Spinach
Strawberries
Turnips

*Cooking may limit the negative effect on thyroid function.

CONVENTIONAL TREATMENT OF LOW THYROID

The conventional approach to correcting hypothyroidism, whether low-grade, moderate, or severe, is to use synthetic levothyroxine (i.e., Levoxyl, Synthroid, Tirosint), which provides T4 (thyroxine) to your system. Synthetic levothyroxine is available in strengths ranging from 13 mcg (micrograms) to 300 mcg, allowing your physician to adjust the dose to achieve normal thyroid levels and also normal levels of thyroid-stimulating hormone (TSH), the pituitary hormone that regulates your thyroid. Because of this, testing levels of TSH is the most precise way to monitor treatment.

The more underactive your thyroid gland is, the higher the dose you'll need to achieve and maintain normal thyroid test results and feel your best. Thyroid hormone is taken daily one hour before breakfast on an empty stomach to avoid interference from foods and minerals. Soy protein, fiber-rich foods, and strong coffee such as espresso can reduce thyroid hormone absorption. Other foods that can also interfere are oranges and grapefruit (due to acidity), dairy (due to calcium), millet, peanuts, and pine nuts.

When your thyroid hormone levels become normal with treatment, you should still get tested every three to six months (depending on how stable your thyroid condition is) to ensure you're neither undertreated nor overtreated. If your physician prescribes too little or too much thyroid hormone, not only will you experience symptoms, you may gain weight. You also need to know that the dose of thyroid medication may need to be lowered as you lose weight. When following my program, regardless of the thyroid hormone treatment you are receiving, your doctor may need to monitor your levels more frequently to adjust the dose accordingly.

HOW THE WRONG TREATMENT OF LOW THYROID
CAN CAUSE WEIGHT GAIN

Many doctors and other health professionals continue to view low-grade hypothyroidism and hypothyroidism with normal blood tests as no big deal. Worse, hypothyroidism, whether low-grade or not, is often not treated with the right amount or type of thyroid medication—this despite the fact that low thyroid leads to poor quality of life, depressive symptoms, fatigue, cardiovascular damage, and weight gain.

- *Too little thyroid hormone* will perpetuate the slowdown of metabolism that I talked about earlier.

- *Too much hormone* in your system will be perceived by your body as a threat to survival and ultimately trigger weight gain once the excess of thyroid hormone is corrected and your thyroid levels are normalized. While too much thyroid hormone can make you lose weight temporarily, it can also make you gain weight even when you still have too much thyroid hormone in your system. Remember that too much thyroid hormone destroys protein, muscle, and bone—and reduced muscle mass, as you now know, slows metabolism. Once your metabolic machinery detects the presence of too much thyroid hormone, your appetite-reducing friend leptin becomes less efficient and you'll be driven to eat more food. You also accumulate free radicals in your body and become resistant to insulin, and the weight-gain cycle worsens.

One of my patients is a good example of what happens when a person is treated with the wrong dose of thyroid hormones. Fifty-year-old Kat flew from Maine to see me about her long-standing weight gain and to make sure her thyroid levels were truly normal, because she didn't feel well even though she'd been taking thyroid medication. Her doctor had prescribed doses of thyroid hormone that were physiologically unsuited to her. Her thyroid condition had been treated incorrectly for many years and her body had suffered immensely. Unfortunately, this incorrect dosage happens quite often.

"I was 130 pounds fifteen years ago. Now I weigh 210. Ever since I had my boy fifteen years ago, the weight has crept onto me. Weird things were also happening, like I was tired and my hair was falling out. One year later, my doctor recognized I was having a thyroid issue. I was put on Synthroid and stopped gaining weight for a while, which seemed good, but then I started gaining again. I couldn't figure out exactly what was wrong. Every time I went back to the doctor, she told me my tests were fine and Synthroid was working fine.

"With the nonstop weight gain all these years, I have other problems. I'm tired and not motivated to do anything. It's harder to exercise. It's like a Catch-22. I'm gaining weight. It's getting worse. It won't stop."

Kat had been getting insufficient amounts of thyroid hormone most of the time. Her TSH levels were in the 3 to 5 range, reflecting a continued thyroid hormone deficit in her system. I found the right dose and ratio of T4/T3 for her and started her on the Protein Boost Diet eating plan along with the supplements I recommend.

At the start, losing eighty pounds was slow but steady. "I was losing maybe one pound a week for the first couple of weeks, and I told myself it may barely be anything but I'm heading in the right direction." As the hormone therapy started working and her metabolism caught up, Kat began to lose about two pounds a week. She also started following my complete mind-body weight-loss program. Ten months after I took over Kat's treatment and monitoring, she'd become a very vibrant-looking 52-year-old, weighing 145 pounds, smiling and flaunting her now-healthy golden locks.

Kat had been taking T4 (levothyroxine) only and at a suboptimal dose. This can result in significant weight gain and lingering symptoms. When you take levothyroxine only to treat hypothyroidism, some of the T4 gets converted in your system to T3, the active form of thyroid hormone. However, the amount of T3 derived from the levothyroxine tablet may not be adequate, in which case you'll continue to experience fatigue, low-grade depression, and sluggish metabolism. For this reason, many patients feel better and manage their weight better when they take medications that include both T4 and T3, a treatment that mimics what a normal thyroid produces.

One of the thyroid medications containing T4 and T3 is Armour thyroid (also called "desiccated thyroid"), an extract of pig thyroid. Desiccated thyroid is the oldest form of thyroid medication on the market. Because it contains both T4 and T3, Armour thyroid continues to be popular and, in fact, many doctors prescribe it alone to their patients. But there's a catch: the amount of T3 in high-dose tablets of Armour thyroid is inappropriate for the human body. Armour thyroid has a high T3-to-T4 ratio, exceeding the normal T3/T4 ratio in humans. If you're prescribed Armour thyroid at higher than 30 mg per dose, for certain your T3 levels will exceed the normal range for a few hours before declining. The surges of T3 during the day caused by taking Armour thyroid as a single high dose result in an imbalance in your body. Even if your blood test results are normal, you may experience the adverse effects of too much thyroid hormone, including weight gain down the road. There are other thyroid medications that have a composition similar to Armour thyroid, including Nature-Throid and Westhroid. Both cause the same imbalance and too much T3 in your system. However, low doses of these medications can be used alone or in conjunction with added T4 (if needed) to restore thyroid balance without overdosing you with T3.

Phyllis, a 44-year-old salesperson, came to see me for low thyroid treatment. Four years earlier, she'd been diagnosed with an overactive thyroid caused by Graves' disease and was treated with radioactive iodine to destroy the overactive thyroid cells (this might sound radical, but it's how we treat some patients with Graves' disease). After the treatment, Phyllis developed hypothyroidism—as most patients do—and was prescribed thyroid hormone in the form of levothyroxine (T4), which restored her test results to normal levels. However, she quickly gained fifteen pounds, a common occurrence after treatment of overactive thyroid. Phyllis had continued to gain weight and was also struggling with low-grade depression and anxiety. Unhappy with her treatment, she'd visited another doctor who prescribed an outrageously high dose of Armour thyroid to be taken once a day to treat the low thyroid. This put high levels of thyroid hormones into her system and caused metabolic chaos—excessive thyroid hormone prompts your body to pack on the pounds, when your thyroid levels become normal again.

Two years later, Phyllis went to yet another doctor, who changed her prescription to levothyroxine-only treatment, and after the new doctor adjusted the dose, her thyroid tests became normal. Yet after that change she'd added another eighteen pounds. By the time she came to me, Phyllis had gained forty-five pounds since the original treatment of her overactive thyroid.

People who have been prescribed too much thyroid hormone, especially in the form of high-dose Armour thyroid or medications containing too much T3, usually suffer a setback in metabolism that will haunt them even after their levels become rebalanced. I changed Phyllis's prescription to a combination of T4 and T3, and she embraced my program in its entirety. This combination enabled her to lose twenty-seven pounds over four months. This is an impressive result, given that too much thyroid hormone almost universally induces a state of weight-loss resistance, difficult to overcome with any other diet.

BEWARE OF MEDICATIONS AND MINERALS THAT CAN LOWER YOUR THYROID LEVELS

Several medications used to treat various medical conditions can affect your thyroid balance by interfering with the gastrointestinal absorption of thyroid hormone. Reduced absorption of thyroid hormone, as a result of taking these medications simultaneously with your thyroid hormone pill, can end up causing low thyroid hormone levels in your body. Medications and supplements that can interfere with thyroid hormone absorption and indirectly result in a slowdown in metabolism should be taken several hours after you take thyroid hormone medication. Medications and minerals (and their brand names) that can produce this effect are listed below.

Medication (Brand Name)	Function
Cholestyramine (Questran)	Lower high cholesterol levels in the blood
Cholesevelan (Welchol)	Reduce cholesterol and fatty substances in the blood
Aluminum hydroxide (Alternagel)	Relief of heartburn, sour stomach, and peptic ulcer
Sucralfate (Carafate, Xactdose)	Treatment of ulcers
Proton pump inhibitors (Losec, Omesec, Prilosec)	Used to treat GERD (gastroesophageal reflux disease)
Sevelamer (RenaGel)	Treats high blood levels of phosphorus in patients with kidney disease
Lanthinum (Fosrenol)	Reduces blood levels of phosphate in patients with kidney disease
Raloxifene (Evista)	Prevents and treats osteoporosis in post-menopausal women
Orlistat (Alli, Xenical)	Used in combination with diet and exercise for weight management
Tyrosine kinase inhibitors (Axitinib, Bosutinib)	Used to treat some cancers
Calcium carbonate (Alka-Mints, Alkets, Maalox)	Calcium supplement or antacid to relieve heartburn, acid indigestion, and upset stomach
Calcium acetate (PhosLo)	Calcium supplement to prevent high blood phosphate levels in dialysis patients
Calcium citrate (Citracal)	Calcium supplement
Ferrous sulfate (Feosol, Fer Iron, Feratab)	Used to treat iron deficiency anemia

If you're taking thyroid hormone medication, don't take vitamins in the morning that contain calcium or iron. It's best to select a calcium-free, iron-free multivitamin and take calcium and iron at least four to six hours after taking thyroid medication.

If you're being treated for hypothyroidism, be aware that the dose of your thyroid medication may require adjustment if you're taking other medications that can affect how your body utilizes thyroid hormones. For example, niacin (to reduce blood levels of cholesterol and fatty substances), testosterone, L-asparaginase (to treat a certain type of acute lymphatic leukemia), danazol (for endometriosis), and glucocorticoids can lower the levels of the protein thyroxine-binding globulin (TBG) that carries thyroid hormone in the blood; this effect in turn requires reducing the dose of thyroid hormone. In contrast, birth control pills and estrogens may make you require a higher dose of thyroid hormone to maintain normal thyroid levels. Your doctor may also need to increase your dose of thyroid hormone if you take barbiturates, carbamazepine or phenytoin (for seizures), or rifampin (for tuberculosis), as these medications make your body break down and lose some of the active form of thyroid hormone.

T4/T3 FOR OPTIMAL METABOLISM

If you're taking levothyroxine (i.e., Synthroid, Levoxyl, Tirosint) for hypothyroidism, your treatment is not duplicating nature. Even if your thyroid test results become perfectly normal with T4-only treatment, you may still be missing the T3 that is crucial for the thyroid to regulate your metabolism. A healthy thyroid gland produces 20 percent of the T3 needed by your body and brain. Though a minute deficit in this potent thyroid hormone may not cause any symptoms or effects, in some people it can affect metabolism as well as mood and appetite. Keep in mind that T3 is the thyroid hormone that works in brain cells to regulate serotonin, noradrenaline, GABA, and dopamine, all involved in balancing mood, emotions, and appetite (more on them later).

Thus, even though your blood test results (including TSH levels) are normal, you may be suffering from "general body" hypothyroidism and its consequences, including anxiety, low mood, hair loss, brittle nails, muscle cramps, fatigue, and weight gain. Including T3 in your treatment may be key to improving your resting metabolic rate (the number of calories you burn when you're just sitting) because it increases your oxygen consumption rate. Research has shown that T3 treatment stimulates you to burn more fat and make your body generate more heat. T3 is the thyroid hormone that can heighten metabolic activity.

Several years ago I was treating a shocking number of patients who had been treated with T4 only and were struggling with lingering symptoms of low thyroid despite having normal blood tests. Treating them with T4 and T3 to duplicate how the thyroid gland naturally functions provided them with spectacular results. Over the years, I have used this same method of treating patients with hypothyroidism when they continue to suffer from symptoms and weight issues. I designed a treatment that combines synthetic T4 and T3, but I've been using a compounded form (a pharmaceutical method of combining ingredients for individualized needs) of T3 rather than the synthetic form. This form of T3 is effective, safe, precise, and practical.

You take the T3 compounded as a single daily dose with levothyroxine. In this way, T3 remains in your system throughout the day and you experience no major surges and troughs in T3 levels as you

How the Protein Boost Diet Supports Balanced Thyroid and Growth Hormones

- It's immune-system-friendly (low in saturated fat, high in monounsaturated and polyunsaturated fat) and makes you less susceptible to an autoimmune attack. This is vital because thyroid imbalance is often the result of an immune system attack on the thyroid. Many cases of growth hormone deficiency are also related to an immune system attack on the pituitary. The best way to prevent an autoimmune disorder is by eating a diet that supports your immune system, and my meal plans also bolster thyroid and pituitary function.

- You'll be eating plenty of proteins containing the amino acids needed for growth hormone production, immune system function, and thyroid hormone manufacturing and efficiency.

- My innovative 20/10 exercise program—along with relaxation techniques, good sleep, and eating in sync with your central clock—makes the thyroid and growth hormone systems work at their peak for optimal metabolism.

- The low-glycemic, multiprotein meal combinations are ideal for leptin efficiency. When you achieve peak leptin sensitivity, your thyroid and growth hormone activity heighten as well as your metabolism.

- Your eating schedule calls for lower-glycemic foods at dinner, ensuring that your insulin levels remain low throughout the night. You want less insulin in your system because it makes your body store fat, whereas growth hormone produced in higher amounts while you sleep encourages your body to burn fat and build muscle. This approach sets you up for the best insulin/growth hormone balance for boosting metabolism.

- The Protein Boost Diet is the only program I know of that emphasizes the importance of proper micronutrients and amino acids necessary for every metabolic function. These include iodine, selenium, and zinc for thyroid hormone manufacturing and arginine for growth hormone production.

do with synthetic T3. Your doctor can adjust the dose of T3 according to your symptoms, your dose requirement, and your age (in contrast to compounded T3, synthetic T3 comes in standard doses of 5, 25, and 50 mcg, which may not be precisely what you need).

Even with this precise form of treatment, you can't expect the fat you've gained because of your thyroid imbalance to melt away. The medications will give you the necessary ingredients, but they aren't sufficient themselves to make you lose weight. You need to do your part, engaging in my complete mind-body program, to reach the results you desire. You need to be proactive and disciplined when it comes to the eating plan and antioxidant supplements I recommend.

HYPERTHYROIDISM: WHEN TOO MUCH HORMONE CRASHES METABOLISM

If weight loss and metabolism were simple matters and too much thyroid hormone were harmless to health, people would take extra thyroid hormone to speed up their metabolisms and lose weight. However, too much thyroid hormone is actually harmful to your metabolism and can make you gain body fat, as Phyllis's case illustrates. Having too much also alters the weight-loss helpers serotonin, noradrenaline, GABA, and beta-endorphins, and can make you become unable to control your cravings. We all know how that ends.

The most common cause of hyperthyroidism is Graves' disease, in which the immune system sends signals to the thyroid to make it produce excessive amounts of thyroid hormone. Other causes include an autonomous thyroid nodule (a growth inside the thyroid gland that takes over the function of the gland and produces excessive amounts of thyroid hormones) and multinodular toxic goiters (several hyperactive growths that produce too much thyroid hormone). Temporary hyperthyroidism, which lasts a few weeks to a few months, can be caused by silent thyroiditis (inflammation caused by the immune system) or by subacute thyroiditis (inflammation caused by a virus).

Too much thyroid hormone in your system makes you burn more calories both at rest and while exercising. Ghrelin, the hormone that makes you feel hungry and slows down your metabolism, is also lower in people who have hyperthyroidism, making their metabolisms speedier. For a significant number of people, the revved-up metabolism overrides eating too much, causing weight loss, a typical symptom of hyperthyroidism.

But individuals react differently to having too much thyroid hormone. You may be among the 20 percent whose metabolism is not energized enough by the excess hormone to lose weight. This 20 percent ends up gaining weight instead of losing it.

If you have hyperthyroidism, you may experience initial weight loss, possibly up to 15 percent of your body weight. However, at the same time many metabolic functions within your body begin to break down. Too much thyroid hormone damages your antioxidant system, increasing inflammation. As your body tries to cope with the inflammation, you become less sensitive to leptin and insulin. Excess thyroid hormone raises blood sugar and insulin to high levels, leading to a buildup of inflammation, and the distortion of your insulin system doesn't stop. One of the end results is the loss of lean muscle, the very tissue that burns energy.

This gradual metabolic dysfunction isn't caused by insulin resistance alone. T3 has energy-boosting qualities similar to another hormone, adiponectin, that tells your body to burn fat for fuel. When you have too much T3 in your system, your body responds by producing less adiponectin in an effort to slow down metabolism. Since your body is suffering from lowered adiponectin, the insulin resistance and leptin resistance are more pronounced, throwing your metabolic activity into chaos.

OVERACTIVE THYROID SYMPTOMS

The most common symptoms are weight loss, restlessness, fatigue, difficulty concentrating, shakiness, rapid heartbeat, hair loss, intolerance of heat, increased sweating, increased frequency of bowel movements, decreased fertility, and irregular periods.

I have patients who chose not to take their hyperthyroid medication because their excess thyroid hormone made them thinner. But even if you have subclinical (low-grade) hyperthyroidism and you're enjoying the increased energy and fat burn, you should begin treatment as soon as possible. Untreated hyperthyroidism can dangerously affect your heart, and your metabolism will eventually crash if you don't get treatment.

You also need to face the fact that many women with overactive thyroid gain weight after their hyperthyroidism is corrected with treatment. The same thing happens when a person suffers from an overactive thyroid as when a person has too much thyroid hormone due to a prescribed overdose of thyroid medication. After the excess thyroid hormone is corrected, leptin levels remain low, making your metabolism slower and your hunger level higher. Too much thyroid hormone in your body is viewed by your hormone system as a threat to survival, and now that your thyroid levels are finally becoming normal, your body begins to encourage you to eat more calories and store more fat.

It's imperative that you not become discouraged and that you continue to treat your overactive thyroid. No matter which treatment you get, weight gain is almost inevitable unless you're proactive and start following an eating plan like the one in this book that promotes leptin efficiency and removes the weight gain–promoting free radicals from your system.

GROWTH HORMONE DEFICIENCY, A CAUSE OF RELENTLESS WEIGHT GAIN

Numerous patients suffer needlessly from years of weight gain simply because their doctors failed to consider GH deficiency as the cause of their symptoms. GH does the opposite of insulin: it encourages fat breakdown by prompting your liver and other tissues to produce the chemical IGF1 (insulin-like growth factor, also called somatomedin-C), which stimulates the growth of cells in the body, making the pancreas produce the right amount of insulin for optimal metabolism of glucose. It makes insulin work more efficiently, so your muscles and liver metabolize glucose properly. If you're deficient in GH, the activity of insulin shifts toward moving sugar into fat in fat cells rather than making your liver convert sugar into other forms of energy.

SYMPTOMS OF GROWTH HORMONE DEFICIENCY

If your body isn't producing enough growth hormone, you'll inevitably gain weight in the form of fat while losing muscle. Symptoms of GH deficiency and low thyroid are remarkably similar, with being overweight a universal symptom. Typically fat accumulates around the abdomen, increasing your waist-to-hip ratio and your risk of metabolic syndrome and insulin resistance. With that, your body can't process insulin effectively, causing high blood sugar and still more fat to be deposited.

Not only do most people with GH deficiency end up with metabolic syndrome, they also tend to have far more abdominal fat than usual, often reflecting a more serious metabolic impairment. GH deficiency also causes high cholesterol and depression, increases cardiovascular disease risk, and impairs quality of life. The impaired metabolism caused by GH deficiency explains why many patients have high blood pressure, insulin resistance, high cholesterol, and high triglycerides. If you have a GH deficiency, the amount of fat you have around your waist correlates with how long you've been deficient.

Here's a list of GH deficiency symptoms in adults:

Excessive fat around the waist
Low energy
Depressive symptoms, moodiness, irritability, and anxiety
Weak muscles
Loss of muscle mass (minimal to significant)
Reduced endurance for exercise
Osteopenia (bone loss)
Sleep problems (insomnia, sleep apnea)

With GH deficiency, you're likely to suffer from a wide range of sleep disturbances. Sixty-three percent of patients with GH deficiency have obstructive sleep apnea, which slows your metabolism (see "Sleep Apnea" in Chapter 5). Having sleep apnea in addition to GH deficiency will accelerate your weight gain and worsen your symptoms. Treatment with growth hormone causes noticeable improvement in sleep within six months.

CAUSES OF GROWTH HORMONE DEFICIENCY

Low growth hormone can be the result of many other common hormone imbalances, including estrogen deficiency and hypothyroidism. Estrogen triggers your pituitary to produce more GH, and when your estrogen levels drop, as they do in menopause, your pituitary slows down its production of GH. This is one reason your metabolism runs slowly and you're likely to gain weight during the transition into menopause. (Taking the right dose of hormones in the form of bioidentical hormone treatment and following my diet will reactivate your GH and make you more likely to succeed in your weight-loss efforts.) Testosterone is another key player in keeping GH levels in the healthy range. Research has shown that men with low testosterone also have low levels of GH, but when they're treated with testosterone, their GH levels rise to normal.

The amount of growth hormone you have also depends on how well-balanced your thyroid system is. If you have low thyroid, your GH levels will be low, too, producing a weight-gain double whammy, since low levels of both hormones cause your metabolism to burn fewer calories. Recent research has shown that even low-grade hypothyroidism can cause a GH deficit, resulting in a sluggish metabolism and weight gain. But there's hopeful news. If you have a thyroid imbalance, when you're treated with thyroid hormone your GH returns to its normal functioning level.

Clear-cut GH deficiency caused by pituitary damage (but not related to other hormone disorders) is not as prevalent as hypothyroidism, and views differ on how common it is. One estimate says about 35,000 adults in the United States have GH deficiency, with approximately 6,000 newly diagnosed adults each year. Another source maintains it's far more common and can be found in one of 3,000 to 4,000 people. These statistics obviously don't include people with other hormone issues such as low thyroid, low estrogen during menopause, or the low testosterone known to reduce GH.

Here's some research that should startle anyone trying to lose extra weight: your pituitary will slow down its manufacture of growth hormone simply because you're overweight or obese. The more fat you've accumulated, the lower your GH is, perpetuating your weight-related GH deficiency and escalating weight gain all over again. It's as though your pituitary responds to your weight gain to reinforce it and make you pursue that trend—as if it were your destiny—by lowering its GH production.

You can see how GH deficiency leads to obesity and obesity to GH deficiency. In fact, once you begin to gain weight, for whatever reason, it becomes a serious struggle to halt the trend and even more so to reverse it. If you want to succeed in your weight-loss program, it is essential to break this cycle of being overweight leading to low GH, which in turn makes you fatter.

A DAMAGED PITUITARY GLAND CAN CAUSE
GROWTH HORMONE DEFICIENCY

The most likely cause of GH deficiency is a defective pituitary gland that isn't producing optimal amounts of growth hormone. Possible reasons include an autoimmune disorder, head injury, or damage to the pituitary gland or hypothalamus from a tumor, surgery, or radiation treatment. Many people, however, have none of these causes but still have impaired GH production. They're diagnosed with what's called an "isolated GH deficiency," related to an impairment of the pituitary cells that normally produce growth hormone.

If you have a GH deficiency caused by impaired pituitary function and your doctor hasn't been able to identify a specific cause, it may be the result of pituitary gland inflammation caused by your own immune system attacking your pituitary (called "autoimmune hypophysitis"), an often-overlooked reason for pituitary impairment.

Depending on the extent of the inflammation, the condition affects the production of GH and other hormones produced by your pituitary (the ones that send signals to other glands such as the adrenals, ovaries/testicles, and thyroid). When pituitary signaling hormones are also deficient, your pituitary is unable to communicate with its target glands, and you'll end up having not only GH deficiency but shortages of other hormones, including cortisol, sex hormones, and thyroid hormones.

Autoimmune hypophysitis affects people with autoimmune thyroid conditions more often—5 percent of patients with Hashimoto's thyroiditis suffer from GH deficiency. A study released in Paris showed that 18 percent of people who had autoimmune hypophysitis also had clinical symptoms of thyroid dysfunction.

For 33-year-old Monica, autoimmune hypophysitis silently packed pounds on her body while it hid behind an obvious thyroid problem. Four years earlier, Monica had been slim, weighing 150 at five-feet-eight. Within those four years she started suffering from worsening symptoms of fatigue, depression, and forgetfulness, and she gained weight on an accelerated schedule—ten pounds, fifteen pounds, and then twenty-five pounds per year. Having a strong family history of autoimmune thyroiditis (Hashimoto's), Monica assumed her thyroid was acting up.

I found she had Hashimoto's thyroiditis and hypothyroidism, and treated her using a well-balanced regimen of T4 and T3. Eight weeks later, she returned and her thyroid function tests showed that her thyroid was perfectly balanced.

"I'm definitely feeling better but still fatigued and not quite right," she said. Monica also still had many of the symptoms she'd had when she first came to me. She still weighed 225 pounds and the symptoms that should have gone away with treatment were still pestering her. I started her on my diet and advised her to begin the 20/10 exercise program. Two months later, Monica was back for a check on her thyroid hormones, but I was shocked that she hadn't lost more than four pounds on my diet with exercise and that her fatigue persisted. She assured me she'd been committed to both.

Suspecting that autoimmunity may have affected her pituitary, I tested her growth hormone and the results indicated GH deficiency. Monica had an autoimmune attack not only on her thyroid, but on her pituitary as well. In fact, an MRI showed an area of inflammation in her pituitary gland that hadn't been severe enough to affect her adrenal glands or ovarian function. Immediately after discovering the cause of her symptoms and persistent weight gain, I started her on growth hormone therapy. Once Monica's levels of growth hormone were balanced, her diet and exercise efforts became effective, and her symptoms gradually resolved. Each month she lost an average of ten pounds, and six months later she was back to her slender build.

BRAIN INJURY IS ANOTHER COMMONLY OVERLOOKED CAUSE OF GROWTH HORMONE DEFICIENCY AND THE RELENTLESS WEIGHT GAIN IT CAUSES

GH deficiency caused by head injury often produces difficulty paying attention, loss of concentration, difficulty learning, and reduced ability to solve problems, as well as phobic anxiety and neuropsychological impairment. If you've experienced a head injury and have these symptoms along with weight gain, your GH should be tested by an endocrinologist (a doctor who specializes in evaluating endocrine— hormone—disorders).

Twenty-five percent of people with traumatic brain injury will end up having GH deficiency. Because the pituitary is a tiny and fragile gland, serious head injury can impair the blood supply and cause inflammation and damage to cells in the hypothalamus. People involved in contact sports, such as boxing and kickboxing, are at high risk of suffering from GH deficiency, as are veterans with traumatic brain injury and others who've suffered brain injury in motor vehicle accidents. The good news is that if you have GH deficiency related to brain injury, your symptoms—particularly your cognitive symptoms—will improve greatly with growth hormone treatment.

Sean, a 48-year-old patient of mine, came to see me about his weight of 280 pounds and multiple symptoms he thought might be related to his thyroid. Twenty-five years before, he'd gradually started to gain weight and quickly noticed more fat accumulation around his waist, which had gotten worse over the years. Around that time, he also started struggling with depression, fatigue, dry skin, and low sex drive, and his cognition was clearly declining. I tested Sean's thyroid and his results were normal. In fact, Sean had had his thyroid evaluated multiple times over the years, and he'd seen many physicians looking for an answer to his weight as well as his crippling symptoms.

I asked him when he'd started noticing his expanding waistline. "A long time ago," he began, "when I had to quit competitive motocross. I was only twenty-five, and I had to give up motocross because I got injured. Motocross was my life and my passion! Without it, I felt like a corporate drone with nothing to look forward to. I stopped caring about working out, and by the time I realized I'd gained a lot of weight, I couldn't work out like I used to. I used to be 160 pounds. Now it's like I lost all of my strength and dexterity. I couldn't tell if it was my lack of motivation or if my body was deteriorating for real."

When I saw Sean for the first time, he appeared to have metabolic syndrome with his protruding waistline, but what was striking was the fact that many of his symptoms were symptoms of low thyroid. Symptoms of low thyroid and low growth hormone are similar, so I questioned him about his motocross years: had he ever had a head injury back in his twenties? "Oh, yeah, quite a few," he said. "Despite precautions I hurt my head maybe six or seven times. Actually on a few occasions they took me to the emergency room, but the CT scans showed my head and brain were okay." Sean's growth hormone test showed that his excess abdominal fat, dramatic weight gain, and muscle loss were actually the outcome of GH deficiency caused by his head injuries.

Sean started receiving growth hormone injections, and two months later he returned for a follow-up, feeling energized and determined to put a dent in his weight. He was shocked at how quickly the growth hormone treatment had unlocked his energy and metabolism. "I'm motivated again. Physical activity seems doable. Just tell me what I need to do so I can get back to normal," said Sean. After we discussed my mind-body program, Sean began following it and continued his growth hormone therapy. One year later he eagerly showed me his new number on the scale: 190 pounds.

A tumor in the region of the hypothalamus or pituitary (or surgery on that same area) can cause damage similar to that of traumatic brain injury and result in GH deficiency. Also, radiation for a pituitary tumor or a brain tumor can damage your pituitary and hypothalamus, triggering GH deficiency and potentially deficiencies of other pituitary hormones.

TESTS FOR GROWTH HORMONE DEFICIENCY

Simple blood tests are not a highly reliable way to test for GH deficiency because growth hormone is released into your bloodstream in pulses and is cleared from your system quickly. Nevertheless, blood tests that look for the GH marker IGF1 (somatomedin C) can be used for quick testing and often will show if you have a GH deficiency. Unfortunately, this blood test can give you false readings, as it can be low just as a result of your being overweight. Growth-hormone-stimulation tests, including the insulin tolerance test, arginine test, and GH-releasing hormone test, are more sophisticated and precise. Insulin tolerance testing can be dangerous, though, because it consists of injecting insulin to cause hypoglycemia. Don't ask for this test if you have a cardiovascular or seizure disorder. The safest and most often performed tests are the GH-releasing hormone test and the arginine-stimulation test.

TREATING GROWTH HORMONE DEFICIENCY

We know that untreated GH deficiency leads to weight gain, cardio-vascular risks, hypertension, high cholesterol and triglycerides, insulin resistance, and inflammation, but two years of GH treatment cut cardiovascular risk by about half.

If your GH deficiency is due to a pituitary disorder, you must be treated with GH injections to reverse the weight-gain trend and regain your quality of life. Treatment with recombinant human growth hormone (examples include Humatrope, Genotropin, Norditropin, Somatropin, Jintropin, Serostim, Saizen) will reduce abdominal fat and increase lean body mass. You'll typically be started at a low dose of GH injected under the skin, visiting your doctor every four to eight weeks to test GH levels and adjust the medication. Once a maintenance dose is established, you'll be monitored every four to six months with blood testing.

People whose low GH is caused by being overweight, not by problems with pituitary inflammation or damage, can't reverse their situation with GH treatment, but can through a weight-loss program that includes a growth-hormone-friendly approach like the one in this book, including sleeping a full eight hours nightly, exercising (exercise is a nice GH booster), eating well-balanced mixes of proteins daily, and enjoying the very-low-glycemic, protein-rich meals, which have GH-boosting effects.

Growth hormone treatment is, generally speaking, safe. Adverse effects include joint stiffness, tingling in the extremities, swelling of the feet and hands, and muscle pains and aches. Concerns that GH treatment increases the risk of cancer or cancerous tumor regrowth are unfounded. Research to date has not shown any evidence that GH treatment promotes cancer. Once you're treated you'll feel better, have more vitality and energy, and drop overall body fat, including the risky visceral fat around your waist. GH treatment will help build more lean muscle, strengthen your bones, and improve heart function as well. However, you also need to follow a diet program that will work with your GH treatment to achieve the best results. Turn to Chapter 9 to get started now.

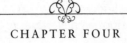

CHAPTER FOUR

MANAGING STRESS TO CONTROL CRAVINGS AND FAT-BOOSTING HORMONES

Central to my weight-loss program is keeping a healthy, stress-free state of mind. Easier said than done, but I can provide some extra motivation. In this chapter, we'll discuss the very real ways stress causes weight gain and also how mood and emotions powerfully affect your cravings, metabolism, and sex life. All this is largely controlled by . . . you guessed it, hormones.

Some diets breezily advise you to stop stressing out, but I'm asking you to recognize that in order to lose weight, you must invest time in relaxation. Let's pause now and take a deep breath through the nose, filling your lungs and blowing it out slowly through your mouth. I've included several techniques here to ease your mind and body from "thinking" that it needs to pack on pounds. Understand that any stress that makes you unhappy will compromise the hormones that keep your metabolism running smoothly. One key to looking good on the outside is being relaxed on the inside.

HOW STRESS MAKES YOU FAT

Stress-induced weight gain comes at you from at least three angles: First, the stress itself meddles with hormones that control appetite. Then your reaction to stress typically sends you to fattening snacks.

Finally, stress compromises sleep, so vital for complete cycling of the hormones essential to weight loss.

Stress comes in many guises. Top sources are money problems, work, the economy, relationships, family responsibility, health problems, job stability, and housing costs. Any of those sound familiar?

When you're stressed, your body responds with a cascade of hormones designed to keep you safe from danger. They're all part of your lifesaving fight-or-flight response, triggered when your hypothalamus (which controls body temperature, fullness, mood, and emotions) sends a "red alert" message to your autonomic (automatic) nervous system and your adrenal glands. When the adrenal glands receive the emergency message, they push out a surge of the hormones adrenaline and noradrenaline to give you a jolt of speed and strength to get away from the threat (the fight-or-flight response is meant to help you fight off the stress or flee from it). Your blood pressure, blood sugar, and heartbeat skyrocket to prep you for action, fighting off a purse snatcher or running from a threat. If you saw a truck barreling toward you at high speed, you'd need to run like the wind to save your life, and you'd be happy these stress hormones were activated to help you move quickly. Their effects prepare your whole body to escape danger. Once the danger has passed, you feel shaky and drained as your system deals with the onslaught of hormones.

But here's where the stress-induced hormonal cascade gets tricky and very destructive to health and weight. Your body doesn't know the difference between a real threat—the purse snatcher or high-speed truck—and the chronic stresses of daily life: stretching a paycheck to cover food and medicine; relationship problems, arguments, breakups; caring for your sick mother; being out of work; children's needs, their carpools, and their homework; piles of laundry; and nothing ready for dinner when you work late.

Your body's response to these constant, lower-level daily stressors is even more complex, hormonally speaking. In addition to triggering periodic spurts of adrenaline, constant daily stress signals the hypothalamus to alert your pituitary to make the adrenal glands release the stress hormone cortisol. With repeated stress—chronic stress—too much cortisol is released, causing fat to accumulate around your waist. That's because too much cortisol swimming around in your system slows metabolism and makes insulin less efficient; this inefficiency boosts fat storage.

Your weight-loss helper leptin starts working poorly, too, when you're generating so much cortisol, so you burn fewer calories and produce less heat. Leptin's job is to tell your brain and body how much body fat you have, limit food intake, and speed metabolism to burn extra fat. You never want to lose the efficiency of this powerful ally, yet when you constantly stress yourself and flood your body with cortisol, this is exactly what happens.

With all the extra cortisol, your immune system suffers as well. You become prone to infection or to antibodies going haywire. Your own body literally attacks your thyroid in an autoimmune disorder. You become susceptible to Graves' disease (an autoimmune condition causing overactive thyroid), autoimmune thyroiditis (Hashimoto's), and low thyroid (which we know leads to weight gain). This cycling of stress leads to lower mood and worsening thyroid dysfunction. The weight gain from excess cortisol and low thyroid hormone can magnify negative self-perception and the inability to cope with stress. Thyroid imbalance itself distorts your perception of stress and the way you handle it. The exacerbated stress, in turn, further affects your thyroid, leading to an escalating cycle of thyroid imbalance/ stress, and you end up having two reasons for weight gain.

Research shows that feeling heavily stressed for just a couple of days results in central hypothyroidism, in which the pituitary stops signaling the thyroid gland to produce its hormones. Your response to stress over time could actually prevent your body from producing enough thyroid hormone. It's all about survival. When your body assumes you're surrounded by threats to survival, it begins its game plan for conserving energy and storing fat.

Another study shows that experiencing stress for just one day reduces production of metabolism-fueling thyroid hormone. Happily, removing the animals in the study from the stressful environment allowed their thyroid hormone levels to return to normal. You can't always control your environment so neatly, but your stress level and coinciding hormone functions rely heavily on your attitude— how you view the stress you're affected by.

HOW YOU PERCEIVE STRESS MATTERS

The way you respond to stress determines your body's biological response to it. A certain boss might make your days miserable with stress, while an unaffected coworker shrugs it off with "C'est la vie—I don't let him get to me." When you hear this boss coming, your stress response is triggered and your body goes into metabolic overdrive. How does it work? Your emotional brain uses *the way you perceive stress* rather than the stress itself to determine how much adrenaline, noradrenaline, and stress hormone cortisol is produced by your adrenal glands and whether your blood pressure rises or not. Also, the way you integrate stress and how you deal with it determine its effect on body fat composition and weight. If you're internally stressed like this regularly, you will overproduce the hormones that make you fat.

If your life is awash in chronic stress, you must address these emotional challenges or your body's physiological response will both hurt your health and make you gain weight. Remember, physiological responses are triggered by hormones in cells that affect your organs and whole body. Stress can cause you to sleep and exercise less, smoke more, and lose control over how much alcohol and food you consume. Extensive research shows that stress is at the root of an extraordinary number of health conditions, including becoming overweight or diabetic. Stress not only can make you take in more calories, it affects your food choices and leads you to eat fattening foods instead of vegetables, meats, and fish. That's because stress can loosen inhibitions and lead to loss of self-control over what you choose to eat and how much. You eat when you're stressed because eating reduces feelings of anxiety or makes you feel better in some way. Gorging on high-calorie snacks temporarily makes you feel better in threatening situations. Stress makes you crave comfort foods that are high in fat, salt, and sugar. Over time, your behavioral response to stress becomes automatic, causing you to seek out the same comfort foods to generate those good feelings again.

Hormonally speaking, the shift of fat to your belly caused by chronic stress is similar to the fat accumulation that occurs in people who have Cushing's syndrome, in which the adrenal glands produce too much of the stress hormone cortisol. The quite rare Cushing's syndrome can be caused by an adrenal gland tumor or pituitary condition that makes the adrenals overproduce cortisol. People who have Cushing's syndrome typically have waistline fat accumulation, insulin resistance, high blood pressure, muscle weakness, and large stretch marks over the abdomen. You'll get almost the same results if you keep your body in a state of constant stress.

CORTISOL OUT OF CONTROL

Before Whitney, 42, became my patient, she'd been able to maintain her weight at around 150 pounds for the previous ten years. At five-feet-seven, she had a healthy weight for her proportions. But in the two years before she came to see me to find answers about why she'd gained so much weight, she'd added fifty pounds and now weighed 200. "This is not normal," she said, standing up to show me her protruding belly. "When I was pregnant with my son, my belly didn't look this bad." She put her hands on a belly bulging out just below her ribs. "I have all this extra here. Doesn't weight usually disperse throughout your body, to your legs and arms? It seems like almost all my weight is going to my abdomen."

Her abdominal fat made me suspect that cortisol had played a role in her weight gain. When I asked Whitney to tell me more about her life, she slumped in the chair and said her father had been diagnosed with brain cancer two years earlier and her estranged husband killed in a car accident a year earlier. "It's been very hard for me and my son, Danny. He saw my own father as his father figure since his dad died. Then my father died a few months ago, and now I'm a single mom with a teenage son who's grieving mightily. Some days I don't think I can cope with anything."

Whitney's stress was compounded by her weight gain, yet she felt losing the weight was not a high priority, given her son's grief. Whitney had begun sleeping less and had no energy or motivation to exercise. She was moving down a path of metabolic dysfunction, and I recommended she take the weight gain as seriously as her son's mental health. We discussed her starting the Protein Boost Diet eating plan as a first step, and I encouraged her to monitor her weight with friends who were dieting. As a next step, Whitney agreed to set aside time to focus on relaxation and her emotional well-being. We reviewed the relaxation techniques I discuss later in this chapter, and she chose to start a yoga class with her friend.

A few weeks later, Whitney returned and thanked me. "I feel like I have a goal to achieve now—something positive—and it's been really helpful to have my friend Debbie help me get back on track when I slip up," Whitney said. "It's been so much easier to feel better about what's happened to me in the past couple of years now that I'm focused on reaching my own goals. Maybe it's my attitude and perception, maybe it's letting go of all that stress. I'm feeling much more motivated, energetic, and happy, and I'm sleeping better, too."

Once Whitney regained her emotional equilibrium, she became even more committed to the full spectrum of my diet and exercise program. Motivated by shared goals and positive reinforcement, she adopted every single aspect of the program for an entire year, by which time her weight was back to a normal 150 pounds. Her attitude completely changed as well. "I feel strong and confident now," she said. "Danny's doing much better. I overcame tragedy, and I got my body back. I feel like, if I can lose fifty pounds while being a single mom, I can do anything!"

BREAKING EMOTIONAL HABITS

Your cognitive brain—your "thinking" brain or executive brain— has no direct control over your appetite, eating impulses, or metabolism. If you try to lose weight by eating less, you'll be constantly challenged by your metabolism and eating impulses. Initially you may lose a few pounds, but you'll stop losing weight because your metabolism quickly plays tricks on you by lowering levels of the helpful hormone leptin, increasing the weight-gain hormone ghrelin, and making your hypothalamus urge you to eat, shifting the hormonal balance that's normally conducive to burning calories. Your eating impulses become more ferocious, and you quickly regain any lost weight. Eventually, your thinking brain will lose in the battle against eating impulses, partly because the habitual memory of reward and pleasure that eating gives you makes you vulnerable to overeating and choosing foods that lead to weight gain. Consuming fattening foods is, in a way, a compensation that resurfaces with every emotional challenge, and this gradually modifies your eating behavior over the long term.

It's a complex system, yet the outcome is straightforward: fat preservation. Your emotional brain generates unconscious feelings, sensed in an area of the brain called the "nuclei accumbens," that motivate you to carry out habitual behaviors appropriate to those emotions ("I feel stressed, I want cookies"). The unconscious feelings are sent to your thinking brain, which recognizes how you feel, but executive control of emotions and drive is heavily regulated by a different part of the brain called the "prefrontal cortical structures." Thus, emotional influences can overpower the executive capacity of your brain to make good choices.

When you're stressed, cortisol affects neurotransmitters such as noradrenaline, serotonin, and dopamine, which are all involved in making your brain respond with a behavior that could lead to satisfaction—for example, the cookies. Your executive, thinking brain has the power to control your emotional brain ("I don't need cookies, I need to eat my healthy afternoon snack"), but under stress your executive brain can easily weaken. This is how cortisol shapes motivation to select certain foods—it affects dopamine levels in the nuclei accumbens. Dopamine is the pleasure seeker (I discuss it further at the end of this chapter). Once you feel stressed, your brain generates an automatic response designed to make you feel better: eating fattening foods.

This unconscious behavioral response to stress is the most crucial link between repetitive stress, gradual weight gain, and ultimately, obesity in so many people. Stress leads your brain to establish a pathway of habits and eating behaviors that become much more powerful than your thinking, executive brain, which works as a smart goal achiever. The irony is that your smart executive brain recognizes these unhealthy drives, but is powerless over eating habits that lead to fat accumulation and obesity.

In simplest terms, when your metabolism registers a threat—and your body perceives stress as a threat—it responds by storing fat. To be truly successful in your weight-loss program, you need a regular program of stress-reduction to help control the impulses generated by stress and your emotional brain.

A DISCONNECT BETWEEN GOALS AND HABITS

Julia, a 26-year-old patient of mine, was struggling with this disconnection between weight loss and emotional eating. It had been three months since her ex had broken up with her, and her plan to get a "hot body" wasn't happening. "I wanted to look better than ever so I could make him feel bad for dumping me," she told me. "It was my only goal at first, and I was focusing pretty well on just losing weight, but then I'd remember why I was trying so hard and I'd feel desperately sad."

During the first month after the breakup, she'd lost five pounds following a strict diet, but she'd had no motivation to get out of bed and exercise. Devastated, she explained "All I want to do is veg out in front of the TV and eat ice cream." In the two months before she came to see me, she'd regained the five pounds plus fifteen more. Rather than working to accept the loss of her boyfriend and achieve that "hot body," Julia had turned to desserts to make herself happy. Once she shifted her focus and started the Protein Boost Diet program—including regular tai chi practice to reduce stress—Julia was able to overcome the effects of stress on her eating impulses. She lost the weight she'd gained and has kept it off to this day.

TRAIN YOUR BRAIN

If like Julia you turn to ice cream (or candy or fries) when you're feeling down, the food choices in the Protein Boost Diet will help you bridge the gap while relaxation techniques teach you to cope with stress more gracefully. Still, you're initially likely to crave unhealthy foods, so it's essential that you identify an alternative behavior for when you feel upset or get a craving. Treat your bad eating habits like the addictions they are, and fight them with a distraction you can always turn to, such as a book, a cup of tea, a game on an electronic device, or a fast walk outdoors. As you grow stronger, you'll remind yourself every time you feel tempted that poor food choices are going to haunt you with excess body fat, further slowing your metabolism and perpetuating the cycle of uncontrollable appetite and weight gain.

One technique that's worked for many of my patients is to train your brain to view sugary, salty, high-carb foods as toxic. Begin to view them not as a treat or reward, but rather as poison for your metabolism. Just like a drug, food gives you an actual rush (it's the blood sugar and dopamine high), and afterward, your body's growing tolerance will make you crave more. You want to conscientiously train your brain to avoid fattening foods, to help you break your food addiction.

I'll be honest with you, though: the process of training your brain to consistently view foods this way is extremely challenging. This is why mindfulness, meditation, and the other stress relievers in this chapter are so supportive in overcoming your emotional, habitual eating response to stress. To make this permanent, you need to

1. *Create a focused inner strength* by embracing all of the components of my weight-loss program (diet, exercise, sleep, and more). This is the ultimate refuge that will enable you to reach a state of mind that makes you feel safe, comfortable, and powerful.

2. *Engage in cognitive behavioral self-therapy* to avoid falling into the trap of stress-induced eating disorders.

3. *Plan relaxing activities* to reduce cortisol levels.

4. *Train your emotional brain* to associate pleasure and satisfaction with eating foods conducive to speedy metabolism (the ones you'll eat on my diet).

5. *Start viewing your poor eating habits as a serious addiction* similar to alcoholism or any other drug addiction.

6. *Boost mood with the good foods in my diet* and address depression with medication or counseling and supplements. If you need an antidepressant, have your doctor select one that doesn't promote weight gain, such as Wellbutrin.

7. *Reduce symptoms of anxiety* by restoring digestive bacterial balance and taking the right relaxing supplements (discussed later in this chapter in "Stress in Your Gut and Probiotics").

Making these changes will help you manipulate your eating impulses and cravings, giving you the ability to lose weight and keep it off permanently. That's what Whitney and Julia did. They embraced my mind-body program, adjusting to an eating plan that they soon came to prefer over ice cream and fries. When you feed your body the foods it needs to stay in perfect hormonal rhythm, this is what actu-

ally happens. Both Julia and Whitney still practice their stress relievers, which, both tell me, helped them relieve the initial out-of-control
cravings. Today when they get stressed, they're supported by the hormonally protective foods in my diet and the centering mindfulness of
relaxation techniques.

DO-IT-YOURSELF COGNITIVE BEHAVIORAL THERAPY

Even if you're not consciously stressed but you're gaining weight as
a result of poor eating habits, getting fat itself can stress you, causing
your pituitary to stimulate the adrenal glands to release even more
cortisol, further enhancing the movement of fat to your abdomen.
Many weight-loss programs incorporate cognitive behavioral therapy, a psychological approach used to treat anxiety disorders, mood
disorders, insomnia, post-traumatic stress disorder, and addictions.
Much research has shown behavioral therapy to be one of the most
effective approaches for weight loss, as well. With my plan, rather
than seeing a therapist you'll practice cognitive behavioral therapy
on your own or with a friend. Here's how it works:

- *Monitor yourself to recognize what stresses you*—deadlines,
  children's homework, meal preparation, etc.—and write down
  how you typically react to it.
- *Ask yourself why the stressors make you feel upset* and how
  you can approach the stressful situation differently.
- *For each stressful situation,* decide on an alternative, health-
  benefiting activity you can do in response, or work toward
  resolving the situation itself.

This do-it-yourself cognitive behavioral therapy should reflect your
way of looking at things for healthier behavioral responses. Many
of my patients keep a diary of triggering situations and possible
solutions. Shopping and preparing meals were stressors for Diane,
an office manager who felt frazzled just about every night because
she had nothing ready for dinner. Diane decided to shop one day
a week, and on the weekends prepare food for the coming week,
freezing quantities so they'd be ready to defrost or microwave anytime. Diane also got other family members involved to offset the

stress of what to have for dinner. Now her sons love cooking soups and chilis on the weekend. Resolving her stress with this approach helped Diane comply more successfully with the Protein Boost Diet eating plans, too.

If you stress because your children's homework isn't getting done, maybe you need to institute a draconian solution, like cutting off all screen time (phone, TV, computer, games) until assignments are completed. Friends who know you and your situation can be enormously helpful. Have a cup of tea with a good pal and ask for feedback. The questions and suggestions friends bring can open your mind to new approaches and help you see when you're overreacting. Have a friend or two along for your de-stressing, weight-loss journey. Relaxation techniques can be even more effective when you include others in your brisk walks, yoga classes, or tai chi.

TO RELEASE STRESS, FOCUS AND RELAX

Lying on the couch staring blankly at the TV at the end of the day may make you feel you're winding down, but to achieve a full stress-relieving effect, your mind needs to be completely focused on an activity. Choose a relaxation technique to practice three times a week, the first step toward relieving stress itself and its hormonal effects on your body and mind. Meditation, tai chi, yoga, massage, muscle relaxation, and visualization are all excellent choices. Honestly, any of the following techniques will help you let go of stress, clear your mind, and raise awareness of your body. I particularly recommend tai chi and yoga to my patients, but as you read through this list, see what appeals to you. The one you choose and enjoy is the one you'll stay with, and that's essential, since stress will always be a part of life.

TAI CHI

A dance-like, gentle martial art, tai chi incorporates concentration and breathing into fluid movements. Consider tai chi a multifunctional relaxation technique. Practicing it regularly can replace feelings of sadness with happiness, remove tension and fear, and encourage better sleep. One study showed that people who practiced tai chi for just twelve weeks experienced significant stress reduction. Even more exciting to me is a study published within the last year that found tai chi reduces inflammation. Perpetual weight gain caused by leptin resistance and insulin resistance worsens with inflammation. By reducing inflammation, tai chi will help you overcome these metabolic setbacks. Practicing tai chi can help you feel more confident, and recent research has shown it boosts quality of life, motivation, vitality, social functioning, and overall mood. The more you practice, the better your mental health and physical function. Classes are widely available even in small communities. Sign up for a series and learn how tai chi can do wonders for stress relief and weight loss.

TAI CHI CHIH

Alternatively, start with a simplified form of tai chi called "tai chi chih," a combination of twenty repetitive nonstrenuous moves and an ending pose. Surprisingly easy and beautifully joyful, tai chi chih will help you focus, limber up, and move intentionally. Google "tai chi chih YouTube" to view videos of the easy, focused movements and get started right now. Or look for a class at a nearby recreation department, hospital, church, or senior center.

YOGA

People who practice yoga regularly often notice they're eating less and more slowly. That makes yoga ideal for gaining control over your food choices while you calm stress. Because there are many different difficulty levels and styles, I recommend you learn yoga with an instructor first in the company of others to make your initial exposure a happy one. Even if you decide against yoga as your primary relaxation technique, it's worth trying for its focus on deep breathing, something you can do while you sit at your desk or on a bus. Yoga has amazing physiological effects. It's been shown to reduce anxiety and depression through its slow stretching and gently held poses. Holding those poses as you breathe deeply increases blood flow, and by "massaging" pressure receptors, you will experience bodily biochemical changes that help depression, pain syndromes, and immune problems.

Key to yoga's stress-relieving power is its ability to drive down levels of the stress hormone cortisol. At least two studies showed enhanced mindfulness with yoga practice, and another revealed an increase in alpha waves in the brain—a sign of relaxation—and reduced levels of cortisol. Scientists studying people with diabetes found that yoga improved energy levels and lowered cortisol. Regular practice will help you achieve a lower body mass index and waist measurement. As a bonus, studies into yoga's effects on sleep disorders such as chronic insomnia show that it improves sleep quality. Like tai chi, yoga instruction is available just about everywhere, offered through community centers and hospitals and by individuals who will welcome you into their classes.

MEDITATION

All forms of meditation require you to sit quietly, clear thoughts from your mind, and focus on an object, sound, or word for ten or twenty minutes. It sounds simple, and it is, though it requires disciplining yourself to slow down and do it (that's what it's all about!). Meditating slows your pulse, slows your breathing, and lowers blood pressure, exactly the opposite of your body's stress response. To get started, Google "relaxation response" or look for Dr. Herbert Benson's book of that name at your library.

TRANSCENDENTAL MEDITATION (TM)

This form of meditation became popular in the United States about fifty years ago, though it has helped people achieve relaxation for thousands of years since its inception in India. All you need to do is sit for twenty minutes, close your eyes, and focus on a single thought—your mantra—that you'll obtain through a TM instructor. The recommended frequency is once or twice daily, in the morning and afternoon, but not too soon before going to bed or after waking up. I find this form of meditation quite practical because you can practice it anytime you have an extra twenty minutes, anywhere. It can also improve sleep.

MASSAGE

Massage relieves stress and reduces muscle tension while lowering the stress hormone cortisol. It also raises levels of dopamine and serotonin, and it's deeply pleasurable and relaxing. Massage, in my opinion, is the best gift you can give yourself, and even if you want a massage regularly, there's no need to splurge at a fancy spa. Look for an accredited massage therapy school where you live. Students often need practice subjects and offer discounts on full-body massages. Or find a qualified massage therapist by Googling the American Massage Therapy Association and using its "find a therapist" tool.

PROGRESSIVE MUSCLE RELAXATION

In this technique, you sequentially tense muscle groups in your arms, legs, face, belly, and chest and then relax them. You focus on the sensation of tension and relaxation, with a simultaneous relaxation of mind and whole body. Google "progressive muscle relaxation" to find an easy step-by-step guide.

VISUALIZATION

This is performed by closing your eyes and using your senses to imagine yourself in a place where you feel relaxed—in the woods, on a lake or beach, in front of a fireplace. Visualization produces a relaxed body, clear mind, and release of tension. In guided visualization, you're guided through the process by a speaker who leads you to calming places in your imagination. There are many fine guided visualizations online. Just search "guided visualization YouTube" to try one.

WHICH STRESS RELIEVER IS RIGHT FOR ME?

Depending on how you experience stress, choose a technique that either calms your mind or enhances energy. Or switch among relaxation techniques, doing some alone and others in groups, depending on your mood. For someone who has trouble falling asleep, tai chi or yoga will help with both the perception of stress and the sleep

An Easy Lunch-Break Stress Reliever

Q. My boss drives me crazy with her constant demands. Every day by about eleven-thirty I can actually feel my heart racing from the stress. Could you recommend an easy stress reliever I can do on my lunch break?

A. A couple of techniques are helpful for stress relief at work. Here's one to dissipate stress while you're sitting at your desk (perhaps when your boss is in a meeting): when you feel your heart racing, focus on taking deep, slow breaths, breathing in through your nose for ten seconds while you concentrate on the air slowly filling your lungs. Then blow out slowly and repeat. You may want to close your eyes and visualize yourself in a peaceful place, such as the top of a beautiful mountain or anywhere you feel empowered or relaxed.

During your lunch break, take the entire time to practice mindfulness. Revel in your physical being, from each bite of food you take to each breath you inhale. Focus on the present—the right now—to release the overwhelming feelings caused by your boss and the work still to do. If possible, step outside for lunch to the nearest park or other green space. Taking a short walk while practicing mindfulness in your breathing and steps will calm your whole mind and body. Notice that focusing on breathing is a feature of both exercises. It may sound simple, but the slower breaths have a powerful ability to calm your heart and your hormonal reactions to stress. Finally, enjoy a cup of tea and take advantage of its L-theanine (see "Sip Your Way to Happiness and Weight Loss" in Chapter 8), a naturally occurring chemical that contributes to calm, relaxed feelings.

issue itself. What's important is that you choose a stress reliever that boosts your mental well-being . . . and do it regularly.

If you experience tension, excitability, or anger in response to stress, try methods that calm, such as meditation or visualization.

If depressive symptoms worsen under stress, making you feel unmotivated or detached, a relaxing yet energy-boosting technique will help you cope. Try rhythmic exercises like walking or jogging, cycling, or a group exercise class while you focus on breathing with every move you make.

If you experience a combination of agitation and depressive symptoms, mindfulness will help you relieve stress as you engage your senses and focus on your present physical being. Mindfulness by definition keeps you from stressing about the past or the future, because you're focusing on the *right now.* Mindfulness acknowledges the present and empties your mind of issues that stimulate stress. Practice mindfulness in all activities throughout your day—walking, eating, and exercising. The idea is to focus on what you're doing in the present moment to relieve you from the distracting effects of stress.

If you prefer practicing relaxation alone, try visualization or meditation. I don't recommend these when you're sleepy because your mind won't fully focus, and falling asleep is a common outcome. Meditation can be done quietly anywhere as long as you use your mind to focus on something, whether a word or a picture. The same applies to visualization. Sit or stand, picturing yourself in a place you'd like to be, whatever that is for you. The more you can make the experience feel real the better, so find an appropriate soundtrack and some relaxing scents like lavender oil. Then get lost picturing yourself walking around your imaginary place.

If you find that socializing and enjoying activities in a group help relieve stress, try a group exercise class. According to a study at Northeastern University, obese women showed a significant change in scores on the Beck Depression Inventory over a six-month period of group exercise and relaxation training. A popular group exercise is Zumba, in which you dance to upbeat Latin music. Games played with groups enhance self-awareness and the positive stress necessary for creativity and learning. Social games and team sports utilize stress in a positive way while they engage your mind in a fun activity. Tai chi done in the park with a group makes you feel part of the greater whole, and the same effect can happen in yoga class.

THE DEPRESSION–WEIGHT CONNECTION: HOW TO INCREASE SEROTONIN

Your eating behavior, appetite, eating impulses, and even your food choices are tightly linked to your mood, emotions, and anxiety level. While it's clear that overweight and obese people have a greater tendency to be depressed, depressed people also tend more to be overweight. It's not understood whether depression is at the root of weight problems or vice versa, but several studies have shown that the two tend to feed off each other in a relentless, self-destructive cycle.

The neurotransmitter serotonin, which shapes your mood and emotions, also influences what you eat. Without the support of serotonin, your ability to regulate how much you eat and which foods you choose becomes impaired. A lack of serotonin has multiple effects on metabolism and appetite that can end up making you fatter and fatter as time goes by.

Serotonin plays a crucial role in regulating mood, temperature, sexual behavior, and sleep. In one of the main areas of the brain, the arcuate nucleus, serotonin also regulates appetite and fullness, and has a say in how much fat we accumulate and store. Serotonin is released by your GI tract when you eat, and the amount released and its efficiency have an effect on the size and duration of your meal. You want healthy serotonin levels, which also speed up metabolism and make you burn calories. Research shows a significant link between the activity of brain serotonin and body weight. Normal serotonin levels allow for optimal function in controlling food intake and experiencing fullness. Low or inefficient serotonin makes you crave junk foods and sweets to self-medicate, eventually leading to weight gain. Hypothyroidism, like estrogen deficiency, throws a heavy blanket on serotonin, damping down levels of this feel-good brain chemical. This triggers cravings for sugars and fats and leads you to eat more in an attempt to boost mood and reduce anxiety.

I'll tell you how my diet increases serotonin activity, which helps you eat less and lose weight, but first a primer on neurotransmitters and depression. Serotonin, noradrenaline, and GABA are the main chemical transmitters involved in depression, and normalizing their levels is essential to maintaining stable mood and behavior. Fascinatingly, thyroid hormone also works closely with these chemicals in your brain to keep mood stable. As you become overweight, your thyroid hormones become less efficient and you set yourself up to become trapped by depression, low thyroid, poor-quality sleep, and weight gain, all related to low serotonin.

Being overweight or obese can bring a poor self-image, low self-esteem, and social isolation, all ultimately leading to depression. Overweight and obese people may find themselves ostracized, stereotyped, and discriminated against. The extra weight can result in chronic joint pain as well as serious diseases like diabetes and hypertension, all of which are linked to depression. Research on obese adolescents showed that in just one year, many became depressed.

While it's clear that a weight disorder can lead to depression, depression also can contribute to weight gain and obesity.

Fluoxetine and sertraline, selective serotonin reuptake inhibitor antidepressants (SSRIs) used to treat depression and anxiety, help curb appetite because they raise serotonin activity in the brain, but SSRIs are not a treatment for long-term weight loss because weight regain often occurs in people taking them.

HOW THE PROTEIN BOOST DIET RAISES SEROTONIN

Exercise stimulates serotonin production and exercising regularly improves mood, depression, anxiety, and perception of stress. Animal studies have shown that exercise increases by two- to threefold growth in the area of the brain (the hippocampus) that regulates mood. You'll also be boosting serotonin with the food choices in my diet. Tryptophan is the essential amino acid needed to produce serotonin, and my diet contains plenty of it. In Chapter 7, I discuss the satisfying tryptophan-rich proteins you'll be eating to boost mood and to optimize feelings of fullness. Among them are game meats, soy, spinach, egg whites, shellfish, fish, whole-grain products, poultry (especially game birds and turkey), seaweed, and sesame seeds. You can also increase serotonin levels and function in your brain by taking more vitamin B_6, vitamin D_3, and inositol, all of which I recommend you take as supplements (see "Essential Antioxidants and Micronutrients to Reshape Hormones for Weight Loss" in Chapter 8). You'll also optimize mood by consuming foods rich in omega-3 fatty acids and by taking the daily omega-3 supplement I recommend.

BOOSTING GABA TO RELIEVE ANXIETY

If you're anxious, you're more likely to binge and overeat the wrong foods. That's because some of the neurotransmitters involved in anxiety are the very same chemicals that affect cravings and eating patterns. One neurotransmitter that plays a central role in this connection is gamma-aminobutyric acid (GABA). If you have low levels, you'll have excessive anxiety, low energy, sleep problems, weight gain, and even metabolic syndrome. Research, in fact, shows GABA supplements dramatically ameliorate metabolic syndrome. GABA deficiency can also lead to diabetes and fibromyalgia. Raising GABA levels will suppress your appetite, boost energy, and help you produce more growth hormone, all vital for weight loss and improving insulin sensitivity. Enhancing GABA levels will decrease your symptoms, improve energy levels, and as a bonus bring a soothing effect.

How the Protein Boost Diet boosts GABA: The highest natural sources of GABA are fish and fava beans, foods you'll be eating on my meal plan. Here are some other GABA-containing foods.

Almonds
Beef liver
Broccoli
Brown rice
Cashews
Citrus fruits
Coconut
Halibut
Hazelnuts
Lentils
Pecans and walnuts
Pistachios
Spinach
Whole grains

STRESS IN YOUR GUT AND PROBIOTICS

If you ever stood up to give a speech and felt butterflies in your stomach, it won't surprise you that your gastrointestinal system—your gut—connects to the part of your brain that senses stress and anxiety. Researchers today are uncovering the powerful effects on your brain of having enough helpful bacteria (probiotics) in your gut. These belly bacteria are the good guys—not the kind that make you feel sick—and having a good balance of bacteria is crucial for weight loss. Friendly flora reduce stress, immune problems, and inflammation in your body, especially in your GI tract. It's becoming clear that eating foods containing live probiotic bacteria—such as live-culture yogurt and kefir—or taking probiotic supplements can decrease anxiety and improve mood, especially in people with stress-related conditions such as weight gain, chronic fatigue, or irritable bowel syndrome.

Curiously, the bacterial strain *Lactobacillus rhamnosus* (*L. rhamnosus*) can directly affect your behavior and physiological responses by sending signals from the intestines through the powerful vagus nerve that connects your gut and brain. *L. rhamnosus* actually enhances GABA activity and as a result reduces anxiety and depression, which in turn modulates your eating impulses for the better. *L. rhamnosus* also knocks down levels of the stress hormone cortisol. Here's how powerful gut bacteria are: researchers studying their effects in mice found that by altering or removing helpful gut bacteria, they could actually change the hypothalamus's signal to the adrenal glands, causing the adrenal glands to release more of the stress hormone cortisol in response to stress and anxiety. Research shows that taking supplements of *Lactobacillus* and *Bifidobacterium* can reverse the outpouring of cortisol in your system in response to stress. Ingesting these bacteria will also enhance your memory and cognitive ability.

HOW THE PROTEIN BOOST DIET ENHANCES HELPFUL BACTERIA

My diet program includes taking a probiotic supplement with *L. rhamnosus* and *Bifidobacterium*, such as Probiotic 7-7, a mix of seven bacterial strains, all crucial for optimizing weight loss (see "Probiotics for Detox and Weight Loss" in Chapter 8).

DOPAMINE AND FOOD ADDICTION

As I discussed at the beginning of this chapter, our eating impulses and eating choices are also regulated by dopamine, the powerful brain neurotransmitter that governs feelings of reward, desire, satisfaction, motivation, and pleasure. You can view dopamine as the pleasure neurotransmitter, designed to deliver positive sensations. People get dopamine bursts from a variety of activities—both good and bad—such as eating, sex, drug use (alcohol, tobacco, illegal drugs), exercise, and gambling. As you might guess, this chemical is implicated in a wide range of addictive behaviors . . . including addiction to food and sex.

Dopamine activity contributes to compulsive overeating and food addiction in a way that's similar to what drug abusers experience. When you eat, dopamine levels rise, producing pleasurable feelings. A dopamine decline makes you want to eat all over again to get more pleasure. In fact, dopamine is the chemical that will make you continue to eat even when you're full. This pleasure response is so powerful it can motivate you to seek out foods that reward you with this good feeling. For many of us, craving foods is a reinforcing behavior to gain more pleasure, an addictive effect that can easily lead to weight gain from eating too much.

Sometime after you finish a meal, your dopamine levels drop and you begin to seek renewed pleasure by eating again. The sad part is that the more you eat, the less efficient dopamine becomes, so you tend to eat even more to produce more dopamine to reach the pleasure you once had. This is a typical addiction scenario. When it comes to food addiction, "users" usually favor fast carbs that quickly turn to glucose, and saturated fats. Animal research supports this idea by finding that when dopamine doesn't work efficiently, animals become obese, and we know that overweight people have lower dopamine levels than their lean counterparts. As you now understand, low dopamine levels or low dopamine sensitivity can make you seek out foods to stimulate dopamine-driven pleasurable feelings. Researchers have postulated that raising dopamine levels might help regulate eating behavior.

Eating carbs and bad fats is definitely an addiction for people struggling with weight gain. While following my diet, you'll be addressing your sugar and fat addiction as seriously as someone trying to quit nicotine or alcohol addiction. And like most addictions, your food-addiction dopamine cycle will take time to break. During the first few weeks on my diet, you're supporting your body and brain with food choices that nourish you and leave you full because they're rich in fiber and selected satiety-fulfilling proteins. The foods in my meal plans are low in simple sugars and saturated fats, helping you slowly but surely rid yourself of sugar and fat addiction. You'll find you're less compelled to crave the foods that made you fatter in the first place and gradually your brain will become conditioned to generate feelings of pleasure when you eat foods that make you slimmer. I can't emphasize enough the importance of empowering your mind with an ultimate goal to get rid of these addictions. Remember, too, that pleasurable activities such as games, sports, and reading will keep dopamine levels high.

How the Protein Boost Diet raises dopamine: Proteins at every meal contain amino acids that make you synthesize neurotransmitters including dopamine, among others. Dopamine is synthesized from the amino acid L-tyrosine, and thus tyrosine-rich foods such as nuts and seeds (particularly almonds, pumpkin, and sesame seeds) will increase dopamine levels. Other food selections in my diet that support beneficial dopamine levels are fava beans, lima beans, avocados, beets, apples, whole grains, soy, and yogurt. Exercise also stimulates dopamine production, and relaxation stimulates dopamine sensitivity, so you're getting nicely rounded coverage. Dopamine levels have a daily cycle, just like many other neurotransmitters and hormones. As my program resets the circadian rhythm of your hormones, you'll optimize dopamine production throughout your day and be rewarded with better mood and satiety.

For my patient Paula, 30, eating junk food was an automatic response to unhappiness. When she was in her late twenties and looking her best at 130 pounds, she married a successful man, but as she started gaining weight rapidly he pushed her to lose it. He started drinking heavily, told her she wasn't the woman he married, and over time became abusive. The nagging and abuse reminded Paula of the abuse her stepfather had doled out and the unhappiness she felt when she was a teenager. Old emotional issues resurfaced, and she quickly lost control over her eating. She told me, "I'd buy a huge amount of fast food, go home, and eat it, but had no idea why." The way she explained it made it seem like eating was a secret obsession, her way of escaping a painful reality, just as when she was growing up.

Paula continued to eat enormous amounts of junk food, which brought the pleasure dopamine provides (that her marriage couldn't) but also zoomed her weight to 220 pounds within a year. At this point, her quality of life diminished severely, and Paula was miserably depressed. Paula said it so clearly to me: "The only pleasure I've had in my life since I married this man is eating, and I simply can't stop." Paula started my eating plan and regular relaxation, and joined a support group. She also discovered a center for abused women.

The physical benefits of my feel-good program and the improvements in Paula's self-esteem laid the foundation for her journey away from food addiction and her abusive husband. She actually began enjoying her conscientious strides toward weight loss, and was able to slim down to 140 pounds in fifteen months. "I feel extremely confident, unlike I've ever felt before," she told me. "I'm so glad I was able to turn my life around! I know I'm still young. I still have my life ahead of me, and I've got a lot going for me now."

CHAPTER FIVE

SLEEP AFFECTS YOUR HORMONES

How to Synchronize Sleep and Food with Your Biological Clocks

Changes in your sleep schedule can make you feel "off." Your body's light/dark–wake/sleep cycle has profound effects on weight. Your body responds differently to foods based on the time of day you eat and what you eat at each meal, so when you eat is important.

I think you'll share my amazement at recent research on the body's rhythms and the science of sleep. I'll show you the extraordinary impact sleep has on your metabolism and sex hormones, what happens to your body during the night, and what happens the following day if you don't sleep enough. We'll also review the various reasons people don't sleep well and how you can fix sleep disorders.

What you eat and don't eat can affect the quality of your sleep. Foods rich in fat can promote insulin resistance and inefficiency of leptin, which can make your respiratory center not function properly, ultimately leading to central sleep apnea. You can gradually improve your sleep naturally by improving your diet. For instance, tryptophan-rich proteins incorporated in my diet promote serotonin production, which helps you experience less collapse of the airway. As your sleep quality begins to improve, your efforts to lose weight start accelerating in the right direction.

YOUR BRAIN'S CIRCADIAN RHYTHM, MELATONIN, AND HORMONES

As with virtually all organisms living on the planet, our biological functions, behavior, and metabolism are influenced by the light/dark cycle. You've probably heard of circadian rhythms. The word "circadian" comes from the Latin *circa*, meaning around, and *diem*, meaning day. Your circadian clock runs on a twenty-four-hour cycle, like a regular clock. Light and darkness are registered by an exquisitely sensitive master clock in your brain called the "central circadian clock." This sophisticated timepiece sends signals to your autonomic nervous system (which controls automatic functions you don't need to think about, like heartbeat, blood pressure, and breathing) and to hormones controlling a vast array of functions including metabolism.

Your central circadian clock does all this in perfect synchrony with your light/dark–wake/sleep pattern. It operates repeatedly in twenty-four-hour cycles, telling you when you should sleep and eat, but it does much more from its location in the hypothalamus, tucked deep inside your brain. Virtually all tissues in your body sense the signals emitted by the hypothalamus, sent via hormones and via the activity of the autonomic nervous system—for optimal metabolism and functioning. Extensive research has shown that interrupted sleep and shift work are significant contributors to obesity and diabetes because they disrupt the hormonal balance related to the delicate central circadian clock.

THE RHYTHM OF YOUR HORMONES

The rhythms of your central circadian clock affect insulin sensitivity, cell metabolism, and hormones linked to hunger and fat burning. They influence your pituitary gland's release of growth hormone, a key player in regulating weight. These rhythms also control other important hormones—thyroid hormones, leptin, ghrelin, sex hormones, and the stress hormone cortisol. If you remember just one thing from this chapter, remember this: poor sleep habits make you lose the coordination of these hormonal systems and ultimately make you fat. Let's look at the circadian rhythms of hormones involved in sleep and metabolism.

MELATONIN IS YOUR MASTER SLEEP CONTROLLER

Melatonin helps trigger sleep. Produced by the pineal gland, a pea-size structure in your brain, it's released by your body in greater amounts when it's dark out, with production dropping when it's light. Melatonin lowers your body temperature to herald the onset of sleep. Your pineal gland starts releasing melatonin when you become surrounded by darkness, at the time when there's a decline in brain noradrenaline (an important neurotransmitter involved in promoting wakefulness), quieting you for the night.

Your body is so exquisitely sensitive that if a light pulse is shone while you're sleeping, your production of melatonin can stop altogether within five minutes, disturbing deep sleep or awakening you. The retina is so sensitive to light that even with your eyes closed, your retina can be stimulated by a weak light pulse. Melatonin helps you go to sleep and continue sleeping when you should sleep—when it's dark outside. Your central circadian clock maintains a constant schedule, and when disruptions like jet lag (see "Coping with Jet Lag" in this chapter) affect melatonin signaling, your body must reset your central circadian clock. In addition to inducing sleep, melatonin slows down the amount of insulin you secrete, a very useful weight-controlling function indeed.

How the Protein Boost Diet supports melatonin: My diet is designed to provide the foods that align best with your central circadian clock hormone profile. Meal timing ensures optimal insulin sensitivity, lower ghrelin activity, and enhanced leptin efficiency. Your highest-protein meal is dinner for a reason. It feeds your body a combination of proteins rich in GABA and tryptophan, conducive to both anxiety relief and serotonin-enhancing effects. They're both beneficial to quality sleep. The last meal of the day is also the one that contains the lowest glycemic load, leading to low insulin levels at night, in synchrony with the effects of melatonin on insulin.

LOW INSULIN MAKES YOU STORE LESS FAT WHILE YOU SLEEP

With melatonin damping down insulin levels during sleep, you can see how your system is designed to shut down insulin's fat storage function and instead allow your body to burn fat. That's why when you head for bed, you want the lowest insulin levels possible.

How the Protein Boost Diet keeps insulin low: My meal plans deliver a steady reduction in low-glycemic carbs as the day unspools. You'll enjoy more carbs in the morning and at lunchtime because you need the energy to move through your day. If you eat too many carbs at night, your blood sugar will be higher, and as a consequence insulin will also be at unwanted high levels, making you store fat rather than burn it.

LEPTIN AT HIGHER LEVELS BURNS UNNEEDED CALORIES DURING SLEEP

Normally, as you sleep, levels of the weight-loss-friendly hormone leptin rise. The highest levels of leptin are actually between midnight and early morning. The purpose of this increase is twofold: suppressing appetite so you can sleep peacefully (and not wake up in the middle of the night with a ferocious hunger) and so leptin can help burn extra, unnecessary calories consumed during the day. Leptin's action while you sleep speeds up your resting metabolic rate (how many calories you burn when doing nothing). It works hard at balancing your metabolism to keep you from gaining extra fat.

How the Protein Boost Diet promotes leptin efficiency: To optimize leptin's function at night, you're providing your system with a highly efficient mix of amino acids at dinner. These maximize leptin efficiency in your cells' mitochondria to increase metabolism. You won't need to think about it much—all the dinner food selections are designed to fulfill this goal.

THYROID HORMONE PREPS TO BURN ENERGY

The pituitary signals the thyroid gland to release more thyroid hormone during sleep by increasing production of thyroid-stimulating hormone (TSH), which rhythmically stimulates your thyroid to produce its hormones. This periodic TSH release ensures the thyroid gland adjusts its function for the very best metabolism. Amazingly, all this goes on for hours until the early morning before you awaken. Thyroid hormone is one of the most crucial hormones in helping you burn fat and calories, even when you're doing nothing. Losing sleep robs you of its powerful weight-loss effects.

How the Protein Boost Diet supports thyroid hormone: The well-balanced schedule of diverse proteins at each meal optimizes the metabolism-boosting effects of thyroid hormone in mitochondria. This complete amino acid profile, with an emphasis on branched-chain amino acids (BCAAs), arginine, and lysine, enhances the ability of leptin and thyroid hormones to energize your metabolism.

GROWTH HORMONE INCREASES DURING SLEEP TO BURN FAT

Here's more positive weight-loss news from your good night's sleep. Growth hormone (GH), which breaks down fats and helps speed up your metabolism, is produced in greater amounts when you sleep. In fact, potent pulses of GH are released from your pituitary during rapid-eye-movement (REM) sleep. You don't want to miss even one of those influential REM periods.

How the Protein Boost Diet keeps GH high: GH is precious for weight loss, and foods containing the amino acid L-arginine prompt your pituitary to release GH. It's for this reason my diet calls for L-arginine-rich foods (see "Protein Variety: The Ultimate Metabolism Enhancer" in Chapter 7) to be eaten at dinner: to help you enhance metabolism as you sleep. All meals are rich in the proteins containing beneficial amino acids that enhance GH secretion, ensuring the symphony of your hormones is perfectly tuned for burning fat during sleep. Getting a full eight hours of sleep will give you optimal GH levels for calorie burning.

CORTISOL HELPS YOU RISE 'N' SHINE

Another hormonal rhythm that your central circadian clock meticulously coordinates is fluctuations in cortisol. You already know that having too much cortisol in your system acts as a stress hormone and increases abdominal fat and cravings for fattening foods. But a normal cortisol level is good and essential. In the early morning hours before sunrise, your central circadian clock signals your cortisol levels to start rising in order to increase blood sugar for use by your organs after you wake up and become physically active. This little example of hormones "talking" to each other illustrates so beautifully why for optimal activity, energy, and metabolism you want to consume higher-glycemic foods in the morning and at lunch rather than in the evening. For a highly efficient metabolism, the diet should reduce, as much as possible, higher-glycemic foods in the evening.

How the Protein Boost Diet powers healthful cortisol: You'll be eating tryptophan- and GABA-rich proteins to minimize your stress levels and to have more restful sleep, both of which will keep your cortisol levels at their lowest in the evening and at night. You will enhance this effect with the right supplements. Low cortisol at night helps the efficiency of insulin and of growth hormone and the speed of your metabolism.

GHRELIN, THE HUNGER HORMONE, ALSO RISES IN THE MORNING

The rhythm of ghrelin is amazing as well. When you awaken, ghrelin levels increase to prompt you to eat breakfast. A few hours later, ghrelin rises again to make you hungry for lunch, and it rises a third time to make you hungry for dinner. Because ghrelin also slows down metabolism, you want to anticipate the hormone's rise and eat breakfast, lunch, and dinner before ghrelin increases to high levels.

How the Protein Boost Diet helps thwart ghrelin: Optimal meal timing and eating high-fiber foods at each meal actually blunt hunger, and also stop the slowing of your metabolism before it happens.

Ask Dr. Arem: Coping with Jet Lag

Q. I travel on business about once a month from Chicago to London, usually working five days before returning. When I get to London, I'm exhausted and can't focus in the afternoons, making work all but impossible. Also, I've gained weight since this travel began. I'm starting to see that wake/sleep cycles are at the center of all this. Can you help me reset my body clock so I am sharper while working abroad and don't keep gaining weight?

A. Use this schedule to reset the synchrony of your clocks (it works for New York to London, too).

TWO NIGHTS BEFORE DEPARTURE

- Go to bed two to three hours before your usual bedtime, eating dinner two to three hours earlier, too.

- Half an hour before going to bed, take melatonin (3 mg) and Relora (250 mg). Melatonin will help initiate sleep and Relora will modulate your cortisol level and also help you sleep.

- If you're anxious about your trip or under other stress, take 250 to 500 mg of GABA as well.

DAY OF DEPARTURE AND ON THE PLANE
- Keep taking the supplements.
- Try to sleep on the plane.

DAY OF ARRIVAL
- Resist taking a nap.
- Go to bed at the same local time as your usual bedtime. For example, if you normally go to bed at 10:00 p.m. Chicago time, go to bed at 10:00 p.m. London time. Bottom line: don't go to bed early.

DURING YOUR STAY
- Continue taking supplements each night until a few days after you get home.
- If you can't be outdoors during the day enjoying the sights, try to be in a brightly lit environment all day. Light will keep sleep hormone melatonin at low levels.
- Make all your meals as low-glycemic as possible (see "Ten Fundamentals of the Protein Boost Diet" in Chapter 10), including breakfast. This helps minimize desynchronization of your central circadian and cellular clocks.

TWO NIGHTS BEFORE RETURNING TO CHICAGO
- Delay your bedtime by a couple of hours.

WHEN YOU ARRIVE IN CHICAGO
- Resist going to bed early, trying hard to stay awake until your usual Chicago bedtime.

YOUR CELLULAR CLOCK: *WHEN* TO EAT *WHAT*

For peak metabolism and biological functions, your central circadian clock and hormone fluctuations need to work in concert with the metabolic activities of your organs. When it comes to metabolism, your body has its own rhythm . . . and its very own clock. Cells and organs are equipped with a cellular clock, which unlike your central circadian clock isn't affected by light/dark signals. Rather, it runs on signals from body temperature, food consumption, the hormone cortisol, and the types of nutrients you deliver to your body (your cells have nutrient sensors that help your cellular clock function properly). Remarkably, because of this clock your cells and organs expect surges in specific nutrients at the times they're accustomed to getting them. The timing and consistency of eating and the types of nutrients you consume help align your two clocks.

Your cellular clock, through "clock genes," tells your cells when they need to undertake activities such as burning fat and how much needs to be burned. Even though your central circadian clock and cellular clocks are controlled separately, they work in harmony when you're well and when you're disciplined about the timing and consistency of your eating schedule. If your clocks are out of sync, you'll begin to have shifts in metabolism and unbalanced hormone activity that doesn't match optimal metabolic activity. This can lead to weight gain, obesity, and diabetes.

Glucose (sugar) metabolism, for instance, is controlled by both your cellular clock and your central circadian clock, the latter causing you to produce more glucose at the beginning of the day—with the dawning of the light—for your muscles to use as energy. At the same time, the cellular clock in your pancreas causes the pancreas to respond to the extra glucose by releasing just the right amount of insulin to process the sugar. If there's a mismatch between the rise of glucose and the pancreas's insulin release, your blood sugar will be higher than normal and you can end up with impaired glucose tolerance. A disrupted cellular clock can bring on obesity. When researchers removed a mouse's cellular clock gene, the mouse became obese, with a fatty liver and high cholesterol, triglyceride fats, and glucose levels. If your two clocks are misaligned as a result of your eating and sleeping at irregular times, the efficiency of calorie-burning leptin will decline, too, resulting in less fat burning. You become insulin resistant, and rhythms of stress hormone cortisol become inverted—increasing rather than decreasing substantially eight to twelve hours after you wake.

NEW RESEARCH REVEALS SLEEP-WEIGHT CONNECTION

In 2012, researchers found that sleep restriction, combined with dis-ruption of the central circadian clock, increases the risk of obesity and diabetes. Because of the clock disruption, the pancreas becomes less responsive to glucose and is unable to release appropriate amounts of insulin. As a consequence, blood sugar levels stay high. The find-ing: circadian disruption and sleep restriction cut your insulin activ-ity by one-third and lower your resting metabolic rate (the number of calories you burn doing nothing) by 8 percent. This apparently small drop from desynchronization of your central circadian clock with your cellular clock converts to an astonishing 12.5 pounds of weight gain in a year.

Even if you were to eat fewer calories, as participants in this experiment did, you still wouldn't be able to metabolize the nutri-ents efficiently, and you wouldn't burn as many calories at rest as you would if you ate at the right times—in alignment with your cen-tral circadian clock.

EATING ON A SCHEDULE SYNCS YOUR CLOCKS

Eating at regular hours during the day—and not at night—ensures the best alignment between your central circadian and cellular clocks. Let me give you an example. Holly, a patient of mine, is a teacher who schedules her meals and snacks according to the fairly rigid timetable of her school day. She's up every morning around five-thirty to walk her dogs, eats breakfast between six and seven, arrives at school before her eight o'clock first class, and takes her school-assigned lunch break at 10:45 a.m. She's more than ready to eat lunch then, and also for her afternoon snack around four. Din-ner's at six-thirty, and then an early bedtime. Holly's schedule is reg-ular and predictable, just the way we want to see it. As she says, "A less-flexible school schedule makes meal timing easy for me."

Now let's look at the effect of unscheduled eating on mice. In one study, mice were fed a high-fat diet during either normal sleep-ing hours or normal waking hours. The mice that ate during sleep-ing hours *gained more than twice as much weight* as the mice eating during regular waking hours. Interestingly, another study showed that genetically obese mice fed exclusively during waking hours had a notable improvement in metabolism. In addition to when you eat, of course you need to be aware of what you eat and avoid too much fat. Mice fed high-fat diets until they became obese had abnormal cellular clocks, clock genes, and metabolisms.

You might be concerned that you don't have a good metabolism due to the genes you inherited. That may be true, but at the same time you can also be hurting your genes with *what* you eat and *when* you eat certain foods. Remember that your cells have nutrient sensors that help your cellular clock function properly. The timing and consistency of eating and the types of nutrients you consume matter very much. In the morning and at lunchtime, your body needs slightly higher-glycemic foods for their glucose and the short-term energy that powers your daily activity. In the evening and at night, your cellular clock expects you to consume much less sugar. Your body also needs metabolism-boosting amino acids at every meal, and more so in the evening, to help regulate your resting metabolic rate in order to burn unnecessary calories during sleep.

I designed my diet specifically to support harmony between the cellular and central circadian clocks so you can reach and maintain the most favorable metabolism for weight loss. By following the eating schedule in Chapter 10, you'll have the energy you need for all daily activities and no extra calories that could boost weight gain at night. For some people, like my 38-year-old patient Wanda, synchronizing the two clocks poses real challenges.

When Wanda came to me, she asked for help with a serious weight gain she'd experienced over the past four years, saying that she was once a petite 120 pounds but had gained twenty-five pounds for no apparent reason. Wanda thought it might be her thyroid underperforming, but she tested normal. I started her on my eating plan, which she needed to modify slightly because the basis for her weight problem was actually her sleep cycle. Wanda was a night supervisor at FedEx and had to work irregular shifts; her schedule varied widely with start times ranging from 9:00 p.m. to 4:00 a.m.

The first step was to establish a regular eating schedule, which meant Wanda would have to request a steady schedule—whatever her nighttime hours, she needed to start at the same time each day. Wanda's request was granted. She could now eat the right meals at the right time for *her* waking hours—different from the waking hours of people who work during the day, but a consistent eating schedule nonetheless. The downside, she said, was that she couldn't eat the same foods as her husband because he was eating breakfast as she was eating her dinner. After he also got on my meal plan, they made sure the morning foods and dinner foods were available to both of them to eat on their different schedules. It paid off. After Wanda followed this scheduled eating for twelve weeks, her weight had dropped to 125 pounds, a healthy weight for her height.

HOW NIGHTTIME EATING MAKES YOU FAT

Eating at night not only disrupts sleep patterns but also causes weight gain and even obesity. If you eat when you should be sleeping—even if you eat the same number of calories as you would in the daytime—you'll gain more weight. Nighttime eating drives down the normal nocturnal rise of energy-burning, appetite-suppressing leptin. Eating at night will misalign your central circadian clock, which wants you to eat when it's light outside, boosting the action of fat-inducing insulin, cortisol, and ghrelin. And it inverts the twenty-four-hour rhythm of blood sugar, which wants you to eat during the day, not at night.

Aligning your eating and sleeping patterns with the daylight cycle is critical for maintaining weight. As you work with my diet, your body will begin to adjust to its new regular meal schedule. The clock genes in essential organs, such as the liver and pancreas, are conditioned by the timing of meals, so if you shift your eating times to a new schedule, the clock genes will adjust their schedule over time to adapt to the new eating pattern. Research shows that when the time of food presentation changes, the expression of clock genes in the liver shifts to adjust to the new schedule.

College students who stay up late and eat after studying or partying can blame their "freshman 15" weight gain on more than just dorm food or higher alcohol consumption. My patient Melissa is a good example of what can happen when you eat out of sync with your central circadian clock. Because she was fearful of getting fat and losing her trim 20-year-old figure (along with the social status she'd worked so hard to achieve), Melissa started fasting. "I wouldn't eat anything all day," said Melissa. "Not even drink water or chew gum. I was so afraid of getting fat. I knew people made fun of girls who gained a lot of weight from drinking too much beer and eating big lunches on campus."

Unfortunately—but predictably—Melissa's hunger kicked in at the worst possible time, and at night she desperately stuffed herself with whatever she could find. "I ate my roommates' leftovers, I ate lunchmeat, I scarfed up whatever was in the kitchen. I was so hungry I couldn't sleep." Guilt kept her from eating the next day, and the cycle of daytime starvation/nighttime eating continued. At the end of her sophomore year, Melissa had gained thirty pounds because of her eating schedule, even though she constantly felt starved.

As a result of her eating when it was dark outside, Melissa's metabolism lost its speed. She became my patient because she thought a thyroid issue must be to blame, but her thyroid function was fine, and there was no other medical reason for her weight gain. After lengthy counseling and learning the importance of scheduled eating—starting in the morning and not eating at night—Melissa began to follow my plan. She also started practicing a regular relaxation technique. Melissa quickly grasped how following the plan would reset her metabolism to burn calories efficiently. She started a regular yoga class and continued to eat my recommended foods on a consistent schedule. In just fifteen weeks, a healthy, nourished, and well-fed Melissa dropped thirty pounds.

If you've been eating at night or skipping any meal of the day, you need to realign your eating patterns to sync with your cellular clock, which expects to eat at certain times, and your central circadian clock, eating when it's light and sleeping when it's dark. My diet plan shows you how. To lose weight as efficiently as possible, you must conscientiously stick to eating three meals and a snack at the designated times each day.

You also need to *sleep well and enough* each night. Once you begin, understand that it takes about nine days to resynchronize your clocks.

MANAGING YOUR SLEEP SCHEDULE: SLEEP WELL . . . AND SLEEP ENOUGH

Synchronizing your meals with your central circadian clock is an important component of my diet program, but it's only part of the plan. Losing weight and building a healthy metabolism rely on the simple and enjoyable act of sleeping. In fact, I recommend an adequate sleep schedule over squeezing extended exercise sessions into your day.

The epidemic of sleep deficiency and sleep disturbances is evolving at the same pace as the epidemic of weight gain. If you're overweight or obese, poor-quality sleep and sleep deprivation are likely to be part of the picture. Lack of sleep strongly correlates with hormone imbalances that slow your metabolism. Unless you address these sleep issues—whether deprivation, fragmentation (interrupted sleep), or poor-quality sleep—your efforts to reset your metabolism through diet and exercise will not fully restore your body's ability to burn fat and lose weight.

SLEEP DEPRIVATION AND SLEEP DISTURBANCES

Over the past half century, there's been a momentous decline in the time we spend sleeping. Many of us sleep fewer than six hours a night, and even children and adolescents who need about nine hours aren't getting enough. Sleep deprivation hurts you from the inside out, opening the floodgates of hormonal disturbances that affect appetite, brain activity, sexual function, energy, and weight. More than likely your bedtime is to blame for sleep shortage. Just as with eating on a schedule, you need to manage your sleep schedule, which may first require reconsidering how much you can do in one day. Rid yourself of the mind-set that by sleeping less you'll accomplish more.

Research has clearly shown that sleeping fewer than seven hours or more than nine hours a night can lead to weight gain and obesity. If you have a sleep-disturbing condition—depression, anxiety, hypothyroidism, enlarged tonsils or adenoids, stress, sleep apnea, or fibromyalgia—you must first address and resolve the medical problem for the best-quality sleep.

Sleep deprivation slows your metabolism and makes you crave sweets. You might assume that you burn more calories just by staying awake longer, but lack of sleep actually works against you. The problem begins deep inside your body where molecules determine your metabolism. When you don't sleep enough or on a regular schedule, your body loses its rhythm and many of your hormone pathways lose their ability to work together and keep your weight in check.

Ask Dr. Arem: How Many Hours Should I Sleep?

Q. How much sleep do I need to give all my hormones a chance to work their weight-loss magic at night? Is it eight hours and, if so, why?

A. Yes, you need eight hours of good deep sleep each night. Research shows an undeniable correlation between being overweight and being short on sleep. And while you might feel fine after six or seven hours, the hormones that support weight loss cannot fully recharge in that time. You'll pay the price with a distortion of the rhythm of more than a couple of important hormones involved in your metabolism. Look what happens with just one or two hours of sleep deprivation.

- *High cortisol:* After a single night of poor sleep, levels of the stress hormone cortisol remain high for twenty-four hours, boosting your appetite for fattening foods, adding pounds (especially around your waist), and leading to insulin resistance and further weight gain.

- *Low serotonin:* Your serotonin level also falls when you don't sleep enough. This indirectly affects your metabolism and weight, as it makes you more susceptible to poor food choices. And once your serotonin level lowers, your sleep quality worsens. Then chronic sleep deprivation puts you in a bind of bad moods, increased appetite, and sluggish metabolism.

- *Loss of precious REM sleep:* Depriving yourself of just a couple of hours of sleep over one night causes your body to produce less growth hormone, thyroid hormone, and leptin, all hormones that supercharge your metabolism.

Don't underestimate the importance of sleeping a full eight hours, even though you might feel functional with six hours and coffee in the morning. If you want peak function of the hormones that speed up metabolism and boost mood, you have got to sleep long enough and you must sleep deeply, without interruption.

Nonrestorative sleep—and this can include poor-quality sleep brought on by sleep disturbances—can easily make you powerless over your cravings. Perhaps the following scenarios will sound familiar. My patient Alicia, 30, may have been tired from restless sleep, but she was determined to work out one to two hours a day six days a week in order to lose weight. Being overweight had been an issue for Alicia's entire life, but it was only relatively recently that she'd become uncomfortably obese, gaining fifty pounds during her pregnancy a year earlier. When she came to see me, she told me she exercised a lot and had cut high-calorie foods out of her diet, yet was able to lose only five pounds in the six months after having her baby. She told me, "I exercise intensely. I drink a lot of water, and I eat strictly 1,500 calories a day. So why am I not losing weight?"

Alicia was certain that she had some form of thyroid or other hormonal imbalance, but as with many of my overweight patients, her test results ended up being normal. Alicia said another concern was how tired she still felt, even though her baby was sleeping through the night. She said she got eight hours every night, adding, "But I do toss and turn all night. I usually don't notice it, though, because it doesn't wake me up much. This might sound silly, but I sleep on an old mattress and I'm used to being uncomfortable."

Like many people who don't realize they're getting poor-quality sleep, Alicia didn't recognize the importance of creating an ideal setting for restful sleep. She agreed to invest in a new mattress, and I gave her the hormone-supporting eating plan laid out in this book. As I was leaving the exam room, she added, "Oh, I also get up two or three times at night to pee, but I have no problem falling asleep afterward." Urinating during the night is another sleep disturbance, but there's an easy fix—fluid restriction, meaning she'd continue drinking lots of water daily, but stop three to four hours before bedtime.

Once Alicia started feeling more rested, with my diet the weight began to come off easily. In just two weeks she lost ten pounds, and now a well-rested Alicia is on the right course to lose the extra weight once and for all.

Emily, 35, had a different set of sleep challenges. A six-months-divorced former ballerina, she'd recently started experiencing mild symptoms of depression. As a new patient, she asked me to help her with balancing her hormones and losing the extra ten pounds she'd gained in the past few months. "I still eat like I did ten years ago when I was 115 pounds. Nothing fattening. Lots of salads, fish, lean meats. I still do my exercises religiously. I know I'm a little older now, but the way I diet and exercise I think I should still look like a ballerina!" said Emily.

When she spoke about the divorce, she began to cry, saying how lonely she felt and how she hated it. To deal with the lonely void in the bedroom, she'd spend her nights on the living room couch watching movies to put her to sleep. "Some of the time I wake up at 2:00 a.m., turn off the TV, and go to bed," she told me. "The other four or five days of the week I can sleep straight through the night on the couch with the DVD title menu playing on repeat. The rhythmic audio track is comforting. I'm a deep sleeper, so even having the sound on doesn't wake me up."

Emily's assumption that she was a deep enough sleeper to ignore the shifting light coming from her TV monitor was wrong. The flicker delayed melatonin production, and the sounds prevented sustained sleep. She was not getting a good night's rest, and this had been going on for six months straight. Her emotional issues were keeping her from falling asleep and she needed a way other than watching old movies to get sleepy. I recommended she start meditating for fifteen to twenty minutes daily as a way of focusing on herself and her health. Emily went online to learn a basic breath meditation, which simply requires clearing your mind, sitting quietly, and noticing your breath as it moves into and out of your body. When she returned to see me six months later, she was back to a healthy weight. "I may not be as skinny as I was when I was 25, but that's okay. I feel great, I adore how centered I feel meditating every afternoon, and I'm much happier than I've been in the past couple years. I wake up feeling ready to take on my life, and I even met a new guy recently who I'm having a lot of fun with."

Alicia and Emily had no idea their sleep environments were compromising quality sleep and causing their weight gain. But as soon as they fixed the environmental factors, they got more sleep and lost weight.

With sleep deprivation or disturbed sleep, your energy balance is destroyed through three pathways: increased appetite, more time to eat, and a slowing of your metabolism.

- While you sleep, weight-loss helper leptin stimulates fat burning. Inadequate or disturbed sleep causes your body to produce more proteins that bind to leptin, leaving you with leptin resistance that makes you burn fewer calories and eat more without receiving signals telling you you're full.

- You also crave fats and sugars during the day as a result of higher levels of ghrelin, the hunger hormone.

- Without adequate sleep, saying "no" to high-carbohydrate snacks becomes more difficult.

Lack of sleep or poor-quality sleep paves yet another path to metabolic syndrome and abdominal fat accumulation. When you're sleep deprived, your cortisol level at dawn—normally high to get you going for the day—becomes blunted. In addition, your cortisol level later in the day, which is supposed to decline as you wind down, rises. Cortisol draws fat to your waist, an unwanted attribute for appearance, metabolism, and health, since abdominal fat promotes insulin resistance.

Sleep deprivation makes your body release and activate more adrenaline and noradrenaline, another state that causes insulin resistance. Not sleeping enough escalates insulin resistance little by little, leading to a cycle of weight gain, more insulin resistance, and metabolic syndrome. Sleep deprivation also makes you produce less fat-burning growth hormone, leading to metabolic dysfunction that in turn affects your sleep.

See if this story sounds familiar. Leslie, a 32-year-old HR manager, came to see me because she couldn't focus and wondered if she had low thyroid because she was gaining weight and having concentration difficulties. Her job was great, keeping her intellectually stimulated and busy, but she'd gained a lot of weight in the past three months, first noticed around her midsection when her trousers wouldn't button. She'd started weighing herself every week, and told me she'd steadily gained one or two pounds a week. We discussed her diet, relationships, and general health. Leslie said even though she had to wake up at 6:00 a.m. to get to work on time, she couldn't stop watching *Law & Order* reruns, which ran until midnight. "They help take my mind off work before I sleep," she told me. "It might sound crazy, but the show transports me to another place where I don't have to think about the politics of my job, even though my boss insists on sending me texts in the middle of the night."

Leslie had been attached to her *Law & Order*–induced sleep deprivation for more than a year, usually sleeping less than six hours a night. At close to 160 pounds (twenty pounds over her normal weight), she continued to unwittingly "feed the beast" by purchasing a new DVD season of the program, which kept her up even later, many nights until after 1:00 a.m. Now with an additional ten pounds under her belt, Leslie was seeking a solution.

Both her weight gain and her focusing problems were the result of sleeping just five or six hours a night. "But I've always only slept five or six hours a night, and I functioned fine in this job for the past couple of years. I don't think my body needs that much sleep. It must be something else giving me these problems," she said.

I explained that good science shows that sleeping too little causes you to have less REM sleep, the very cycles during which your pituitary releases potent bursts of the fat-burning, metabolism-revving growth hormone. Her body was not getting a chance to fully rest, and her hormone balance reflected that, having gradually changed from keeping her system healthy to packing on the pounds.

Leslie's prescription was lights out and audio off by 10:00 p.m. Shutting down all light-emitting devices (TV, computer, phone) along with their audio pings was crucial for her hormone levels and thus her weight. Leslie was actually glad to have a "doctor's note" for why she wouldn't be seeing those 1:00 a.m. texts from her boss. I also wanted her to eat according to my diet plan to help her restore her hormonal balance and the overall condition of her metabolism. The next time we met, she said, "It must be the combination of the healthier diet and the extra sleep. Within a week I was already focusing better at work." Two weeks after that, her weight started moving in the right direction—down. And in six months she returned to her ideal weight and felt like her confident self again.

BEWARE OF SLEEP FRAGMENTATION

Even if you're sleeping eight hours a night and you think you don't have a sleep disorder, you may still be affected by sleep fragmentation, which can affect your metabolism as unfavorably as sleep deprivation. Sleep fragmentation is anything that disrupts your sleep and wakes you up during the night, including an alert from your phone or a siren from an emergency vehicle. Even if you consciously ignore these disturbances and fall back to sleep quickly, sleep fragmentation is still affecting you. This is because your body responds to the distraction by waking up, which disturbs REM sleep and thereby deprives you of deep sleep.

Chelsea was a bright 22-year-old new mom with a mission: to restore her prepregnancy figure as soon as possible after giving birth to Shawna. She did everything she thought she needed to do to achieve a great body again—hired a personal trainer who made her exercise five times a week and met with a nutritionist weekly to ensure her diet was optimal. But rather than slowly losing her pregnancy weight, she saw the scale move in the opposite direction. Ten months after giving birth, she asked me to help solve her weight problem. "I'm doing everything I can, Dr. Arem. I used to be so thin, too. One baby shouldn't make me gain this much weight, and I'm only twenty-two! Other women who have children in their thirties are able to lose the pregnancy weight. Why can't I?" she asked.

Her thyroid hormone levels were normal, so I asked Chelsea about the possibility of sleep fragmentation, as most new moms wake up constantly to feed and tend to their infants. Chelsea said, "But I'm a stay-at-home mom, so I'm sure I sleep plenty. During the day, I nap while Shawna naps if I feel tired. The only problem is at night when my husband and I are both trying to sleep. She's colicky and wakes up and cries a lot. My husband works days, so I'm the one who always goes to Shawna. There have been times when it felt like I woke up every hour on the hour, but I catch up during the day."

Clearly, Chelsea's hormonal rhythms had been disturbed by sleep fragmentation due to Shawna's cries. As Shawna grew, the colic lessened and she began sleeping more quietly throughout the night, leaving Chelsea to sleep without disturbance. And after just five weeks of sleeping deeply, Chelsea finally started to lose weight. With her good diet, exercise, and restful sleep, she easily lost the weight that had been plaguing her.

REM sleep can also become fragmented as a result of sleep-disrupting stimuli like sleep-disordered breathing, sleep apnea, pain, or prostate disorders leading to frequent urination, all of which cause poor-quality sleep. Disturbing noises such as a distant car alarm or a television's white noise can reduce how much REM sleep you get. Remember that even if you don't notice a difference in your sleep, the slightest fragmentation can be another factor affecting your weight.

SLEEP APNEA

Sleep apnea is brief and frequent interruptions of normal breathing during sleep. In obstructive sleep apnea, these interruptions are caused by a collapse of the air passages, leading to a block in airflow for ten seconds or more. Central sleep apnea is repetitive, brief cessations of breathing caused by poor signaling from the brain to the diaphragm, rather than obstruction of air passages. Some people have both types of sleep apnea.

During the shallow or paused breathing, you move out of deep REM sleep into a lighter, poorer-quality sleep state. In obstructive sleep apnea, the collapse of the upper airway—usually at the pharynx—is often caused by reduced muscle tone or coordination, enlarged tonsils and adenoids, or a close-down of the breathing passage due to interference by the tongue and soft palate. Sleep apnea causes repetitive hypoxia (a drop in oxygen levels), which results in disruption of hormones that regulate metabolism. Lack of oxygen also disturbs neurotransmitters in the brain and makes your body produce stress chemicals that affect your health and overall well-being.

Erik, 47, had snored all his life, according to feedback from his mother, roommates at school, and wife. Yet Erik's weight gain hadn't begun until his early twenties. "Since college, I've put on weight

Symptoms and Health Effects of Sleep Apnea

Anxiety

Attention deficit/hyperactivity disorder, uncontrolled urination at night (enuresis), and depression in children

Daytime sleepiness

Disturbed sleep

Fatigue

Gastric reflux

Headache

High blood pressure

High LDL cholesterol and low HDL cholesterol

Insomnia, depression, and leg pain in women

Insulin resistance and diabetes

Irregular heartbeat

Nighttime urination

Sexual dysfunction in men

Weight gain

steadily. I just can't lose weight, even though I run marathons. I could run ten miles a day, it seems, and my weight wouldn't budge."

Erik came to see me for a thyroid evaluation, thinking his thyroid might be to blame for the extra weight, but it tested normal. But when he told me about the snoring, he added, "After a while my wife stopped commenting on it. I guess she learned to live with it. I know that at home or on a plane I still wake up sometimes short of breath and gasping for air."

He tested positive for obstructive sleep apnea, which is common in overweight people. Erik could finally overcome his weight-loss resistance by treating the sleep apnea using a continuous positive airway pressure (CPAP) machine while he slept. This device uses mild pressure to push air through any blockage. Two months after he started using it, Erik no longer woke up gasping for air, and he felt he was getting much better quality sleep. "It's only been a couple months, but I feel fresher, probably in a better mood, too, when I wake up." And because he'd also started on the Protein Boost Diet, Erik lost weight for the first time in twenty years—fourteen pounds.

Correcting Erik's sleep apnea issue and following my diet solved his weight problem by restoring the balance of hormones that would speed up his metabolism and help him burn fat.

HOW SLEEP APNEA MAKES YOU FAT

Sleep apnea is actually a common reason for metabolism slowdowns and the relentless weight gain they cause. Sleep apnea causes the stress hormone cortisol to rise at night, a time when it should be low. High cortisol levels make leptin work poorly, gradually leading you down a path of weight gain, metabolic syndrome, and diabetes. Inefficiency of weight-loss helper leptin escalates weight gain and makes your breathing even more difficult, as a result of its effect on your ability to respond to carbon dioxide. When you have sleep apnea, the intermittent lack of oxygen makes your body produce reactive oxygen species and inflammatory chemicals called "cytokines" that make you tired, cranky, and sleepy during the day. These chemicals also contribute to a slowdown in metabolism. Leptin inefficiency and the burden of inflammation can cause your mitochondria, which normally burn fat, to become sluggish. The result is fewer calories burned and a cooler body temperature.

Sleep apnea also stimulates neuropeptide Y, a powerful chemical produced by the hypothalamus that magnifies hunger. Growth hormone (GH), so helpful to a speedy metabolism, is produced in higher amounts during REM sleep, but sleep apnea lowers your GH levels because of reduced REM sleep and the periodic drops in oxygen. Low GH in turn makes insulin resistance worse and slows your metabolism further. One study found that 32 percent of people who have disordered breathing during sleep have metabolic syndrome.

Being overweight can cause sleep apnea, and even mild weight gain can trigger it. When this happens, a cycle begins in which weight gain leads to sleep apnea and sleep apnea leads to further weight gain. The sad part is that once you start on a weight gain/sleep apnea cycle, the numerous metabolic disturbances induced by sleep apnea will make it even more difficult for you to lose weight. If you've been trying to lose weight but haven't been successful despite every effort, you must consider sleep apnea a major piece of the puzzle and restore nighttime breathing and deep sleep as a first step.

Obstructive sleep apnea can even affect children, especially obese children. But even children who aren't overweight can have it, and it will then gradually make them overweight or obese as they enter the endless weight gain/sleep apnea cycle. Both aging and gaining body fat make you more likely to have sleep apnea. One study found that a mere 10 percent increase in body weight over four years increased the risk of sleep apnea sixfold. More fat in the neck area as a result of being overweight puts more pressure on the airway, which is why overweight and obese people are more likely to have obstructive sleep apnea.

OTHER TRIGGERS FOR SLEEP APNEA

Smoking leads to inflammation of your airways and makes you more vulnerable to sleep apnea. Also, if you smoke, your sleep will be further disturbed by waking when nicotine levels drop during sleep.

In addition to being overweight, menopause seems to be a major trigger of sleep apnea. Many women who have never had a sleep disorder experience sleep apnea as they go through the menopause transition. Underlying this is a hormonal imbalance during and after menopause that causes fat to move to the waist, chest, and neck, placing more pressure on the upper airways and slowing metabolism.

Having menopause-related sleep apnea often precipitates an impressive, dramatic, and seemingly unexplainable weight gain, understandably disturbing to women going through hormone-imbalance-driven emotional upheaval. Also, serotonin levels drop as a result of low estrogen during menopause, and serotonin plays an important role in regulating the muscle tone that opens the airways as you sleep. Without adequate serotonin to keep muscles toned enough to hold upper airways open, the airway collapse disrupts breathing and you start having sleep apnea. Those with low brain levels of serotonin, including people with depression, have a tendency to suffer from sleep apnea and weight gain. You also have a higher risk of sleep apnea if you have hypothyroidism, diabetes, heart or kidney disorders, PCOS, or insulin resistance.

DIAGNOSING AND TREATING SLEEP APNEA

Suspect sleep apnea if you gradually accumulate fat, especially in your abdominal area, and also if you notice that your daily performance of tasks and creativity have become impaired. You can have sleep apnea even without snoring. Snoring, in fact, is an indication that you have only a partial collapse of the airways. A long-lasting lack of oxygenated air from a partial airway collapse results in a syndrome called "hypopnea," and that's what makes you snore.

Having sleep apnea impairs your ability to lose weight because your hormone system is imbalanced as a result. Treatments, which require a specialist's diagnosis, include surgery or the continuous positive airway pressure (CPAP) machine.

Oral appliances show a 60 to 80 percent success rate for obstructive sleep apnea. Patients who use them experience less daytime sleepiness, improved cognition, and better results on simulated driving performance tests. They also have lower nighttime blood pressure and lower cholesterol and triglyceride levels. You can get an oral appliance from an experienced dentist.

Ask your physician about medications that have been shown to improve sleep apnea and associated symptoms. Metformin, a type 2 diabetes drug, can help because it reduces insulin resistance. SSRI antidepressants such as fluoxetine (Prozac) can also decrease sleep apnea by holding the upper airways open while you sleep.

SOLUTIONS FOR INSOMNIA

If you suffer from insomnia—difficulty falling asleep or staying asleep—take a melatonin supplement thirty minutes before bedtime to induce sleep and advance the dark phase of your central circadian clock. Doses ranging from 1 mg to 3 mg half an hour before bedtime are sufficient and safe. Avoid taking higher doses of melatonin because too much can lead to infertility or accelerate the course of Parkinson's disease.

Anything that relaxes you should become a nightly routine. Watching TV and staring at a computer or handheld device might seem relaxing, but they aren't helpful. The bright light inhibits melatonin production. Dim your lights in the late evening, and try different forms of relaxation, from stretching to exchanging massages with your partner, until you find one that works best for you. These easy sleep inducers can also help.

- The relaxation techniques described in Chapter 4 are my best prescription for improving sleep.
- Evening exercise is followed by a drop in body temperature, which can actually help you fall asleep.
- If you're following my plan and exercising during the day, that too will help you sleep better at night.
- Take a warm bath before you go to bed. Returning to room temperature after heating up in the bath gives you a cooling sensation and the drop in your body temperature after bathing encourages sleep.

If you're still having trouble falling asleep, perhaps it's because you're feeling you haven't accomplished enough during the day. Challenge yourself with mentally stimulating activities throughout the day, but quiet down before dinnertime.

By following the Protein Boost Diet, you'll be eating proteins and taking probiotics, so the good bacteria in your gut will promote GABA activity in your brain, easing anxiety and ushering in sleep. Going to sleep by 10:00 p.m. also gives your body enough time to produce optimal amounts of metabolism-boosting hormones and rest before sunrise. But if you're reworking your sleep routine, don't go to bed too early. Start by being in bed exactly eight hours before you need to wake up, and soon you will figure out when the best bedtime is for you.

SLEEP MEDICATIONS

If you have insomnia, you may need to use a sleep medication, but sleep drugs are only a temporary solution. Always try melatonin first, along with regular yoga or tai chi practice. If this isn't helpful, talk to your doctor about using a sleeping pill, but know that some prescription sleeping drugs can cause you to lose conscious control over your actions. Even the safest ones should be taken for only six to eight weeks. You may need a medication to overcome chronic insomnia initially, but as you nourish your body and remove stress with my program, you'll see positive changes in your sleep patterns.

Tips for Improved Sleep

Many of my patients are driven to succeed at both work and weight loss, and yet they have trouble in both areas because they're not sleeping well . . . or enough. Here are some tips.

Straight eight: Start on a sleep schedule that ensures you get eight hours every night. Your hormones require eight hours to restore their weight-limiting power.

Cool and comfortable: Make sure your room is cool and your mattress comfortable.

Don't go into the light: Eliminate all light sources to make your sleeping room as dark as possible. Any amount of light—even the tiniest—interferes with production of melatonin, your sleep hormone, and causes weight gain. Cover the lights on your alarm clock. By 10:00 p.m. turn off the TV, computer, phone, and all lit devices. Remember your iPad, or other reading device, is backlit, so if you read on one, stop by 10:00 p.m.

Quiet it down: To avoid fragmented sleep, eliminate disturbing sounds including TV, radio, and the ping that sounds when you get a text (turn off your phone, leave it in another room, and know you can return those messages tomorrow).

CHAPTER SIX

BALANCING ESTROGEN AND TESTOSTERONE HORMONES TO LOSE WEIGHT

Putting your hormones in perfect balance at every level will make you feel you've upgraded your life. Any imbalance has effects on weight, but sex hormones are crucial in defining body fat composition and distribution. In previous chapters, I introduced the major hormone players that directly and indirectly affect weight, body fat, and metabolism—leptin, ghrelin, insulin, cortisol, growth hormone, and thyroid hormone. In this chapter we'll look at how sex hormones—estrogen, progesterone, testosterone, and DHEA—regulate growth hormone and the efficiency of insulin and leptin, and thus your appetite and body fat. We'll also discuss hormone replacement therapy for menopause, and how to choose the right hormones to succeed with weight loss and prevent further weight gain. As part of aging, every woman faces menopause and every man a decline in testosterone and the inevitable shifts of metabolism they produce.

POLYCYSTIC OVARY SYNDROME

A common cause of weight gain is the hormone disorder polycystic ovary syndrome (PCOS), which affects 6 to 10 percent of women of reproductive age. The ovaries of women with PCOS produce imbalanced amounts of estrogen, progesterone, and testosterone. The combination of imbalanced estrogens and too much testosterone in their system causes fat to accumulate, particularly in the abdominal area, in turn leading to insulin resistance.

Your doctor will test you for PCOS if you have an abnormal menstrual cycle, unwanted hair growth on your face or other parts of your body, acne, and insulin resistance. Other clues are high fasting insulin levels, impaired glucose tolerance, a high testosterone level, high LH (luteinizing hormone) compared with FSH (follicle-stimulating hormone), and ovarian cysts, which can be found with an ultrasound of your ovaries.

Thirty to 75 percent of women with PCOS become overweight or obese. If you have it, your condition will never go away, but you can lose weight and reverse your symptoms by following my diet and using the right hormones and other medication. Women with PCOS find it challenging to lose weight on conventional diets because they're typically trapped in a vicious cycle of resistance to leptin and insulin. Around the world, 12 to 46 percent of women with PCOS also have metabolic syndrome.

If you have PCOS, whether it was recognized during your reproductive years or not, its effects on weight and metabolism will continue to haunt you after menopause. Your testosterone levels will continue to be high and you're likely to gain even more weight and to have more abdominal fat and metabolic syndrome than if you didn't have PCOS.

RESTORING HORMONAL BALANCE WITH DIET

Overweight women with PCOS need to make serious, long-term adjustments in order to be able to lose weight. Recent research shows that losing as little as 10 percent of your body weight makes ovulation occur more frequently and increases your chances of conception. Losing weight also lowers testosterone levels and decreases insulin resistance. Women with PCOS who followed a low-calorie, low-carb, high-protein diet lost more fat than those who were on a low-calorie diet supplemented with simple sugars.

My low-glycemic modified Mediterranean diet is ideal for any woman with PCOS because it enhances insulin sensitivity and can reverse the many metabolic and hormonal imbalances that perpetuate symptoms and weight gain. My diet will eventually make you less hungry and reduce overeating. Follow the 20/10 exercise program, too, and stay away from fad and starvation diets. They'll threaten your immune system and slam the brakes on your metabolism.

METFORMIN AND BIRTH CONTROL PILLS CAN ALSO HELP

To optimize weight loss, discuss with your doctor whether you should take metformin in conjunction with following my diet. Metformin, a type 2 diabetes drug, decreases insulin resistance, lowers testosterone levels, and helps restore normal periods. Taking an oral contraceptive can also help restore hormonal balance and break the cycle of insulin resistance and high testosterone levels. Birth control pills are usually a combination of estrogen and progestin (a synthetic derivative resembling progesterone). Work with your doctor to choose a birth control pill containing the right type of progestin (preferably a newer-generation pill having the least male hormone and glucocorticoid effects) to decrease symptoms and make weight loss easier. Yasmin, Femcon, and Ovcon are some of my suggested choices for PCOS because they help with acne, unwanted facial hair and body hair growth, menstrual cramping, and weight issues.

MENOPAUSE: HOW LOW ESTROGEN AFFECTS WEIGHT AND METABOLISM

The decline in the sex hormones estrogen and progesterone that occurs before and during menopause causes weight gain in most women. Menopause is the point in a woman's life when she no longer has periods. Perimenopause is the five- to ten-year period preceding menopause. During perimenopause, women experience hormone fluctuations and then a gradual decline of sex hormones. This imbalance can easily trigger a slowdown of metabolism and a gradual, seemingly inexplicable weight gain most women find extraordinarily frustrating.

Menopause is a normal part of aging and occurs on average around age 51, though it can happen sooner or a few years later. With estrogen levels running low at menopause, you have less serotonin in your brain to keep mood and emotions stable. Serotonin is the neurotransmitter that also suppresses cravings and helps you breathe well while sleeping. As a result of altered neurotransmitter activity during menopause, you might have trouble sleeping or wake up several times during the night, anxious or covered with sweat from night sweats, leading you to feeling sleepy and fatigued the next day. Low estrogen also leaves skin thin and dry and can impair cognition. Some symptoms start during perimenopause, worsening as you reach menopause.

Weight gain also often begins during perimenopause, becoming more obvious when your periods stop altogether and estrogen plunges to its lowest levels. The more rapid your decline in estrogen during menopause, the more weight gain you'll experience. Women who go through menopause as a result of surgical removal of the ovaries are 78 percent more likely to become obese, and have a five times greater chance of becoming severely obese.

EXTRA FAT BRINGS EXTRA SYMPTOMS

If you're already overweight when you reach actual menopause (meaning you've not had a menstrual period for twelve months), you're more likely to suffer from menopause symptoms, including hot flashes and night sweats. The good news is that losing weight can ease menopausal symptoms.

This is what happened to Laurie, a 51-year-old executive who came to see me because of menopause symptoms that made her quite debilitated in daily life at work. She said, "I don't know how I'm going to keep my position as CFO if I'm bent out of shape with hot flashes every time I hold a meeting. They seem to hit me at the most inconvenient times! My days are already difficult. I'm tired and nervous, not myself. I went from superconfident to overemotional, and I think it's obvious to the people at the office. They've been asking me, 'Are you okay?' For the past year, I've also gained weight."

Laurie started to gain weight at age 40, while she was taking care of her mother, who was fighting breast cancer. Laurie began feeling depressed. She could barely cope with both work and her mother's cancer, and then her daughter started getting in trouble at school. Laurie was so overwhelmed that she let her weight grow from 155 pounds at age 40 to 210 pounds by the time she was 51. She'd become menopausal a year earlier and gained ten more pounds since. "My hot flashes have gotten a lot more frequent in the past few months," she said. "For three hours a night I'm constantly covering myself with my comforter and then taking it off. I also wake up with aching muscles at night."

Her thyroid test was normal and I could find no other medical condition that could be slowing her metabolism except for the recent onset of menopause. Laurie felt that hormone replacement therapy wasn't an option for her. She had a history of thrombophlebitis at age 35 while she was taking birth control pills and also feared taking hormones, since her mother had breast cancer. Instead, she worked with my program until she lost forty pounds. Fascinatingly, all of Laurie's menopause symptoms disappeared when she reached a healthy weight. Laurie's story shows how being overweight itself can contribute to menopause symptoms and how losing weight can resolve them.

ESTRADIOL DROPS DRAMATICALLY DURING MENOPAUSE, AFFECTING HUNGER HORMONES AND METABOLISM

Estrogen affects many tissues in the body, including your reproductive organs, bones, liver, nervous system, immune system, gastrointestinal tract, and heart. This all-important female hormone protects against bone loss, so when menopause occurs and estrogen levels drop, you lose bone density and your risk for osteoporosis increases. Your body produces different kinds of estrogens, but estradiol (E2) is the hormone that has the biggest impact on metabolism and fat distribution. Take a look at what this powerful hormone does.

- Before menopause, estradiol keeps your pancreas healthy and producing just the right amount of insulin.

- When estradiol levels start to decline during perimenopause and become very low at menopause, the pancreas becomes infiltrated with fat and, as a result, can become unable to compensate for the insulin resistance. The result may be metabolic syndrome and diabetes.

- Additionally, estradiol influences growth hormone (GH), which helps you burn fat and preserve lean muscle mass. A lack of estrogen makes you deficient in GH, adding yet another culprit to your slowing metabolism and fat accumulation.

There's more sorry news regarding the effect of falling estradiol levels on the weight-loss helper leptin. During the transition into menopause, estrogen deficiency promotes leptin resistance, making you hungrier and further slowing metabolism. Before menopause, normal levels of estrogen activate receptors in the hypothalamus that increase the chemical that suppresses appetite (pro-opiomelanocortin) and decrease the chemical that promotes hunger (neuropeptide-Y). This explains why at menopause, when estradiol falls, women tend to crave sugary and fatty foods—another reason for weight gain. Poor-quality nutrition in combination with declining hormones makes women who have gone through menopause even more vulnerable to weight gain and obesity. Researchers evaluating the diet quality of women past menopause found that only 3 percent of study participants were eating a high-quality diet. Fully half the women were eating junk foods, with high consumption of refined carbs, sugars, and saturated fats. For anyone, a diet rich in refined carbs and saturated fats leads to cardiovascular disease, but this is especially true of women after menopause. I cannot emphasize enough the health benefits of my diet if you're nearing menopause or you've already gone through it. Happily, if you're past menopause, taking estradiol via hormone replacement therapy will help control hunger and restore the effects of leptin efficiency and GH activity on your metabolism to prevent further weight gain and to help you lose weight.

MORE BELLY FAT AT MENOPAUSE

Before menopause, estradiol causes women to lay down more fat under the skin rather than around the abdomen, while men tend to naturally accumulate more belly fat. Fat tissue under the skin contains more receptors for estradiol, while visceral fat (which collects around the abdomen and vital internal organs) contains more receptors for the male hormone testosterone. This explains why at menopause women tend to have a shift in body fat from the buttocks and thighs to the abdomen. Belly fat excess is a harbinger of insulin resistance and high cholesterol.

Now you understand why estradiol's decline affects so many aspects of your metabolism and the way you look and feel. You might also wonder why your cholesterol, which has been in a normal range for years, is suddenly abnormally high. All these changes are consequences of low estradiol levels. The redistribution of fat to your waistline now makes you vulnerable to heart disease, high blood pressure, metabolic syndrome, osteoarthritis, and diabetes. Suddenly, after menopause, cardiovascular disease becomes a major cause of death.

TESTOSTERONE IMBALANCE DURING MENOPAUSE

As estradiol levels drop during menopause, the manufacture of testosterone by the ovaries declines as well. The proteins that bind and carry sex hormones (including estrogens and testosterone) in the bloodstream decline as well. This has to do with the liver reducing its manufacture of these proteins. The end result is a low total testosterone level and imbalanced testosterone activity. This means it's not only low estrogen levels that slow metabolism and cause insulin resistance during perimenopause and menopause. Imbalanced testosterone activity could contribute to these metabolic malfunctions during menopause.

LOW THYROID DURING MENOPAUSE

When you're transitioning into menopause, you become vulnerable to thyroid problems, and menopause can also worsen an existing thyroid issue. The frequency of hypothyroidism jumps to one in every eight women at menopause. The hormonal shift makes your immune system more likely to attack and hurt your thyroid (see "Hashimoto's Thyroiditis as a Cause of Low Thyroid" in Chapter 3) as if it were a foreign object, and this leads to low thyroid. Not only does thyroid imbalance exacerbate the symptoms of menopause, it can also make the menopause transition more stressful. Thyroid imbalances slam the brakes on metabolism even further, worsening cravings and bringing on dramatic weight gain. In recent years researchers have begun to understand that estradiol helps maintain the foundation of metabolism that thyroid hormones hold, with estrogen levels and estrogen receptors apparently playing a role in the health of thyroid cells. To lose weight through a healthy metabolism at menopause, you must get your thyroid hormones balanced and working efficiently.

With low thyroid, you may have fatigue, dry skin, cold intolerance, hot flashes, anxiety, mood swings, sleep problems, depressive symptoms, and the concurrent cravings for food from lowered serotonin. But wait—you already had these symptoms when your estrogen dropped just before menopause. Menopausal symptoms actually worsen when your thyroid is unbalanced because the symptoms are similar and build on each other. Once your hormones stress your mental well-being, life can become extremely hard to manage. Losing weight is out of the question for many women during this clamorous transition until both hormone issues are meticulously resolved.

Lucy, 53, whom I'd treated for hypothyroidism for eight years, became menopausal two years ago. She told me one day, "I know my thyroid's off, and I need my thyroid hormones adjusted. I can tell whether it's my thyroid or menopause. I've learned in the past couple of years which is what. Many symptoms caused by thyroid and menopause are the same, but when my thyroid is off even a little, I can feel it. The symptoms are much more intense."

Lucy was absolutely right. Thyroid testing showed that she'd become a little more deficient in thyroid hormone than when she'd seen me six months prior, and she needed more medication to reach perfect thyroid balance. Since her last visit, the function of her thyroid gland had declined further as a result of the autoimmune thyroid condition Hashimoto's thyroiditis. Low thyroid and estradiol deficiency have quite a few overlapping symptoms. For women, balanced thyroid hormones and estrogens are crucial for a healthy and stable serotonin system in the brain. When both sex hormones and thyroid are unbalanced, the effects feed each other and your emotional well-being is seriously hammered. If, like Lucy's, your symptoms become more intense, make sure your thyroid isn't at the root of it all.

COMMON SYMPTOMS OF HYPOTHYROIDISM AND MENOPAUSE
Anger
Anxiety
Decreased tolerance for stress
Depression
Fatigue
Irritability
Lack of motivation and lack of interest

Low sex drive
Mood swings
Sadness; crying spells
Sleep disturbances
Thin, dry skin
Weight gain

You'll have a difficult time stalling weight gain without correcting any thyroid hormone imbalance and/or estradiol deficiency. For this reason, I suggest your thyroid be tested when you start having irregular periods and when you reach menopause. I also believe that menopause is one of the periods in a woman's life during which annual thyroid testing should be conducted. Even low-grade hypothyroidism can worsen hot flashes, sleep problems, mood issues, and weight gain during this time. View TSH levels greater than 2 mIU/L with suspicion, even if your test still falls in the normal range. If you're already being treated for a thyroid imbalance, your thyroid hormone treatment may need to be adjusted. As I explained in Chapter 3, an ultrasound of your thyroid and a test for Hashimoto's thyroiditis (anti-TPO antibody testing) can be helpful in diagnosing Hashimoto's thyroiditis.

SLEEP APNEA DURING MENOPAUSE

In addition to low thyroid, sleep issues such as sleep apnea often add to symptoms of menopause and make the weight struggle worse, because sleep apnea itself slows metabolism. Imagine the hormonal chaos already occurring as you transition into menopause. Add a failing thyroid gland, and on top of it all, sleep apnea. Now you have three major slowdowns in metabolism working against you simultaneously, triggering your body to accumulate outrageous amounts of fat in a short period of time.

Tracy, 53, like so many other patients, came to see me to find out whether her chronic symptoms and significant weight gain could be explained by hormones. She'd been struggling with fatigue, forgetfulness, feeling cold, and low mood for three years, and she was having issues with interrupted sleep for two years. Tracy cried when she told me about her weight, explaining that when she was 40, she was slim for her frame at 135 pounds. She said, "Dr. Arem, I feel deformed and horrible, and I now weigh 215 pounds. There is definitely something wrong with me and my hormones!"

Tracy was distressed, struggling with her sense of self and quality of life. I tested Tracy's thyroid and found she had low-grade hypothyroidism (a slightly underactive thyroid; see "Thyroid Gland: Metabolism Energizer" in Chapter 3), which contributed to her weight gain. But the primary causes were her menopause-triggered declining estrogen levels and sleep apnea.

I reestablished Tracy's thyroid and estrogen balance with hormone treatment. She also started using a CPAP machine and following my eating plan for better hormone balance. The newly healthy levels of estrogen and thyroid, along with correcting the metabolism-slowing effect of the sleep apnea, did the trick. With her hormones back to normal, she felt much better and gradually saw her body return to a fitter profile than she'd had in years.

SYMPTOM RELIEF WITH HORMONE REPLACEMENT THERAPY (HRT)

In addition to gaining weight, 75 to 80 percent of menopausal women experience classic symptoms of menopause: hot flashes, night sweats, sleep disturbances, cognitive changes, vaginal dryness, and anxiety. Many women also undergo metabolic changes that increase their risk of having metabolic syndrome, high cholesterol, diabetes, and heart disease. In my opinion, the most effective way to alleviate symptoms and prevent a metabolic disorder is to take hormones via bioidentical HRT.

- The sooner you start HRT during your menopause transition, the more heart-protective benefits you'll reap: taking HRT cuts your risk of coronary heart disease by nearly half. Hormones also lower blood pressure and reduce inflammatory chemicals that promote cardiovascular disease.

- Supplementing with estradiol also helps your brain stay sharp. The protective properties of estradiol on the brain work to minimize chemical damage and inflammation, helping prevent Alzheimer's and Parkinson's diseases. Prolonging the presence of estradiol in your system seems to lessen the overall likelihood of neurodegenerative diseases. A healthy level of estrogen also enhances dopamine activity.

- Estradiol improves insulin sensitivity and fat metabolism. Taking hormones to lift estradiol levels can help you lose weight by suppressing cravings and speeding up metabolism. This is because estradiol boosts the weight-loss helper leptin so it works more effectively, making you feel full after eating and helping your metabolism burn calories briskly. An analysis of research conducted over several years clearly demonstrated that nondiabetic menopausal women who take hormones gain more lean muscle mass and lose more of their waist circumference and abdominal fat than women who don't take hormones.

- Estradiol improves your physical capacity and physical activity. The benefits of estradiol for your metabolism are also greater when you are physically active and you exercise. One study looked at the effects of HRT and physical activity on body mass index and metabolic profile changes in postmenopausal women of similar age. It found that, after four months of HRT, the HRT-taking women who were physically active had lower body fat compared with women who were less physically active. Even in inactive women, though, HRT caused a significant reduction in belly fat and shrank the waist-to-hip ratio (see "Are You Overweight or Obese?" in Chapter 1).

HOW PROGESTIN IN HRT HELPS . . . AND HINDERS

For women whose uterus is intact, progesterone should be added to HRT to protect against cancer of the uterus and thickening of the endometrium, the inner lining of the uterus. Progesterone is often prescribed in a synthetic derivative form called "progestin." Some progestins, however, have male hormone and glucocorticoid effects. Progestins are not exactly the same molecule that your body produces. They are molecules having a structure similar to progesterone and mimic some of the effects of the natural hormone progesterone. Unfortunately, taking a progestin with estrogen reduces many of estrogen's benefits, including the weight benefits and improvement in insulin sensitivity. Women who've had a hysterectomy who take estrogens alone experience more improvement in insulin sensitivity than women who take both estrogen and a progestin. It makes sense that if you've had a hysterectomy, you don't want to add a progestin to your treatment. Progestins simply negate the beneficial metabolic effects of estrogen, though for women with a uterus, progestins are an essential protection against uterine cancer.

Progestins decrease blood flow to the brain, so taking an estrogen with a progestin doesn't benefit cognition as well as cyclic progesterone (see "My HRT Advice" in this chapter) or estrogen taken alone. A study conducted by the Women's Health Initiative showed that women taking Provera along with Premarin had an increased risk of dementia and stroke as they got older.

CHOOSE NATURAL PROGESTERONE RATHER THAN A PROGESTIN

As you transition into menopause, the more testosterone you have in your system, the more likely it is you'll have insulin resistance and weight gain. If you're including some form of progesterone in your HRT, choose one that has the fewest androgenic properties (meaning the hormone acts less like the male hormone testosterone), and preferably as an FDA-approved bioidentical progesterone pill or a vaginal gel. Natural progesterone, the same molecule that your body normally produces, actually has no androgenic properties, and for this reason I recommend only natural progesterone be used as part of your HRT rather than a progestin with male hormone or glucocorticoid properties.

MY HRT ADVICE

- Take bioidentical estrogen (estradiol) in the form of a transdermal patch or an FDA-approved gel.

  If you have a uterus you need to take progesterone, which is available in various FDA-approved forms or compounded (made with combined ingredients for individualized needs). To enhance the weight-loss benefits of estrogen in HRT, take the progesterone in a cyclic fashion—ten days every month or every two months.

- One of my best choices for progesterone is Prometrium, as it has no androgen or glucocorticoid properties. Avoid taking medroxy progesterone (Provera), since it's a progestin that has some androgenic and glucocorticoid effects.

> ### Ask Dr. Arem: How Do I Decide on HRT?
>
> **Q.** What about studies that link taking some types of HRT to heart attacks, cancer, and stroke? How do I figure out the risks?
>
> **A.** Before you start taking hormones, weigh the risks against the benefits based on your medical history. Avoid HRT if you're diabetic, have cardiovascular disease, or have a history of blood clotting.
>
> Always start with the smallest dose possible to relieve menopause symptoms and address weight issues. Keep in mind that you may be predisposed to risks such as breast cancer (although scientific research has not been conducted on bioidentical hormones), so get a mammogram first. I also recommend ultrasound tests if needed, because they provide you with a more accurate evaluation of your breast cancer risk. A family history of breast cancer is a factor against taking HRT.
>
> Start eating well and adopt a healthy, active lifestyle like the one in my program. Aim to ameliorate blood pressure, blood sugar, and cholesterol problems.

KEEP HRT DOSE AS LOW AS POSSIBLE

Standard doses of estrogen are too high for many women and may unnecessarily increase the risk of breast cancer, blood clots, and stroke. When it comes to hormones, your goal is to get maximum benefit with minimal risk. My recommendation is to use the lowest dose possible of both estradiol and progesterone for symptom relief and reversing insulin resistance. The dose needs to be tailored to your needs as I have advocated for thyroid treatments. HRT can be continued with the consent of your doctor as long as you are benefiting from it and have no side effects.

The Women's Health Osteoporosis, Progestin, Estrogen (HOPE) study evaluated conjugated equine estrogen (Premarin) combined with medroxyprogesterone acetate (MPA) and found that low doses were as effective in reducing the number and intensity of hot flashes as standard doses. Another study found that low doses of Premarin were as effective as standard doses in lowering cholesterol and triglycerides and improving health of blood vessel lining. This research indicates that low doses of hormones may be all you need to get all the benefits you're seeking while minimizing the health risks.

I RECOMMEND BIOIDENTICAL HRT RATHER THAN
SYNTHETIC HORMONE DERIVATIVES

Over the years, I've changed my HRT prescription patterns. I now believe the hormones a woman should take ought to be the same hormones her body naturally produces—the kind found in bioidentical hormones. Concerns about hormone safety were triggered by the release of the Women's Health Initiative (WHI) study in 2002, in which researchers concluded that the risks of taking conventional HRT (Premarin and Provera) outweighed the beneficial effects. But this study and other research tested hormones that your body does not naturally produce. The WHI research did not address whether bioidentical hormones can cause harm.

Bioidentical hormones used for HRT are the same hormone molecules produced naturally by your body and must be taken in a way to mimic their natural release into your system by the ovaries. When you take a hormone in the form of a tablet, like Premarin and Provera, the hormones first pass through your liver, where they change as they're metabolized. Compare this with a hormone released by your ovaries and distributed throughout your body before it reaches the liver. The best way to mimic what and how your body delivers its hormones is in the form of a transdermal patch or a gel, because it's able to enter your bloodstream without changing at all from being metabolized by your liver. Using the transdermal (skin patch) form of estradiol decreases your risk for venous thromboembolism (blood clots) by 30 percent, compared with taking an oral estrogen—showing the power of how your medicine is delivered.

Bioidentical estradiol is available in FDA-approved forms (patch or gel) and in a compounded form such as a cream. The main disadvantage of the patch is possible skin reactions. Compounded creams, however, may cause unstable estradiol levels, but it's still an option for some. Some of the most popular pharmaceutical forms of bioidentical estradiol are Vivelle, Vivelle-DOT, Climara, FemPatch, Estrace, Estraderm, EstroGel, Elestrin, and Divigel.

TO HELP WITH WEIGHT,
WHEN SHOULD I START TAKING HORMONES?

When it comes to weight, research supports hormone treatment early in menopause. The best time to initiate HRT, I suggest, is within the first year after you stop menstruating, or even sooner if your gynecologist agrees. One study compared the weight outcome of women who started taking hormones twelve months before they stopped having menstrual periods with that of women who started taking hormones later, and showed that the effect on weight was virtually the same. Both groups of women had the same rate of obesity later on. The problem with this research is that women who sought out HRT early on because of menopausal symptoms could be the ones who are more likely to have weight issues. The other problem with the study is that the women studied did not take bioidentical HRT.

Taking hormones in your first menopausal years (within one to three years of menopause), however, has clearly been shown to reduce abdominal fat and both total and LDL cholesterol, and to improve cardiovascular health and fat metabolism. From my own experience with patients, the sooner you start taking hormones, the better your chances of controlling your weight-gain trend and the more weight you'll be able to lose.

We talked earlier about the heart and brain protection HRT confers. Again, taking hormones early seems to make a difference. As years progress, especially after menopause, cognition can decline, but taking hormones can preserve your brain's productivity. Animal studies show that rodents that received HRT within three months after the removal of their ovaries (to induce menopause) had better results on problem-solving tests compared with rodents that received hormones ten months after surgery-induced menopause. Early treatment of menopausal rats with estradiol significantly enhanced cognitive tasks. Humans who have taken hormones sooner in menopause, rather than later, have much better productivity in the long run. You can stay sharp mentally and control your weight by timing your treatment. Because menopause symptoms lessen with physical activity and weight loss, it's ideal to also start following my program early in your transition to menopause.

GET HELP WITH PHYTOESTROGENS

I believe plant estrogens (called "isoflavones") can help alleviate the effects of low estrogen while giving you benefits for weight and menopause symptoms. Recent research, however, shows that plant estrogens don't confer the same magnitude of protection as HRT for cognition or against hot flashes. Even though the chemical structure of isoflavones resembles the estrogens in your body, they're often not a sufficient alternative on their own. Scientists have shown that plant isoflavones can help women past menopause reduce the loss of bone density, lower LDL cholesterol, and help relieve hot flash symptoms. Isoflavones from soy, red clover, and black cohosh imitate the activity of your body's natural estrogens. These ingredients found in many natural supplements can help you with your menopausal symptoms and weight if you elect to not take HRT.

TESTOSTERONE TREATMENT FOR WOMEN

After you've learned that testosterone promotes insulin resistance and fat redistribution to your abdominal area, it may sound paradoxical to suggest adding testosterone to your bioidentical hormone replacement regimen. The reality is that women's testosterone levels decline during perimenopause and menopause. When you take estradiol to balance your hormones, the free or bioactive form of testosterone becomes lower, and taking supplemental testosterone at a low dose actually may help with well-being and weight loss in women.

Testosterone treatment in women who are going through menopause also helps with sexual problems often experienced as a result of declining testosterone levels. Treatment enhances sexual desire, pleasure from intercourse, and frequency of sex. Side effects of testosterone are hair growth, acne, and headaches, but they're not likely with low-dose treatment. You can take testosterone by injection, implant, cream, or patch, or in sublingual form. I advise my patients to use a patch or a sublingual form. Some women have a skin reaction to testosterone patches or creams at the application site, though it's typically mild. Testosterone replacement may help those whose ovaries have been removed surgically; it also provides great benefits, when taken in the right amount, to women who have had a natural menopause.

Here's proof that using the right dose counts. Testosterone patches at a dose of 300 mcg per day were shown to ameliorate sexual dysfunction and help with weight loss in surgically menopausal women. Taking 150 mcg per day did not result in lessening of sexual dysfunction or improvement in weight loss. Taking 400 mcg per day can cause side effects, and the positive effects on weight are minimal. If you decide on the patch, take 300 mcg per day.

DHEA AND DHEA-S

Hormones with androgenic properties (hormones having effects like the male hormones testosterone or androsterone) in women can promote weight gain, insulin resistance, and a shift of fat tissue toward the waistline. Dehydroepiandrosterone (DHEA), however, can help with your weight when taken in the right amount. DHEA and dehydroepiandrosterone sulfate (DHEA-S, a by-product of DHEA) are the most abundant hormones circulating in your body, and are major male hormones produced by the adrenal glands. DHEA works to improve fat distribution and insulin sensitivity by virtue of its hormonal by-products, including estradiol. It also helps lower the amount of the stress hormone cortisol you have in your system. Finally, DHEA enhances the efficiency of adiponectin, the hormone that tells your body to burn fat for fuel and that improves the efficiency of insulin.

The amount of DHEA and DHEA-S your adrenal glands produce gradually rises starting when you are about age 6 to 8 and continues until you're 20 to 30, when levels begin to gradually decline (this is in contrast to the adrenal hormone cortisol, which is produced in the same amounts throughout life). If you're overweight, it gets worse: high insulin and insulin resistance drive down DHEA levels even further. Therefore the decline in DHEA as a result of weight gain causes even more weight gain.

DHEA regulates your metabolism along with immune and cognitive function, and declining levels can lead to impaired cognitive function and poor physical health in older people. A well-conducted study showed that older overweight adults who took 50 mg of DHEA daily had fat loss around their abdomens and decreased insulin resistance. Taking DHEA reduced both visceral fat and fat under the skin, even though participants didn't change their diet or exercise. Your doctor can check your DHEA-S levels with a blood test. If your level is low, consider asking your doctor about taking DHEA in physiological doses to help break the vicious cycle of fat accumulation and insulin resistance.

TESTOSTERONE IN MEN

Importantly, testosterone in men promotes lean body mass and prevents fat accumulation. Testosterone begins to drop at age 30 and continues its decline with age. Low testosterone levels in men are quite common, affecting 50 percent of men over 60. This is significant because men can easily gain weight and find weight loss difficult as their testosterone levels fall. Men generally tend to accumulate more visceral fat than women. With low testosterone, even more abdominal fat accumulates. Low testosterone also sets the scene for insulin resistance, which encourages still more fat accumulation, metabolic syndrome, and even diabetes. Animal research has shown that the insulin resistance caused by low testosterone can be reversed with testosterone replacement.

If you have low testosterone, you're more likely to have too much body fat as well as high insulin levels, high triglyceride levels, and low HDL cholesterol (the helpful type). Research has repeatedly shown that the lower testosterone levels are in men, the higher their body mass index and the greater their waist-to-hip ratio and waist circumference. Excessive body fat itself will drive down testosterone levels, further accelerating weight gain. Low testosterone can also be caused by sleep apnea, dysfunction of the hypothalamus or pituitary, testicular damage, or surgical removal of the testicles. In addition to weight gain, low testosterone can cause a loss of sexual desire and erectile dysfunction. It can also reduce energy and motivation, make you feel depressed and sad, and cause a loss of self-confidence.

To find out if you have low testosterone, ask your doctor to measure it with a blood test. Be aware, though, that the range for normal levels is so broad that it may not be easy to establish a connection between your symptoms, weight gain, and the low testosterone level. Testosterone replacement therapy will improve your sense of well-being, sleep, mood, erectile function, and libido. It will also help you lose body fat, lower insulin levels, and decrease abnormal levels of triglycerides, cholesterol, and other fats, and thus help prevent cardiovascular disease. However, hormone therapy can worsen sleep apnea. For this reason, before starting treatment you may want to have an overnight sleep study to see if sleep apnea is contributing to your weight issue and low testosterone.

Testosterone treatment is available in different forms: intramuscular injection every one to two weeks, oral, sublingual, pellet under the skin, skin patch, and gel. The best form, in my opinion, is the gel (Testim, Androgel, First Testosterone) applied daily, which provides more steady blood levels. Also, the dose can be adjusted according to blood levels. Just as for women, bioidentical testosterone is available at compounding pharmacies.

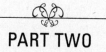

PART TWO

EATING FOR A BRISK METABOLISM

The Fundamentals of the Protein Boost Diet

CHAPTER SEVEN

THE PROTEIN BOOST DIET FOODS THAT RESET YOUR HORMONES AND BOOST METABOLISM

In this chapter I reveal the secret foods that make my diet the best approach to losing weight. Certain foods have the power to help you shed pounds, chief among them my carefully selected array of proteins. The Protein Boost Diet emphasizes specific proteins—not just lots of protein—throughout the day to help you overcome metabolism slowdowns and weight gain and to control low mood, poor energy, and ravenous appetite. The multiple protein sources I've chosen for each of your meals contain precisely the right combination of specific amino acids (the molecular units of protein) to help the master weight-controllers leptin and thyroid hormone work at peak efficiency. These amino acids also promote vigorous production of growth hormone, your fat-burning, muscle-building friend.

Over the past decade, many dieters committed to high-protein diets were eating chicken and egg whites at almost every meal. That's not only tedious; it's not nearly as beneficial as mixing diverse proteins. On my plan, *you'll be enjoying two or three different protein sources at each meal,* which will enhance feelings of fullness, burn energy, reduce hunger, and prompt your metabolism to operate faster. The Protein Boost Diet combines protein mixing with beneficial carbs and fats, in order to help you heal your hormones and supercharge your metabolism. You won't have to remember specifics: my weight-loss diet prescription is clearly presented in Chapter 10, and in the pages that follow you'll find concise reminders of how I developed each component of my meal plan to make choosing the right foods an effortless proposition for you.

With most diets, you lose some weight but preventing regain is tricky. Your body's natural response to calorie restriction is to protect itself from starvation by slowing its calorie burn and making you hungry ("Eat!" your body tells you, a message from hunger hormones). That's why people who try to lose weight by starving themselves drop a few pounds initially but inevitably regain them. You simply cannot lose weight by severely restricting calories.

Statistics show that, after following commercial diets such as Weight Watchers, Jenny Craig, LA Weight Loss, Medifast, or Optifast, you'll probably regain at least half of what you lose within one to two years. Many of my patients tried these plans and did lose weight initially, but eventually regained it. Most of those same patients are now on my diet, feeling energetic and healthier all around, and are happy with their long-term results.

Other popular low-carb diets like South Beach and Atkins tend to focus on a single facet of the food spectrum, wanting you to believe that eliminating a particular food or food group is the golden key to weight loss. As you know from earlier chapters, effective weight loss is possible only if you address every factor contributing to your weight-gain disorder—sleep problems, stress, poor food choices—and the skewed hormone activity at the center of each of these. Ignoring one or more will prevent you from losing weight, and will contribute to regaining the weight after you stop a diet. You need to restore the efficiency of all your hormones and reverse the imbalances that feed into the cycle of continuous weight gain.

Unlike most diets that cause you to plateau after a few weeks or months and then regain, the Protein Boost Diet's eating plan is designed to maximize the efficiency of your metabolism from the inside out. You lose the weight and set yourself up for successful long-term weight-loss maintenance without starving.

HOW I MODIFIED THE TWO BEST DIETS
TO MAKE THEM BETTER

The Protein Boost Diet is adapted from both the Mediterranean diet and the high-protein diet principles for weight loss and optimal health, and it is based on the latest hormone discoveries.

The Mediterranean diet is far closer to the way our ancestors ate than the refined, processed, high-sugar, and high-saturated-fat foods most people eat today. Its menu includes fresh and locally grown whole, unrefined plant foods such as fruits, vegetables, beans, nuts, and seeds; fewer than four eggs a week; very small amounts of red meat; and virtually no processed foods. Sweets in the Mediterranean diet are made from nuts, modest amounts of concentrated sugars (such as honey), dairy products (cheese and yogurt), and olive oil. A moderate amount of wine is enjoyed with meals.

The Mediterranean diet has numerous health benefits. Adopting its general principles can make you lose weight, lower blood pressure and LDL cholesterol, reduce your cardiovascular risk, and reduce symptoms of rheumatoid arthritis and neurodegenerative disorders such as Alzheimer's disease and dementia. The Mediterranean diet is not a low-fat plan, but it helps reverse metabolic syndrome and glucose intolerance by incorporating good fats from nuts and olive oil. It includes high amounts of good monounsaturated fatty acids and low amounts of unhealthful saturated and trans fats. If you have diabetes, the Mediterranean diet will give you the best control of your blood sugar.

Besides incorporating many aspects of the Mediterranean diet into the Protein Boost Diet, I also used the principles of a high-protein diet similar to the principles embraced by the Protein-Rich Oriental Diet (the PRO diet), developed by Korean researchers, with well-documented, lasting effectiveness. On the PRO, you eat low-glycemic, low-saturated-fat, high-protein foods made up of legumes, soybean curd (tofu), soy milk, mushrooms, nuts, seafood, fish, chicken breast, other lean meats, and vegetables. You do not eat any foods that are high in simple sugars, refined grains, or saturated fats. The PRO diet results in twice the weight loss of, and a greater reduction in waist circumference than, calorie-restrictive diets.

Here are a few highlights of the Protein Boost Diet.

IT IS ADAPTED FROM THE MEDITERRANEAN DIET, BUT IS UNIQUE

The Mediterranean diet doesn't offer guidance as clearly as this plan does. The Mediterranean diet gives no produce selections for each meal, no advice on when to eat certain foods throughout the day, and no specific protein mixing recommendations.

On the Protein Boost Diet you'll be eating more proteins than in the Mediterranean diet, with specific protein mixes for each meal, making the diet unique, combining the Mediterranean and PRO diet properties. In addition, it is higher in fiber than the Mediterranean diet. You'll also consistently be eating low-glycemic and high-fiber meals. These properties uniquely beneficial to health and metabolism explain why the Protein Boost Diet will help:

BOOST YOUR METABOLISM

My approach combines low-glycemic, low-saturated-fat foods with beneficial fiber and proteins specifically chosen for their ability to enhance metabolism. Yes, the foods you eat on my plan dramatically affect your hormones and the way your body burns calories. Hundreds of my patients have had what they call "miraculous results." Most recently, one woman lost an astonishing seventeen pounds in a mere five weeks—in a completely healthy way.

MEND YOUR METABOLISM

This diet progressively helps you mend your metabolism, correcting all the hormonal imbalances you've developed as you gained weight, and reverses this trend and brings your weight down. My protein choices for each meal actually reduce hunger and make your fat-burning hormones (leptin, thyroid hormone, and growth hormone) more balanced and efficient. The foods in my diet are also rich in other nutrients that promote thyroid activity and boost metabolism, such as inositol (from kidney, green, and lima beans, brown rice, artichokes, okra, grapefruit, limes, and blackberries). Essential for maintaining healthy cells, inositol is also crucial for peak thyroid function and for the pituitary gland to "talk" to the thyroid so you have the most powerful weight-burning thyroid balance possible. Getting enough choline—another essential nutrient well represented in foods such as salmon, turkey, chicken, soy, beef liver, veal, almonds, kidney beans, eggs, quinoa, spinach, and cauliflower in my eating plan—has also been shown to reduce body fat.

QUICKEN CALORIE BURN RATE

By eating my carefully chosen nutrient-rich foods and eliminating foods that trigger and perpetuate a lethargic burn rate, you'll be moving toward a crucial goal: accelerating your metabolism. At the same time, my foods curb appetite without making you count calories or feel unsatisfied—they reduce the hunger that's been haunting you. The food selections for each meal throughout your day will quickly become routine, and your scale and measuring tape will provide all the proof you need of food's action on the systems that determine how much body fat you carry.

IMPROVE MOOD WITH FOOD

You will (literally) eat up the mood-boosting food selections in my meal plans, which directly affect the hypothalamus by producing the feel-good chemicals GABA, serotonin, and dopamine—all of which enhance fullness. Improving your psychological state is vital to keeping stress from triggering hunger and fat accumulation. I also want you to feel optimistic as your weight starts dropping. It's optimism, after all, that confers the motivation to continue with the diet and your workouts, with stress reduction, and with your sleep schedule.

SUPPORT YOUR IMMUNE SYSTEM

A robust immune system is important for everyone, but people with autoimmune conditions need to be especially conscious of foods that are friendly to their systems. Being overweight, you are likely to have high leptin levels but your body is probably also resistant to leptin, meaning that it can't hear the helpful "I'm full" signal that leptin provides. Remember that too much leptin can trigger your body to attack itself, leading to autoimmune conditions like Hashimoto's thyroiditis (see "Hashimoto's Thyroiditis as a Cause of Low

Thyroid" in Chapter 3). Reversing high leptin levels and leptin inefficiency with the Protein Boost Diet helps prevent future autoimmune disorders.

As you read on, don't be concerned with memorizing which proteins confer what benefits. In Chapter 10, I offer a complete list of favorite foods, with easy charts showing which proteins to eat at breakfast, lunch, and dinner.

PROTEIN VARIETY: THE ULTIMATE METABOLISM ENHANCER

If you've traditionally eaten a lot of refined carbs—the ones in breads, crackers, and sugary baked goods—you know that once you've eaten them, you quickly want more. These foods rapidly turn to glucose in your body, spiking blood sugar, which then crashes and makes you hungry all over again. Here's the part where we're going to change your eating habits, but in a most delicious way. You'll start every meal with proteins from at least two sources, and the protein choices will change from one meal to the next.

You'll eat a mix of proteins, because they contain amino acids—the building blocks of protein—that play many vital roles, including regulating how your genes keep you healthy or change in ways that make you susceptible to illness. But they're also essential for the body to manufacture powerful hormones and chemicals, including the ones that control weight: thyroid hormones, leptin, growth hormone, insulin, adrenaline, adiponectin, histamine, serotonin, and melatonin.

Eating this protein mix is a central pillar of my diet because there's no question that eating balanced amounts of amino acids is essential to your weight-loss effort. All types of protein help you retain nice lean muscle mass as you lower your calorie intake and as you get older, but my plan takes this a step further. Eating more of certain amino acids is key to losing weight when you diet. The *quality* of the protein and its proportion to carbs and fats is central to enhancing your metabolism and curbing appetite.

PROTEIN AND ITS AMINOS HELP YOU FEEL FULL
AND BURN MORE CALORIES

Eating protein makes you feel full in two ways. First, proteins affect appetite by directly influencing GI tract hormones and chemicals. Individual proteins work differently on the GI tract. Rapidly digested proteins such as the dairy protein whey, for instance, quickly cause the release of cholecystokinin, a hormone that makes you feel full. This leads to a delay in the emptying of your stomach and suppresses appetite. A slowly digested dairy protein, casein, clots in the stomach, prompting a cutback in your body's release of the potent hunger hormone ghrelin. Other slowly digested proteins, such as egg whites and soy, have similarly potent effects on ghrelin. With ghrelin lowered, you experience a prolonged feeling of fullness and won't keep eating.

At the same time, protein's amino acids stimulate thyroid hormone's effect on mitochondria—your cellular power plants—to generate more heat, causing you to burn more calories even when sitting. Your hypothalamus senses this heat and sends out the "I'm full" signal. Take a bow, amino acids. This remarkably helpful hormone cascade begins when you simply eat a mix of different proteins with their metabolism-boosting aminos at every meal.

The unique amino acid compositions of different proteins have varying but significant effects on either suppressing appetite or igniting calorie burn. For instance, fish induces more satiety than beef or chicken, and this is why I recommend fish four to five times a week for dinner. You want to feel as full as possible in the evening, when most of us struggle with cravings for sugar and other fattening foods after a stressful workday. Also, you'll achieve better satiety from casein, more calories burned from soy, and improved fat burn from whey, another example of the benefits of mixing proteins and their diverse amino acid structure.

I've selected for my diet the best protein sources with the highest content of the amino acids that are the most effective in activating mitochondria to burn fat, abate hunger, and support your hormone system. Most of these aminos are essential amino acids, meaning our bodies can't manufacture them and we get them only from foods. These are the ones that are crucial for activating mitochondria to burn fat. Here's a quick review of the most powerful aminos.

- *Branched-chain amino acids (BCAAs),* the queens of weight-loss aminos, are leucine, isoleucine, and valine—essential amino acids found in high amounts in a range of foods including beans, meats, fish, grains, and cottage cheese. BCAAs speed up metabolism and help regulate blood sugar. Eating more BCAAs was linked to a lower prevalence of obesity in middle-aged East Asian and Western adults.

- *Lysine* reduces anxiety and calms stress, helping with cravings and stress-related eating. It is found in fish, which I recommend you have for dinner several times a week. Other foods rich in lysine, among my favorite picks, are quinoa, beans, lentils, and egg whites. In a related action, it regulates production of the fat-promoting stress hormone cortisol and reduces overactivity of serotonin receptors, effectively de-stressing your brain. It also helps leptin do a more efficient job of making you burn fat. In your body, lysine is converted to L-carnitine, which promotes fat burning.

- *Methionine* aids in fat breakdown and digestion. From turkey to quinoa, many choices on my Favorite Foods lists contain high amounts of methionine, so you'll be supercharging thyroid hormone activity to achieve a fat-burning metabolism. People who took methionine supplements improved their insulin sensitivity and started to burn fat instead of storing it in the liver. Because methionine boosts the effect of thyroid hormone, which fosters calorie-burning heat production, eating foods rich in this amino acid can heighten metabolism.

- *L-arginine* helps you achieve a leaner body by reducing the amount of stored fat you carry and substantially increasing your metabolism's power source: the mitochondria in cells. It also prevents fat accumulation and prompts your pituitary to release growth hormone, a precious weight-loss supporter. As you age, you produce far less growth hormone and, as a result, lose muscle and tend to gain fat. Arginine-rich proteins found in eggs, fish, turkey, chickpeas, soybeans, beans, and quinoa can slow this process. This amino also helps reduce blood pressure, lowers blood sugar and triglyceride fats, and helps insulin work more efficiently.

- *Taurine* and *tryptophan* define emotional rescue. Taurine is the amino your brain uses to manufacture GABA, the neurotransmitter that naturally eases anxiety, depression, irritability, agitation, and insomnia. Its calming effect helps you cope with stress and eating impulses. Found in seafood and meat, taurine also helps insulin work more efficiently. Your body uses tryptophan to manufacture serotonin, the feel-good neurotransmitter that enhances mood and controls sleep, memory, and appetite. Tryptophan-rich foods help you sleep better, burn more calories, and keep cravings at bay. They include egg whites, cod, soybeans, sesame seeds, pumpkin seeds, pistachios, almonds, Parmesan cheese, turkey, beef, salmon, and cheddar cheese. If you are lactose intolerant, you could be deficient in tryptophan because lactose intolerance impairs its gastrointestinal absorption.

- *Histidine* and *tyrosine* ensure proper function of your endocrine (hormone) system and immune system. Histidine is needed by the body to produce histamine, vital for the immune system to respond competently to foreign agents and protect you against infection. Histamine also helps you release gastrin, a hormone that regulates digestive function. It also helps eliminate heavy metal toxins (see "Detox from Heavy Metal

---

Dr. Arem's Weight-Loss Quick Tip: Protein First, with Fiber

When you start a meal, eat protein first, along with belly-filling fiber. This duo fills you up quickly (much sooner than if you'd eaten carbs). Follow my meal plans and you'll see.

- You'll be well-fed at every meal with two or three specific proteins, chosen because they contain precisely the right amino acid combinations for peak leptin and thyroid hormone efficiency and vigorous production of growth hormone, your fat-burning, muscle-building friend.

- The right protein choices actually rev up metabolism, burn calories, and reduce hunger.

- Dinner has the most protein . . . so you get the aminos that optimize leptin and growth hormone, priming you to burn fat while you sleep.

Exposure" in Chapter 8) such as mercury that may have contributed to your weight gain. Foods with generous histidine levels include game meats, beef, turkey, lamb, chicken, soy foods and tofu, fish, seaweed, pork, and kidney beans. Tyrosine is also hugely important for healthy metabolic function. Your body uses it to manufacture several key neurotransmitters and hormones, among them adrenaline, noradrenaline, dopamine, and all-important weight-controlling thyroid hormones. Foods rich in tyrosine are chicken, turkey, fish, peanuts, almonds, soy, avocados, bananas, milk, cheese, yogurt, cottage cheese, lima beans, pumpkin seeds, and sesame seeds.

Dr. Arem's Weight-Loss Quick Tip: Stress-Calming Menu Rx

The amino acid lysine eases anxiety and stress. Keep levels high all day with this lysine food prescription: Eat three lysine-rich proteins daily to improve mood and anxiety—eggs for breakfast, lima beans for lunch, and fish for dinner. You're already feeling calmer. My meal plans will show you how.

WHERE DO THE DIET'S MIXED PROTEINS COME FROM?

Many people believe protein from meat is the most nutritious, but that's not true. Meat has smaller portions of usable protein than some vegetables and legumes. Whether a protein is easily usable by your body depends on its amino acid composition, the configuration of the protein molecule, the quantity of branched-chain amino acids (BCAAs), how the protein interacts with the other constituents of your meal, and its enzyme content. As you follow my diet, you will:

- *Eat fish, turkey, chicken, and veal more than red meats.* The major benefit of meat proteins is that they're complete, meaning they contain all the amino acids you need to get from food. But because red meats are high in saturated fats, I don't recommend eating them often. When you do eat them, you must pay attention to portion size. Fish, turkey, chicken, and veal—fish especially—contain fewer calories and less saturated fat while delivering top-quality amino acids that make

How My Diet Mixes Proteins and Their Amino Acids

To enable you to get the complete and consistent amino acid profile you need to lose weight, my diet embraces all the main protein sources every day. Just follow my meal plans in Chapter 10; they're a foolproof way to get high amounts of all the aminos you need. Here's an example of a balanced day's mixed protein.

Breakfast

1. Egg whites or lean meat such as turkey or salmon or tuna (canned or cooked fresh)

2. Low-fat cheese, to provide you with satiating casein and whey

Lunch

1. Lean meat or fish

2. Legumes (beans and lentils) with filling fiber and good carbs

3. Alternative proteins such as low-fat cheese or quinoa

Dinner

1. Fish or lean meat

2. Low-fat cheese

3. Protein-rich, low-carb vegetables

---

mitochondria burn more calories. Lean meats and fish are also rich in arginine.

- *Eat eggs and egg whites* for an excellent complete protein rich in all the amino acids you need to optimize weight loss—a good substitute for lean meat at lunchtime.

- *Eat reduced-fat dairy proteins.* Dairy is a valuable source of high-quality proteins with beneficial weight loss properties. As discussed earlier, whey protein and casein, found in milk, cheese, and yogurt, have potent satiating effects. In addition, whey protein is quite rich in BCAAs, which have the powerful effects of rapidly suppressing your appetite, making you feel full, and energizing mitochondria to burn fat. Dairy, however, contains lactose (milk sugar), to which many people are intolerant, and casein can worsen gluten sensitivity. For these reasons I am selective about dairy products. I include reduced-fat cheeses and yogurts in small amounts. Dairy sources I recommend the most, because of their higher whey protein content, are fat-free and low-fat cottage cheese, reduced-fat ricotta or feta, low-fat or fat-free yogurt, and goat cheese.

- *Eat protein-rich vegetables.* Vegetable proteins are as nutritionally good as those in meat, but vegetable proteins should be consumed with meat and fish for the best possible effects on your metabolism. By combining two or three protein-rich vegetables in a meal (which I recommend you do at dinner), you'll get all the essential amino acids and L-arginine in the right amounts for successful weight loss. If you eat chicken and two or three protein-rich vegetables, you'll achieve a better amino acid profile than if you'd eaten a large portion of beef.

- *Eat soy.* The PRO diet's success is probably due to its high levels of soy protein and the very favorable amino acid composition of the soybean and its many derivatives (including tofu and soy milk). Soy is extremely rich in BCAAs as well as in glutamine and arginine, which build muscle. This amino acid profile helps you lose body fat. Soybeans' protein content ranges from 36 to 56 percent, making it one of the highest-protein foods known. Research demonstrates that it's soy's specific amino acid composition that has the most influence on metabolism. Don't eat too much, though, as it contains a lot of fat—healthy fat, but fat nonetheless. Follow my meal plans, which limit soy to three servings weekly, and you'll be fine.

- *Eat lentil and bean protein.* These two have an excellent amino composition that enhances metabolism and curbs appetite. Through my research on legumes, I've identified the ones that deliver the greatest weight-loss benefits. You'll enjoy them mostly at lunch and breakfast (they're a delicious, sustaining addition to your first meal of the day), but not at dinner as they're rich in carbohydrates.

- *Eat quinoa and grain proteins.* Grains often lack lysine, the calm-producing amino you don't want to be short of, but quinoa is a notable exception. It provides excellent-quality protein and may be one of the most wholesome, nutritious foods known. Quinoa is rich in the amino acids conducive to weight loss, including lysine, methionine, and arginine. It also fuels the production of the feel-good neurotransmitter serotonin because it contains nearly six times as much tryptophan as wheat. Quinoa is also gluten free. Brown rice and whole wheat have benefits similar to, but not as great as, quinoa's. They're both high in protein and have a lower sugar content than most other grains. When you reintroduce grains in Phase 2, you'll choose selected whole grains high in protein and fiber.

CARBS AND FATS SHAPE YOUR BODY AND HEALTH

Eating a moderate amount of good carbohydrates and fats is central to my eating plan. Carnivores who eat meat only are rarely fat and, in fact, have very little fat tissue. Animals like the hippopotamus, which eat rice, millet, and sugarcane, on the other hand, have ample fat tissue. A body conforms to its contents: you are what you eat. Carbs are an essential source of energy, but some benefit the body more than others. Your body metabolizes any type of carbohydrate more easily than it does fats and proteins, but because it can't store them in very large quantities in comparison with fats, they're not a reliable long-term energy source for survival. However, completely eliminating carbohydrates is neither realistic nor healthy.

CARBS AND THE GLYCEMIC INDEX

How high your blood sugar spikes and how long it stays elevated after you eat a particular food define where that food falls on the glycemic index (GI). Carbohydrates that are digested quickly have a high GI, and the higher the GI, the more insulin your pancreas releases, triggering a lay-down of fat. High-GI foods are usually refined and processed, such as any bread not made of whole grains (including white and wheat bread), white rice, white pasta, chips, waffles, doughnuts, bagels, pretzels, and french fries. You need to eliminate them from your diet along with extremely high-GI foods such as sugar-laden fruit juices, ice cream, sweetened cereals, and cookies.

Carbs that release glucose at a slower rate have a low GI. These foods, typically high in fiber and protein, include whole oats, chickpeas, kidney beans, artichokes, broccoli, celery, cucumbers, peppers, spinach, tomatoes, many fruits, carrots, yams, peanuts, lentils, rye, and unsweetened yogurt. The GI of what you eat has a tremendous effect on the hormones involved in regulating how much fat you store. Eating high-GI foods leads to weight gain first and then to insulin resistance, metabolic syndrome, obesity, and diabetes. Metabolism-wrecking high-GI foods and the repeated blood sugar spikes they trigger cause inflammation and free radicals to surge in your body. They also damage your cardiovascular system. The inflammation they cause targets all organs, including your hypothalamus, where the signals from the "I'm full" hormone leptin are compromised. You want leptin to be heard loud and clear because it limits food intake and makes your metabolism burn fat faster. Clearly you need to select foods that will give you the least rise in blood sugar and that have the lowest sugar content.

The Protein Boost Diet Embraces Healthy Carbs

I very intentionally shifted your carb intake to meals eaten early in the day so your body can burn them off when you're most active and when your hormones are primed to process them most efficiently. You'll also adjust the order of what you eat, starting first with appetite-suppressing protein and fiber, and continuing with a good selection of superhealthy carb foods that don't load you with sugar.

My Favorite Food lists keep sugars low, with dinnertime foods the very lowest. If you're overweight, you're almost certainly insulin resistant, meaning insulin levels are higher than they should be because your pancreas—producer of insulin—is trying to compensate for the inefficiency of insulin in your liver and muscles. For this reason I recommend low-sugar dinner foods, which push fat-storing insulin down to its lowest levels while you sleep and thus maximize the efficiency of calorie-burning leptin. Even with low-sugar foods at dinner, you'll still enjoy lean meats and fish and generous amounts of vegetables from my low-sugar vegetable list. But at dinner you won't eat legumes or fruits because they are rich in carbs.

ARE YOU A GOOD STARCH OR A BAD STARCH?

Starches are the sugar reserves of plant and grain carbohydrates, and they have vastly different properties. Starches are made up of amylopectin and amylose—both complex carbohydrates—but amylopectin-rich foods are bad starches that are quickly digested and raise your blood sugar dramatically. Foods rich in amylopectin broadly parallel the high-GI list: tortillas, white rice, white and wheat breads, potato chips, potatoes, cornmeal, pretzels, sweet corn, crackers, french fries, and all processed wheat products. On the other hand, amylose does not easily get digested and broken down in the GI tract. Because of this, foods containing amylose don't spike your blood sugar. It's a good starch whose effects on your system are a little like fiber's.

The Protein Boost Diet Is Starch-Selective

The Protein Boost Diet contains no bad starches but draws generously from foods high in beneficial resistant starches, such as beans. You'll enjoy these good starches at breakfast and lunch and avoid most of them at dinnertime, because they're still sugar sources and we don't want your body turning that sugar into fat while you snooze. My meal plans include generous amounts of resistant starches to help you with weight loss and keep your blood sugar levels constant. Foods rich in resistant starch include lentils, adzuki beans, black beans, black-eyed peas, chickpeas, kidney beans, pinto beans, soybeans, quinoa, long-grain brown rice, whole oats, whole-grain wheat, and yams.

FIBER, YOUR PARTNER IN WEIGHT LOSS

Dietary fiber is the indigestible carbohydrate found in plant foods such as vegetables, fruits, legumes, and nuts. Eating high-fiber foods at every meal is an essential component of the plan, because fiber has amazing effects on your body, not the least of which is helping you lose weight and improving your general health. The secret to fiber's central role in weight loss? It contains no calories because your body can't digest it to produce any usable form of energy. However, fiber is absolutely packed with micronutrients. Its antioxidants, including selenium and zinc, help protect against tissue damage. For weight loss, clinical and epidemiological research strongly supports the use of high-fiber diets and fiber supplements, though you shouldn't require a fiber supplement if you're following my meal plans.

Fiber also suppresses appetite. One study showed that people of normal weight ate significantly more fiber than obese people. A high-fiber diet decreases blood sugar in diabetics and helps mend the conditions involved in metabolic syndrome. High-fiber eating also helps prevent cancer, lowers cardiovascular risk, and ameliorates diabetes, high blood pressure, constipation, diverticulitis, and irritable bowel syndrome. There are two types of fiber, each with specific benefits.

- *Soluble fiber readily dissolves in water.* Pectin, mucilage, and gum are all soluble fibers, and they form a viscous gel in your gastrointestinal tract that slows the stomach in emptying its contents. This in turn slows down the absorption of macronutrients and helps you feel fuller longer. Soluble fiber is like a sponge that swells as it passes through your GI tract. Its impact on hormones is just what we like to see. With your stomach full of swollen fiber, you automatically produce less of the metabolism-slowing hunger hormone ghrelin. Fiber slows down the whole process of digestion and also helps you eat less at your next meal.

- *Insoluble fiber, or roughage, passes through your GI tract without disintegrating.* Examples are lignin (found in strawberries and root vegetables), cellulose (cabbage, apples, and legumes), and hemicellulose (whole grains and bran). Insoluble fiber helps food and toxins pass through your GI tract and encourages regular bowel movements.

The Protein Boost Diet Incorporates Fiber

Fiber is so beneficial to weight loss that you'll be eating specific high-fiber foods (both soluble and insoluble) at every meal, a proportionally high amount of fiber relative to total calories. Your daily consumption is roughly 35 to 40 grams, broken down like this:

Breakfast: 5 to 8 grams, from vegetables, beans, whole grains, and fruits

Lunch: 15 to 17 grams, from legumes, whole grains, vegetables, and fruits

Dinner: 15 to 18 grams, from vegetables, salad greens, and occasionally quinoa and brown rice

---

HIGH FRUCTOSE CORN SYRUP (HFCS) AND FRUCTOSE

On my diet you won't be adding any sugar, and yet I want you to understand how the highly potent sugars fructose and high fructose corn syrup (HFCS) act on your system. Fructose is immediately converted into an outrageous amount of glucose after you consume foods containing it. This high sugar load causes inflammation and makes you store more fat.

But fructose's contribution to weight gain doesn't end there. Rats or mice fed a fructose-enriched diet ended up with an enhanced ability to absorb fructose through their intestines. Think about this. Your body falls in love with fructose's ability to provide massive amounts of energy and finds a way to encourage fructose absorption by increasing transporters in your GI tract. It's almost sci-fi spooky. HFCS is added to astonishing array of deli items, including potato salad and baked beans, as well as the obvious sources like candy, baked goods (cookies, pies), and sugared drinks. Avoid it, period.

You also must be careful about high-fructose foods that you might have thought were healthful. To lower fructose intake, avoid canned fruits, canned vegetables, ketchup, and fruit juices. Dried fruits like dates, raisins, figs, and prunes contain such high amounts of fructose they're comparable to consuming high fructose corn syrup.

FRUITS AND VEGETABLES HIGH AND LOW IN FRUCTOSE

Fruits are nature's own source of fructose, even though they contain beneficial fiber to slow sugar absorption. If you want to drop weight and keep it off, you must avoid even fresh fruit that's high in fructose. On the table of My Favorite Fruits in Chapter 10, you'll find a thorough list of fruits that contain less fructose and sugar than others. Eating fruit at the beginning of a meal will make you crave sugar. By enjoying small portions at the end of breakfast or lunch—after you've eaten protein and fiber—you'll be mostly full before you take your first bite of sugar. Think of fruit as dessert for breakfast and lunch. Optimistically, you can enjoy a rainbow of fruits for dessert every day, *twice* a day.

To reap maximum benefits of fiber-rich, vitamin-rich vegetables without contributing to sugar intake, my meal plans include vegetable selections lowest in fructose. In general, fresh vegetables have far less fructose than fruit does, so you can still consume plenty of them without worrying about sugar overload. To lose weight as efficiently as possible on my diet, you'll eat vegetables with a higher fructose content less often. Canned, juiced, and packaged veggies have considerably more fructose than fresh. Please don't overcook vegetables, because cooking converts complex carbs of vegetables into more simple sugars. A light steam is ideal. See the table in Chapter 10 for my favorite vegetables.

ARTIFICIAL SWEETENERS

Because table sugar (saccharose, a simple carb) readily spikes blood sugar and insulin levels and leads to weight gain, artificial sweeteners and sugar substitutes are replacing it in processed foods and beverages more and more these days. But I want you to stay away from artificial sweeteners. There are indications that consuming them in high amounts may lead to bloating and even bladder cancer. Many of my patients who turned to artificial sweeteners to satisfy a sweet tooth developed cravings for sweets, and research backs up this observation. Scientists tracking more than 450 people who drank diet soda for nearly ten years found the diet soda drinkers' waistlines expanded a stunning 70 percent more than those of people who didn't drink diet soda. Artificial sweeteners make your brain experience hunger without delivering any real nutrients to calm appetite.

WHAT ABOUT "NATURAL" SUGAR SUBSTITUTES?

Before you jump onto this bandwagon, check out the fructose content. My patients have been asking me lately about agave nectar, whose fructose content is actually extremely high. Same goes for honey, molasses, and anything else containing fructose. These are "high fructose corn syrup alternatives," and you should avoid them all. If you choose to use an alternative sugar, use stevia in moderation. It's a plant-derived sweetener that has positive effects on blood sugar compared with table sugar, and also has antioxidant properties. A little goes a long way. For fun, grow a stevia plant and use tiny amounts of its intensely sweet leaves.

LACTOSE (MILK SUGAR) IN MILK AND MILK ALTERNATIVES

Instead of cutting out milk entirely, dieters often choose fat-free or reduced-fat milk, but they're missing the fact that the lactose remains. Lactose is milk's naturally occurring sugar and a glass of low-fat milk still contains a lot of it. When you digest milk, large amounts of milk sugars are absorbed quickly into your bloodstream and stored as fat. In my diet, I recommend milk alternatives that contain the same or even higher values of essential nutrients and have low sugar and fat content as well. Soy and almond milks, even with added cane sugar, contain half the sugars of dairy. But please don't drink the sweetened versions. Replace dairy milk with *un*sweetened soy or almond milk. My favorite is unsweetened soy milk at breakfast because of its low sugar and high protein content.

Some studies suggest that the lactose in milk helps with weight loss. Predictably, the National Dairy Council supports this claim, but in my view the studies remain inconclusive and the claim is somewhat misleading. The component of milk that does help you lose weight is the calcium (see "Calcium and Weight" in Chapter 8), which helps limit fat absorption. There's no scientific proof that lactose promotes weight loss. There is, however, plenty of information supporting the fact that lactose, just like other sugars, will increase weight gain if you don't monitor your milk intake carefully.

Coconut milk is not an option because of its high saturated fat and calorie content. Rice milk isn't included in my diet because it is much higher in simple carbohydrates but lower in proteins than other milk options. Whichever milk alternative you choose, make it unsweetened and be mindful of serving size recommendations.

FATS

There's a common misconception that all fats are bad for you and will make you fat. The reality is that some types of fat are important for your health. Fats in general are crucial for the growth and development of healthy cells and nerves and for manufacturing hormones. It's important to monitor the specific types of fat you eat daily, though I manage this for you in my meal plans, which include oily fish (sardine, herring, anchovy, salmon, trout, and mackerel), nuts (walnuts and almonds), and plant-derived oils (olive oil and grapeseed oil) in proper balance. I also recommend you use organic oils, so you're not getting a side order of pesticides with your fats.

The American Heart Association recommends that a 25 to 35 percent total fat intake is appropriate for a healthy diet. However, the American Association of Clinical Endocrinologists (AACE) advises as low as 15 percent total fat intake for overweight people. I recommend your diet include 15 to 25 percent of the good fats that will help energize your metabolism and give you the best cardiovascular and other health benefits. Cutting out simple sugars and bad carbs will help drive down your insulin levels, to enhance fat breakdown and elimination. But if you reduce your bad carb intake and then eat too much fat to compensate, you'll still gain weight. That's because fats get stored as fat—they're not converted into a readily usable form of energy. High-fat diets have been shown to enhance fat accumulation. Too much animal fat in your diet is also likely to cause insulin resistance and leptin resistance in your brain and muscles, slowing metabolism and increasing appetite. Too much fat also causes inflammation in your body and brain, as well as heart disease and negative immune system responses. The brain inflammation can compromise your cognitive capacity and reduce brain cell longevity, effects similar to those seen in the brains of depressed people.

Fats are made up of fatty acids, either saturated or unsaturated, and each type of fat contains a different fatty acid composition. Saturated and trans fatty acids are unhealthy fats that raise total cholesterol and low-density lipoprotein (LDL) levels. Unsaturated fatty acids have been shown to lower total and LDL cholesterol, raise high-density lipoprotein (HDL, the helpful kind) cholesterol, and decrease cardiovascular risk. Limiting saturated fat and cholesterol while eating unsaturated fats is an important component of my weight-loss diet.

Saturated fats encourage appetite. Eating too much saturated fat leads to a chemical effect on your brain that will make you want to eat more of it. Fats can damage and inflame areas of the hypothalamus that respond to the weight-loss helper leptin, precisely what we want to avoid to reset metabolism and lose weight.

Red meats, full-fat milk, and whole dairy products are loaded with saturated fat. Lauric acid, myristic acid, and palmitic acid (found in cow's milk, meat, and palm oil) are three types of saturated fats that raise cholesterol levels. Stearic acid (found in cocoa butter and red meats) doesn't have this effect. A beefsteak contains both palmitic and stearic acid, and some diet plans believe that the benefits of stearic acid "cancel out" the disadvantage of palmitic acid. Although this may be true for stearic acid's effects on cholesterol levels, it's not clear that the weight-promoting effects of these saturated fats are actually canceled out. This is why I don't recommend eating much red meat. There are so many healthful sources of proteins that are more helpful to weight loss.

Because cheese is also high in saturated fat, I recommend that you eat only cheeses that deliver the least amount of saturated fat and calories: low-fat and fat-free cottage cheese, low-fat and fat-free cream cheese, and fat-free string cheese. You can also eat fat-free mozzarella, low-fat ricotta, reduced-fat feta, and goat cheese, but in small amounts. Yogurt should be a low-fat or fat-free dairy or soy version with no added sugar.

Trans fatty acids (trans fats) promote weight gain in addition to increasing the risk of coronary heart disease in the same way as saturated fats. Pastries, chips, pizza, fried foods, and fast foods are quite rich in trans fats. You won't find them on my diet.

Monounsaturated fats lower your total cholesterol and LDL cholesterol levels and raise your HDL cholesterol. On my diet you'll be eating a nice percentage of monounsaturated fats, such as those found in olive oil.

Polyunsaturated fats also offer tremendous health benefits. They lower LDL cholesterol and triglycerides and reduce cardiovascular disease and inflammation. Foods rich in polyunsaturated fats include olive oil, salmon, almonds, natural peanut butter, and avocado. In high amounts they cause your body to produce toxic fats that can slow metabolism and induce inflammation. On my food plan you'll enjoy a well-balanced amount of polyunsaturated fat that won't harm you in any way.

The Protein Boost Diet Balances Fats

In my daily meal plans, a perfectly balanced mix of healthful, weight-loss-promoting fats replaces those that lead to weight gain, such as saturated and trans fats. Following the Protein Boost Diet makes it easy to track your daily fat intake, since I've done the calculating for you. You'll be eating foods with good fats at every meal—an average of 15 to 20 percent of your calorie intake, including plenty of omega-3s in the fish you'll enjoy four or five times weekly. Here are some examples.

Breakfast: avocado, olive or other vegetable oil, olives, ground flaxseed, nuts, nut butter

Lunch: tofu, avocado, olives, olive or vegetable oil

Dinner: tofu, avocado, olives, fish, olive or vegetable oil

Omega-3 fatty acids, found in oily fish and some plants, encourage calorie burn and feelings of fullness. Omega-3s also unequivocally lower blood pressure, reduce triglyceride fat levels, prevent abnormal heartbeats, and lower the overall risk of cardiovascular disease. Getting enough omega-3s is essential for stable mood because your brain cells require these fats for peak function of serotonin, the neurotransmitter that protects against stress and depression, bolstering your weight-loss effort. Omega-3s also help keep dopamine levels in a healthy range, support your immune system, and provide potential anticancer benefits.

Many foods in my meal plans also contain the omega-3s called eicosapentaenoic acid (EPA) and docosahexaenoic acid (DHA), which support weight loss. Omega-3s reduce appetite and make you burn fat more efficiently. They also increase a chemical in the brain that makes you feel full and stop wanting to eat more. Omega-3s enhance the function of mitochondria by burning calories and raising body temperature. If you're overweight and have insulin resistance, you're likely to have a fatty liver and an accumulation of fats in your system. Omega-3s make thyroid hormone work more efficiently at clearing fat from your liver. Consuming omega-3s will help speed your recovery from insulin resistance, leptin resistance, and metabolic syndrome. Omega-3s lower triglyceride levels and fat stores while increasing oxygen consumption, all indications of heightened metabolic activity.

Because diet alone might not provide enough precious omega-3s, my program also adds a daily supplement (see the chart in "My Favorite Vitamin-Antioxidant-Micronutrient Regimen" in Chapter 8 for details).

Omega-6s: Flaxseed oil, hemp oil, and grapeseed oil all contain either omega-3s or omega-6 fatty acids, but none of them contains EPA/DHA. They contain mostly omega-6s, which are helpful in lowering glucose levels. Some researchers proclaim astonishing benefits from gamma linoleic acid, an omega-6, for cancer and other health issues. However, omega-6s promote inflammation, counteracting the benefits of omega-3s. The optimal ratio of omega-3s to omega-6s is 2 to 1. You probably get more than enough omega-6s from meats, eggs, and oils used for cooking. In fact, the average American diet provides fifteen to thirty times more omega-6 than omega-3. When your ratios are out of order from eating too many omega-6s, your immune system goes into defense mode, making you more likely to have inflammation, blood clots, and autoimmune disorders.

Coconut oil is a healthy fat that helps stimulate metabolism and aids weight loss. It's been used for thousands of years in tropical coastal areas and is also a popular traditional remedy among Asian and Pacific populations. People in the tropics who use coconut oil (primarily for cooking) are generally less afflicted with heart disease and cancer. Coconut oil is rich in medium-chain fatty acids (MCFAs), which are quickly burned in the body for energy rather than stored as fat, enhancing metabolism and making you burn more fat. If you consumed the same number of calories from MCFAs as another dieter consumed of saturated fat, you'd gain much less weight. One study even showed that taking coconut oil as a supplement decreases waist size. After losing your unwanted weight, you'll regain far less if you get some of your daily fats from coconut oil. Coconut oil also strengthens the immune system, improves digestion, helps you absorb essential nutrients, and improves feelings of fullness.

Coconut oil also contains conjugated linoleic acid (CLA), a fatty acid that can reduce body fat and enhance metabolism, increase lean muscle mass, and reduce abdominal fat. CLA is more effective when you exercise regularly. However, like all oils, coconut oil is rich in calories—one tablespoon contains 120 calories. Thus I can only recommend you take one teaspoon of coconut oil in the morning before breakfast every day to enhance weight loss . . . but only if and when you're faithfully following my 20/10 exercise program.

CHAPTER EIGHT

DETOX YOUR METABOLISM

Food and Supplements as Medicine

You can't lose weight and keep it off successfully unless you get rid of toxins. For this reason, I encourage regular detoxification using food, drink, and supplements (and a few spices and herbs, too). Toxins alter levels and/or efficiency of weight-controlling hormones, such as thyroid hormones, estrogens, testosterone, cortisol, insulin, growth hormone, and leptin. Toxins also alter the function of neurotransmitters like dopamine, noradrenaline, and serotonin, all of which play key roles in regulating metabolism. In short, toxins affect how your body controls weight, altering fat levels and making your body store more fat. They compromise suppression of fat cravings, ability to burn fat stores, and physical activity levels.

DETOX, DEFINED

A food detox eliminates harmful chemicals from your body and helps you learn how to gain control of your nutritional choices to improve health, diet, stress, and weight. Calorie-restrictive detox diets are popular among Hollywood celebrities who want to shed pounds fast before filming. But because the body responds to calorie restriction by holding on to fat, using any detox method as your sole approach to weight loss will eventually crash your metabolic machinery, extending the time it takes to reset your metabolism to normal afterward. By using my Sensational Detox Smoothie and raw fennel as part of your program from Day 1, you'll naturally cleanse your body of the harmful toxins that can contribute to setbacks in metabolism and restrict your weight loss efforts. To effectively detox, you also need to address any food allergies and sensitivities, *Candida* yeast, and bacterial imbalance in your GI tract.

SENSATIONAL DETOX SMOOTHIE + RAW FENNEL

To detoxify your body, you need an abundance of antioxidants and plenty of water to flush out toxins and free radicals (see "Antioxidants Protect Your Body from Oxidative Stress" later in this chapter). My smoothie combines the most effective detoxifying ingredients to draw toxins out of your body and keep you fighting free radicals all day. I've chosen ingredients that have substantial health benefits, so you're also preparing your body for good health and weight loss. To keep your detox flush on full blast, drink this blend twice daily for the first seven days of the diet (during Phase 1; see Chapter 10).

Let's look at the smoothie ingredient list.

Citrus juices contain an abundance of antioxidants; special phytonutrients found in them called "limonoids" can clear your liver and slowly break down carcinogens. On top of its reputation as a well-known source of antioxidant vitamins, grapefruit contains lycopene, the antioxidant found in tomatoes. Together grapefruit and lime can improve insulin and cholesterol levels. If you can't eat grapefruit, the lime will suffice.

Strawberries have anticarcinogenic flavonoids, reduce LDL cholesterol, and help lower your risk of cardiovascular disease, stroke, and diabetes. They're also an excellent source of vitamin C, B vitamins, potassium, and phosphorus, and their ability to scavenge free radicals prevents damage to the cell. Use organic strawberries, as the conventionally grown berries are more likely to have a high pesticide load.

Celery protects you from oxidative stress with its rich source of vitamins. Celery's two best aspects: it's an organic source of sodium to hydrate you and its alkalizing properties help antioxidants work more efficiently in your body.

Spinach helps blood pressure and blood flow with its ability to decrease cell damage and to increase oxygen delivery to your cells.

Garlic and *parsley* are powerful detoxifiers. The antibiotic properties of garlic boost the immune system and benefit cardiovascular health. It's a super spice that can ameliorate oxidative stress. I've offset the bad-breath possibility with parsley, which freshens breath and aids digestion. Parsley's chief role, though, is to protect your mitochondria from oxidative damage. Parsley also contains vitamins C and A, calcium, magnesium, iron, and organic sodium.

Detox begins when you wake up. Sip the smoothie before you eat breakfast and again before dinner to jump-start your detox system. Consider drinking the smoothie even after you've achieved your weight goal, as some of my patients do because it helps them maintain their weight. If you choose to start drinking the detox smoothie before you begin the diet or drink it for more than seven days, no worries—it is safe and beneficial. To make it, blend these seven beneficial ingredients together.

Strawberries: 4 small
Celery: 2 stalks, with leaves, coarsely chopped
Spinach: 1 cup fresh
Grapefruit: ½ small
Lime: ½
Garlic: 1 clove, crushed
Parsley: 1 cup, chopped

Then eat raw fennel. My patients always ask me why. Fennel boosts your immune system, and its weight-loss capabilities date as far back as ancient Greek times. Fennel has strong antioxidant benefits and also aids digestion. Its appetite-suppressing potential will help you lose weight. Originally used to treat ailments including cough, asthma, uterine cramps, and gout, fennel reduces inflammation and purifies your blood, bladder, and liver.

In the morning, follow your smoothie with a chopped raw fennel bulb (half a bulb if it's large) to set you up for a day of good digestion and disease defense. Do not try to blend the fennel with your smoothie because it will not cooperate with your blender. If you wake up with headaches or migraines, fennel in the morning is especially advantageous because it can relieve them. It's also helpful for menstrual cramps. The flavor of fennel is probably quite different from what you'd normally eat for breakfast—a bit like licorice—but many of my patients love it. If you live in an area where fennel isn't available year-round, buy fennel bulbs in bulk, chop them, and freeze in portions for later use. But because fennel is not always available, do not stress about its absence. The smoothie alone will adequately flush out free radicals.

HONOR YOUR BODY'S OWN DETOX DEFENSES

Your body has its own natural defense system to expel harmful toxins. First, the vast organ we know as skin acts as a direct barrier that prevents harmful substances from gaining entry to your body. Your liver is another frontline detox player, processing toxic chemicals including those in food (pesticides) and drinks (alcohol, sugar). It's also one of your body's major fat burners. Your liver starts by neutralizing or altering the composition of toxins, fats, and sugars and then transforms them into water-soluble substances so they can be eliminated from the body. If your liver is impaired, overworked, or congested with toxins, it can't break down fats efficiently, and you'll end up storing more fat. The smoothie and fennel help protect the liver and help it detox your body.

Your body itself produces toxins from cellular processes needed to sustain life, but, if you're healthy, your elimination system efficiently clears these chemicals from your body, with a little help from antioxidants (see "Antioxidants Protect Your Body from Oxidative Stress" in this chapter).

FOOD SENSITIVITIES

A food sensitivity is best thought of as a subtle form of food allergy. Full-blown food allergies are most often related to shellfish, fish, tree nuts (cashews, walnuts, almonds, and pecans, among others), and peanuts (which are legumes). Bona fide food allergies cause dramatic symptoms (such as mouth and throat itching, hives and itchy skin, or even a life-threatening closing of the airway), whereas food sensitivities usually don't bring on such noticeable symptoms. Allergic reactions to food affect 3 to 4 percent of adults, but food sensitivities are far more common, affecting about half the population. When you're sensitive to a specific food, your immune system produces antibodies against components of that food, and the interaction in your system generates inflammation that can slow your metabolism and increase hunger. One study found levels of antibodies to food components (indicating inflammation) to be much higher in obese children than normal-weight children; this suggests that food sensitivities, by generating inflammation, can contribute to weight gain.

The foods most often causing sensitivities are dairy products and eggs, though egg whites provoke less sensitivity than yolks (my diet includes limited dairy products because they contain a lot of saturated fats and milk sugar). If you know you have a sensitivity to certain foods, remove them from your diet to help you lose pounds and enhance your overall energy and mood—even cravings for fattening foods will diminish. Food sensitivities can cause bloating, impair gastrointestinal (GI) function, and contribute to damaging inflammation in your GI tract. Your doctor can test you for food sensitivities using several methods, but there's an easier way. To understand how following my program can help you uncover any food sensitivities see "The Protein Boost Diet Food Sensitivity Program."

SENSITIVITY TO GLUTEN

Gluten is a protein in wheat, rye, and barley to which many people are sensitive. Severe sensitivity to gluten is called "celiac disease," an autoimmune disorder that causes flattening of the tissues lining your digestive tract, inhibiting your ability to absorb nutrients. Celiac disease affects just 1 percent of the population, primarily women of European ancestry. While some people with celiac disease don't have symptoms, the most common are abdominal pain, bloating, gas, fatigue, headaches, joint pain, and decreased appetite. Your doctor can perform blood tests to make a proper diagnosis. While there's currently no cure, you can manage celiac disease by following a strict gluten-free diet.

With gluten sensitivity, there's no test to say for certain that you have it. Unlike the impaired nutrient absorption of celiac disease, sensitivity to gluten generates inflammation that promotes weight gain similar to that caused by sensitivities to other foods. The fix is easy: avoid obvious gluten in your diet and don't eat processed foods, gluten-free or not. Phase 1 of my eating plan is a naturally gluten-free diet (check the footnotes in the food charts in Chapter 10 if you have celiac disease) that you can use for life if you're gluten sensitive or suspect you might be.

CANDIDA YEAST OVERGROWTH

Your weight problem may have been aggravated by an overgrowth of *Candida*, a yeast that can easily survive and grow on skin and in your mucous membranes, respiratory tract, and vagina. While a moderate amount of yeast can live in happy balance with normal body bacteria and not affect health, too much yeast in any part of your body causes symptoms such as a white-coated tongue, abdominal discomfort, unexplained persistent coughing or sore throat, recurring urinary tract infections, irritability, mood swings, and sensitivity to odors. When you harbor too much yeast, its sheer strength in numbers can tempt your body into eating more and you'll have cravings for alcohol, sweets, and other simple carbohydrates. Yeast thrives on sugar and produces a chemical that makes the body crave anything sweet. The more yeast overgrowth, the more intense your cravings will be. Amazing, isn't it?

Yeast overgrowth can result from overwhelming your body with antibiotics. It often occurs in people who have chronic sinusitis or bladder infections for which they've taken repeated antibiotics. However, antibiotics enter your system not only via prescriptions, but also in the foods you eat, including factory-raised meats and vegetables that are treated with large amounts of antibiotics to promote growth of the animal or plant. Too many antibiotics also cause your body to lose the helpful bacteria that fight off yeast. Women who take oral contraceptives for extended periods are also at risk for yeast overgrowth. The best way to fight overgrowth is to avoid antibiotics and oral contraceptives and cut sugar from your diet. Probiotics are extremely helpful in fighting any yeast currently in your system as they restore your body's helpful bacteria to normal levels.

THE PROTEIN BOOST DIET FOOD SENSITIVITY PROGRAM

Given that half of the population may have some type of food sensitivity leading to inflammation and weight-loss resistance, you need to address this possibility in a practical way. The foods that most irritate and inflame our bodies are grains and processed foods. For this reason, you'll eliminate them for the six weeks of Phase 1 (see the Meal Plans in Chapter 10) and periodically thereafter (though I don't encourage eating processed foods again once you start the diet).

Phase 1 is intended to annihilate inflammation in your system while treating the sugar addiction that almost surely underlies your weight gain. During these six grain-free weeks, you're permitted to eat quinoa, which is gluten-free and nutritionally behaves as a legume rather than a grain. After Phase 1, you can gradually reintroduce certain whole grains, but always in moderation. On my plan, every three months you'll go grain-free for two weeks. If you're like many of my patients, you might find that after eliminating grains for six weeks, you feel so good you want to maintain a diet without them. This is fine. Either way, my food sensitivity detox will drive down inflammation and make your long-term weight management successful and permanent.

PROBIOTICS FOR DETOX AND WEIGHT LOSS

Healthy GI bacteria are part of your circle of friends for healthy weight loss. Recent studies show that bacterial imbalance in the gut can cause a number of symptoms, including constipation, gas, and bloating. Eating a poor diet influences gut bacteria and can also make you gain weight—some types of bacteria break down unusable nutrients (polysaccharides) into digestible sugars, so the presence of these bacteria can actually cause you to absorb more calories. Growth of bad bacteria and depletion of the good in your gut also affect metabolism, causing weight gain by promoting inflammation in your GI tract and body.

Good bacteria or probiotics proliferate and remain healthy when you consume a lot of fiber and foods rich in oligofructose, found in asparagus, chicory root, garlic, onion, wheat, and barley. By eating low-fat or fat-free plain yogurt, you'll also be taking in friendly bacteria.

Antibiotics are a principal cause of bacterial imbalance. When you take them, they eradicate bacteria, including the helpful ones. Use them only when absolutely necessary. To restore bacterial balance, take a probiotic supplement and you'll have a support team helping you control hunger and reduce fat storage. Choose a probiotic that includes several helpful bacteria. For more on probiotics and their ability to thwart stress, see Chapter 4.

DETOX FROM HEAVY METAL EXPOSURE

About eighty years ago, physicians began noticing heavy metals in their patients' bodies. These highly toxic metals damage cell membranes. Some alter and destroy mitochondria and damage the lining of blood vessels. Heavy metals even at low levels are unsafe. Hair strand testing can be the most accurate method for detecting heavy metals because it reflects accumulation over time, but consult with your doctor about how to get a reliable test and before you use any over-the-counter detoxing products.

EAT LOW-MERCURY FISH

Mercury can trigger autoimmune thyroiditis, which can initiate other complications, including a slowing of metabolism and weight gain. Mercury can also cause fatigue and headaches that can affect your ability to stay on track with my diet program. Pregnant women especially should avoid eating high-mercury fish. Fish is a major component of my diet because of its healthful omega-3 fats and because its potent amino acid profile boosts metabolism. Because of the preservatives and high salt content in most canned fish, I recommend that you eat fresh, wild-caught fish that are low in mercury.

Fish with low mercury: Wild-caught salmon, scallop, cod, tilapia, sardine, haddock, anchovy, herring, Atlantic or Pacific mackerel, whitefish, trout
Fish with medium mercury: Spanish mackerel, snapper, halibut, fresh tuna
Fish with high mercury: Grouper, orange roughy, king mackerel, swordfish, shark, tilefish

One of my favorite foods, salmon, is sold both as wild-caught and as farm-raised. Wild-caught is a far better option. Farm-raised salmon contains a lot of obesogens (see "Our Hidden Toxic Environment" in Chapter 2) and is lower in omega-3 fatty acids. It also has added toxins like pesticides and antibiotics and artificial color. Wild salmon is healthier because the fish eat omega-3-rich ocean creatures while farm-raised salmon is fed grains.

DETOX WITH FOOD AND DRINK

One of the best and safest ways to detox regularly is by eating and drinking well. My diet program is an effortless way to begin. Junk foods, soft drinks, fruit juices, refined carbohydrates, and alcohol all place a heavy toxic load on your digestive system and metabolism. Alcohol, with its high sugar content, for example, breaks down into toxins and free radicals in your blood while decreasing nutrient absorption. Wean yourself off alcohol and ideally stop altogether if you're serious about losing weight. Reduce caffeine to one cup of coffee during the first half of your day. Decaffeinated green tea is widely available and makes an ideal substitute. You can maintain a lifelong detox by eating the food selections in my diet, which are high in cleansing antioxidants and fiber. Here are some more detox recommendations.

STAY HYDRATED

Drink more than the minimum eight glasses of water daily if you're exercising (and I know you are). Water flushes toxins and curbs appetite. Begin your day with a cup of warm water and a squeeze of fresh lemon juice or capful of cider vinegar. You'll be cleansing your liver and encouraging fat metabolism.

AVOID PROCESSED FOODS

Processed foods are loaded with harmful additives, dyes, preservatives, and artificial sweeteners, which can disrupt your body's weight-regulating pathways.

SELECT ORGANIC PRODUCE WHEN POSSIBLE

The reason for choosing organic is not simply that it contains better nutrients. Commercially grown produce has pesticides and hormone-disrupting chemicals, which over time can negatively affect your health even in small traces. Even though research might suggest that the effects of organic foods and nonorganic foods are not clinically significant, the added chemicals can affect the activity of hormones, and the effects creep up on you. You cannot control the amount of toxicants you inhale through air pollution or by other unnoticeable means, but you can minimize your toxic chemical intake by eating organic.

SELECT MEAT AND MILK CAREFULLY

Meat from factory-raised animals can be extremely harmful to your weight-loss efforts because these animals are given antibiotics and synthetic hormones to increase their growth. Just as you can build up resistance to antibiotic drugs from prolonged use, you also build up weight-loss resistance by eating antibiotic-laced meat. The only way to ensure your meat isn't contaminated by antibiotics is to eat organic meat or meat from a farm that raises animals responsibly and cleanly.

Since conventional milk comes from genetically modified, hormone-infused cows, choose organic reduced-fat milk that comes from cows that aren't treated with hormones that induce obesity. Better yet, look for milk from cows raised on grass instead of proinflammatory grains. Dairy milk is not included in my favorite foods list, but you'll want to choose organic versions of the low-fat and nonfat cheeses and yogurt I do include. While they can cost more, the health impact is far too beneficial to ignore.

GENETICALLY MODIFIED FOODS

Some meat, milk, fruits, and vegetables are genetically modified to increase growth and production. In most states, there's no way to tell if you're eating food containing genetically modified organisms (GMOs), but the vast majority of organics are not genetically modified. While the effects of GMOs aren't entirely understood, we do know that they promote super germs to which our bodies have no resistance. Growing genetically modified produce also requires more pesticides, adding to the toxic load that's so harmful to health. Eating organic foods or foods from a trusted local farmer is the only way to ensure that your food is in its purest state possible.

PRO-DETOX CHOICES

Many fruits and vegetables help you with detoxification because of their action as a diuretic, antioxidant, or antibacterial, or because the food has unique qualities that aid the detox process, such as fiber that helps clean your digestive tract. These foods are an integral part of my diet, making it easy to know which foods will keep you free of inflammation and help you feel rejuvenated.

ANTIOXIDANT/MICRONUTRIENT SUPPLEMENTS, SPICES, AND HERBS

Antioxidants and micronutrient supplements are essential additions to your healthy diet. Based on my extensive research on the dozens of supplements available, this section will tell you which ones will work and why you need to take them to support your body during weight loss and beyond. As your body reshapes itself and you reset your metabolism, you're undergoing thousands of changes at the molecular level. You need extra antioxidants to clear the by-products of these chemical reactions. Many of the micronutrients discussed in this chapter you'll also be getting in the foods that make up my diet. But you need more nutrients than even the most nutritious food supply can provide to support the amazing changes happening inside your body. Supplements will decrease your insulin and leptin resistance, pushing your metabolism up to optimal speed.

For best results, be diligent about taking a well-balanced antioxidant mix to reduce inflammation and fully energize your metabolism. Along with the specific micronutrients and my favorite weight-loss herbal supplement discussed below, antioxidants form an arsenal powerful enough to put aging—and fattening—free radicals in check.

Plus, liberally using fresh spices in your meals will rev up your energy levels and mood. Doesn't that sound like a delicious prescription?

Ask Dr. Arem: What About Diet Pills?

Q. Is there any safe and effective diet pill?

A. I'm doubtful an easy weight-loss solution will ever come in pill form. The majority of diet pills have no scientific research to support their claims and any brief benefit you get is outweighed by the downright harmful effects they have on your long-term weight and overall health. Phentermine, for example, can be highly habit-forming and drives down levels of the weight-loss helper serotonin, a neurotransmitter that keeps mood strong and positive so you can more easily withstand cravings (you don't want less serotonin—you want more). The drug orlistat, which promotes weight loss by inhibiting fat absorption, has horrible gastrointestinal side effects. My advice is to stay away from them all. Instead, choose safe, effective supplements that balance your hormones to help you lose weight. You'll find them listed later in this chapter, in "My Favorite Vitamin-Antioxidant Micronutrient Regimen." For maximum benefit, combine them with the eating and exercise plans in this book.

ANTIOXIDANTS PROTECT YOUR BODY FROM OXIDATIVE STRESS

Oxidative stress is the sum of all the free radicals you produce as a result of just living and breathing . . . and also the ones brought on by exhausting exercise, stress, sleep deprivation, depression, and excessive consumption of fats and carbohydrates. As the trillions of cells in your body perform their many functions, by-products of chemical reactions leave behind highly oxygenated compounds called "free radicals," potentially toxic if they accumulate in cells. When the balance of free radicals and your natural antioxidant system (which clears free radicals) is out of sync, you get oxidative stress and cell damage. Poor nutritional choices burden your body even further. Alcohol, medications, too much radiation from the sun, inflammation caused by infection or allergies, and iron overload all gear your body toward oxidative stress. Smog, cigarette smoke, and industrial chemicals increase your body's volume of free radicals and oxidative stress.

Oxidative stress from normal, day-to-day body metabolism and outside sources harms the genes that tell your cells what to do, damages organs (including your cardiovascular system and brain), and leads to accelerated aging, cancer, heart disease, infertility, Alzheimer's, Parkinson's, kidney disease, nerve damage, and cataracts. It also weakens the immune system and can damage your thyroid. So how do you thwart ever-present oxidative stress? You need antioxidants—vitamins C, D, and E, carotenoids (vitamin A), polyphenols, and trace elements such as selenium, zinc, and others. Taking the right amounts of vitamins, minerals, and other antioxidants minimizes free radical buildup and oxidative stress, improving overall cellular health because cells live longer and are healthier. As a result, antioxidants slow premature aging.

HOW EXACTLY DO ANTIOXIDANTS HELP WITH WEIGHT LOSS?

If you're overweight or obese, it's a virtual certainty you have high levels of oxidative stress in your body and a great deal of inflammation in your fat tissue. Oxidative stress can cause the weight-controlling hormones leptin and insulin to work inefficiently. Taking antioxidants helps clear a path toward successful weight loss by improving metabolic efficiency. Antioxidants such as glutathione, vitamins C and E, and coenzyme Q-10 relieve and prevent high levels of oxidative stress in mitochondria. Keeping your mitochondrial oxidative stress/antioxidant system shipshape with a complete antioxidant regimen allows mitochondria to continuously burn energy and boost metabolism.

Some antioxidants are vitamins, but not all. *Trace minerals* like vanadium, copper, manganese, and molybdenum work like antioxidants to protect you from free radicals. *Polyphenols* and *flavonoids* are other types of antioxidants you get from tea and coffee and from eating the fruit and vegetable selections in my diet. The effects of polyphenols and flavonoids are similar to those of vitamins in that they transport free radicals out of your body.

ESSENTIAL ANTIOXIDANTS AND MICRONUTRIENTS
TO RESHAPE HORMONES FOR WEIGHT LOSS

When your body is inflamed from metabolic dysfunction—as it is when you're overweight—you're even more in need of a diverse antioxidant-micronutrient mix to protect you from further oxidative stress and other weight-promoting factors. Damaged proteins, as a result of too much oxidative stress, cause cells to become dysfunctional and die. This accelerates aging and can lead to inefficient thyroid hormone, leptin, and insulin. Antioxidants and micronutrients can also indirectly boost your metabolism by elevating emotions. Jump to the charts "My Favorite Vitamin-Antioxidant-Micronutrient Regimen" and "Other Supplements" to check the specific recommended doses for each of the following.

Alpha lipoic acid (ALA) enhances L-glutathione's ability to clear toxins from your liver. ALA works like opening a high-speed lane in congested traffic: it clears several unique free radicals from your body while protecting cells' mitochondria and raising the activity of glutathione. ALA's powerful antioxidant activity can reduce diabetic nerve damage and insulin resistance. When you take ALA, you should see improvements in insulin sensitivity in as little as eight weeks.

Chromium helps weight loss by enhancing insulin efficiency. Chromium supplements in the form of chromium picolinate decrease insulin resistance and improve blood sugar control, triglyceride levels, and HDL. In a ten-year study, obese men taking chromium lost nearly twice as much weight as obese men who didn't take it. Niacin-bound chromium reduces fat by activating genes that promote lean muscle development and the breakdown of sugars. However, stick to the recommended dosage in the chart at the end of this chapter. Don't take more than that, because too much chromium can up your risk of muscle breakdown and kidney failure.

Coenzyme Q-10 (CoQ-10 or ubiquinone) works like an antioxidant and is needed by cells to generate energy and keep metabolism humming. Your body naturally produces CoQ-10 but begins to lose the ability to produce it from food by age 35 or 40. The resulting low levels decrease the metabolic function of your cells' mitochondria and deficiency can contribute to thyroid imbalance, thyroid hormone inefficiency, and thyroid cancer. Beware of stress, infection, and poor eating habits, for they lower CoQ-10.

Vitamin A is used to convert the thyroid hormone T4 to T3. Deficiency is linked to lower production of thyroid hormone, decreased uptake of vital iodine by the thyroid gland, underactive thyroid, and thyroid enlargement (goiter). You also need vitamin A for memory and good cognitive (thinking) function under stress. Different forms of vitamin A include alpha-carotene, beta-carotene, lutein, beta-cryptoxanthin, and lycopene. In vegetables and fruits, you can spot vitamin A by color—the orange of carrots comes from beta-carotene, and lycopene infuses grapefruit and tomatoes with pink and red coloring. Beta-carotene is nontoxic and one of the most potent antioxidants in food. Avoid animal-derived vitamin A (C20 apocarotenoid, but labeled as vitamin A) because it has six times the amount of vitamin A in plant-based beta-carotene and other carotenoids, and high amounts can be toxic to the liver.

B vitamins are essential to health and their effect on brain and mood helps with weight loss, as positive mood helps control cravings.

> *Vitamin B_1 (thiamine)* facilitates the brain's use of glucose and is necessary to metabolize sugar. Deficiency for just six days can bring on impaired cognitive function and depression, and even slight deficiencies can cause mood swings in women.
>
> *Vitamin B_2 (riboflavin)* balances the powerful effects of B_1 and B_3.
>
> *Vitamin B_3 (niacin* and *niacinamide)* helps calm the brain and reduce anxiety. Niacin can reduce cholesterol, but taking more than 1,000 mg daily can cause tingling and flushing.
>
> *Vitamin B_6 (pyroxidine)* regulates blood glucose levels and helps you lose weight. You must restore B_6 levels daily through supplements because your body flushes it out in urine rather than storing it.
>
> *Vitamins B_9 (folic acid)* and *B_{12}* support positive mood by aiding homocysteine metabolism, and can ease symptoms of depression. These two Bs actually improve the effect of antidepressants because they're needed to manufacture neurotransmitters.
>
> *Vitamin B_{12}* helps your body produce energy from the fats and proteins you eat while improving memory. Vegetarians are at especially high risk of B_{12} deficiency, which causes anemia,

muscle weakness, depression, memory loss, pain, low blood pressure, and disturbances in metabolism.

Vitamin C, an energizing antioxidant, helps damp down stress levels, and when taken at higher doses (over 2,500 mg) reduces blood pressure and levels of the stress hormone cortisol, and improves your response to stress. Increasing vitamin C intake decreases body mass. As a bonus, exercising with adequate amounts of vitamin C (500 mg was used in a study) can increase fat burn by 30 percent. Vitamin C also supports good brain function, cognition, and mood because neurotransmitters need it to function—for example, in transforming dopamine to norepinephrine.

Vitamin D's effects include better mood and a decrease in anxiety and depression. This mighty vitamin supports effective insulin secretion and helps balance blood sugar. Vitamin D receptors are found in more than thirty-five tissues, including those involved in regulating calcium. In fact, the duet of vitamin D and calcium (see "Calcium and Weight" in this chapter) have wonderfully beneficial effects on weight loss. You get vitamin D naturally when your skin is exposed to sun, but with the risks of premature aging and skin cancer from sun exposure you're better off taking a supplement.

Vitamin E slows aging caused by free-radical damage, especially in the brain. Research shows taking vitamin E supplements can protect against cognitive impairment and dementia in older adults. However, taking too much can offset its benefits. To keep your antioxidant system well-balanced, it's essential that you not take more than 400 IU of vitamin E daily.

Iodine is essential for peak thyroid function, key to a healthy metabolism. Deficiency lowers thyroid hormone production, and therefore escalates metabolic problems. Nearly one-third of the US population is iodine-deficient. You get some iodine from iodized salt and seaweed, but you may not get enough given that many salts are not iodized. Beware of supplements containing too much iodine, as a total daily intake exceeding 1 to 2 grams can activate autoimmunity (in which your body attacks itself) and disturb thyroid function, causing either underactive or overactive thyroid.

L-glutathione is essential for achieving optimal weight loss with my program. Antioxidant L-glutathione, which cleans your liver of oxidative stress, makes the liver more efficient at flushing free radicals.

Magnesium is needed to metabolize carbohydrates, fats, and proteins. Deficiency reduces the effectiveness of glucose and insulin metabolism. Your body is easily depleted of magnesium via sweat during exercise and by drinking too much alcohol.

Para-aminobenzoic acid (PABA) is uniquely suited to my eating plan. Because PABA increases the utilization of proteins and preserves mitochondria, the beneficial effect on metabolism of all the proteins in your diet is even more impressive.

Selenium is vital for mood stability and thyroid function. Thyroid hormones need enough selenium to convert T4 to T3 (the most active form of thyroid hormone), and T3 enhances metabolism, regulates organ function, and slows the effects of aging. Selenium's effect on immunity makes it a requirement for your body to survive. Working with your immune system, it helps shield you from viral infections, autoimmune attacks on the thyroid, inflammation caused by Hashimoto's thyroiditis, thyroid cancer, and damage from free radicals. But don't overdo it. Excessive selenium (more than 400 mcg/day for adults and much less for children) can cause thyroid damage, fatigue, abdominal pain, diarrhea, and nerve damage. Because selenium blocks the destructive effects of free radicals on muscle, deficiency causes muscle damage and hinders muscle performance—important to know as you begin my workout.

Zinc's effects on serotonin positively affect mood and behavior, and zinc also helps prevent autoimmune disease and infection. Low serotonin from zinc deficiency actually worsens your cravings, makes you unhappy, and weakens your immune system. People with major depression also tend to have low zinc levels. If you have an overactive thyroid, you can easily be short of zinc because you lose it via urine, as a consequence of hyperthyroidism. Also, zinc levels are often low in obese people. In fact, in the past, doctors have prescribed zinc to treat obesity.

ANTIOXIDANTS: WEIGHT-LOSS BENEFITS AND BEST FOOD PICKS

This chart shows the weight-loss benefits of various antioxidants along with foods included in the Protein Boost Diet containing good amounts of these micronutrients.

Antioxidant	Weight-Loss Benefits	Main Food Sources
Vitamin A	Supports thyroid function, improves brain function and mood during stress	Eggs, fish, broccoli, carrots, spinach, squash, peas
Thiamine	Improves mood and sugar metabolism	Chicken, turkey, fish, whole grains, peanuts, lentils, lima beans, eggs
Riboflavin	Aids in metabolism of nutrients	Chicken, turkey, fish, whole grains, peanuts, lentils, lima beans, eggs
Niacin	Lowers cholesterol	Chicken, turkey, fish, whole grains, peanuts, lentils, lima beans, eggs
Vitamin B_6	Helps metabolize sugar and fat, aids in synthesis of serotonin, epinephrine, dopamine, and GABA	Garlic, tuna, cauliflower, broccoli, asparagus, brussels sprouts, turkey, salmon, leafy greens
Folate	Improves mood	Fortified grains such as quinoa or brown rice
Vitamin B_{12}	Helps derive energy from fats and proteins	Beans, whole grains, green peas, broccoli, avocado, asparagus, chickpeas, almonds, lentils, leafy greens
Vitamin C	Protects against heavy metal toxicity, lowers stress, increases fat burn	Red peppers, cauliflower, broccoli, peas, leafy green vegetables, citrus fruits, parsley, melons, strawberries, tomatoes
Vitamin D_3	Improves sugar metabolism	Fortified milk and sunlight on bare skin (nonfood source)
Vitamin E	Reverses oxidative damage	Whole grains, almonds, soybeans, leafy green vegetables, asparagus
Biotin	Improves blood sugar and nutrition metabolism	Swiss chard, romaine lettuce, carrots, tomatoes
Pantothenic acid	Lowers stress and anxiety levels, helps sugar metabolism	Yogurt, avocado, milk, chicken, lentils, sweet potato, split peas
Selenium	Balances neurotransmitters, thyroid, and other hormones affecting mood	Whole grains, wheat germ, oatmeal, mushrooms, garlic, soybeans, Brazil nuts, walnuts, cashews, lean beef, tuna, eggs
Zinc	Boosts serotonin	Shellfish, lean beef, turkey, wheat bran and whole grains, soybeans, green vegetables, ginger, cashews
Copper	Antioxidant	Shellfish, whole grains, beans, nuts
Manganese	Antioxidant	Whole grains, nuts, leafy vegetables, tea
Molybdenum	Antioxidant	Legumes, whole grains, nuts
Quercetin	Improves sugar metabolism and blood pressure	Citrus fruits, parsley, sage, tea, olive oil, dark berries
L-glutathione*	Cleans liver of toxins	Avocado, asparagus, garlic, spinach, tomatoes, curcumin (turmeric)
Alpha-lipoic acid	Increases glutathione levels, helps vitamins C and E work more efficiently	Red meat, organ meat, yeast

(continued on next page)

Antioxidant	Weight-Loss Benefits	Main Food Sources
PABA	Protects mitochondria, metabolizes protein	Whole grains, mushrooms, spinach
Lycopene	Antioxidant, improves cholesterol levels, increases energy	Tomatoes, pink grapefruit
Vanadium	Improves insulin sensitivity and cholesterol levels	Black pepper, dill, parsley, mushrooms, shellfish

*Not found in food, but the foods listed help your body produce L-glutathione.

SIP YOUR WAY TO HAPPINESS AND WEIGHT LOSS

If I told you a drink could make you happier, you might assume I was suggesting a cocktail, but in fact tea has properties that boost mood and also help with weight loss. Caffeine, L-theanine, and polyphenols are major components of tea. L-theanine, a naturally occurring amino acid in tea, is the main contributor to the calm, relaxed feelings tea elicits. It also enhances brain activity, helps regulate anxiety, and has brain-protective properties.

When you're acutely challenged by stress, taking 200 mg of L-theanine can drive down your stress level, helping you avoid the unwanted abdominal fat and cravings for high-calorie foods triggered by the stress hormone cortisol. L-theanine also relaxes your mind without making you drowsy. Electrical brainwave activity studies reveal it sharpens focus and attention, decreases mental fatigue and tiredness, relieves anxiety, and enhances performance on high-level cognitive tasks.

Polyphenols are potent antioxidants found in tea and coffee, and their effects are stronger in these drinks than in a serving of berries, another rich polyphenol source. Because drinking caffeinated sources of polyphenols can lead to dehydration, consider white tea, decaffeinated green tea, or vervain (verbena) tea, with less caffeine and generous polyphenols. Grapeseed extract, pomegranate, and blueberry are rich in polyphenols as well. Research shows that grapeseed extract increases insulin sensitivity, and administering grapeseed extract to mice after a high-fructose meal alleviated inflammation and oxidative stress.

For weight loss, green tea has numerous benefits including increasing calorie burn, and this effect isn't solely caffeine derived. The potent flavonol characteristic of green tea, epigallocatechin gallate (EGCG), is responsible. EGCG has been shown to decrease body fat accumulation and alleviate symptoms of metabolic syndrome. One study showed that people who took decaffeinated green tea extract lost weight while those who took a placebo gained.

On top of all this, green tea benefits insulin sensitivity, aiding your body's fight against metabolic slowdown. Green tea, containing more than 60 percent polyphenols, is a powerful aid for reducing both oxidative stress and weight. Its catechins also support the detoxification process by protecting your liver from harmful toxins.

I know sweet tea and green tea with honey are popular, but you must not sweeten your tea while you're on my diet. Honey contains high levels of fructose, and most bottled teas contain high fructose corn syrup (which like any sugar has devastating consequences for blood sugar levels and weight). Green tea is traditionally consumed without sweeteners after a meal to aid metabolism, boost energy, and keep you from feeling sluggish. A hot cup of tea with a squeeze of lemon helps detoxify your body, too. Make unsweetened tea one of your go-to drinks to heighten antioxidant activity.

PROMOTE SLEEP WITH MY FAVORITE DETOX TEA

Sip a bedtime cup of vervain tea featuring the herb verbena (*Verbena officinalis*), admired for thousands of years for its health-promoting properties. A cup of vervain tea between dinner and bedtime is your go-to tonic for detox preservation while you're resting. You already know green tea as a popular antioxidant drink, but a lemon verbena infusion holds superior antioxidant catechins with double the free radical–scavenging power of many other antioxidant drinks. The powerful antioxidants in verbena have a much higher activity than ascorbic acid, the source of vitamin C. Lemon verbena tea will help lower the inflammation that hinders the efficiency of your metabolism-boosting hormones. That means you'll wake up the next day feeling fresher and with your metabolism working at a higher level.

MY FAVORITE SLIM-AND-TRIM HERB MIX

For many weight-loss herbs, the efficacy and safety remain uncertain, but I wholeheartedly recommend one supplemental herb: Relora. Take 500–750 mg daily in divided doses during your weight-loss program for an extra edge in fighting body fat. Consider Relora especially if you tend to overeat in response to stress. Relora provides a patented extract from *Magnolia officinalis* and a proprietary extract from *Phellodendron amurense*. The marker compounds from these botanicals help reduce stress and balance cortisol, the stress hormone that causes fat to accumulate in the belly. People who eat in response to stress typically gain weight because of both the extra calories and the raised cortisol levels from anxiety.

Although it's not a solution to longstanding feelings of anxiety or depression, Relora can temporarily reduce transitory anxiety and enhance feelings of well-being. If you've read Chapter 4, you understand the importance of having a regular stress-reducing practice. So when you need to even out a spiked stress level, Relora can reduce surges in cortisol and prevent stress-triggered eating. I often recommend that my patients taking Relora add *Garcinia cambogia* (500 mg) daily, which reduces fat production, raspberry ketones, which promote fat burn, and yerba maté (150 to 200 mg) daily, an herb with high polyphenol and antioxidant content. Yerba maté enhances calorie burn by affecting the activity of genes that cause weight gain. You can find a mix of all these wonderful ingredients in Body Slim Mediterranean.

SPICE UP YOUR FAT-BURNING ENERGY LEVEL

Fresh and dried herbs and spices that act as stimulants not only make food delectable, they can also increase your resting metabolic rate and help you exercise more efficiently. With a stimulated energy level, you'll burn calories more efficiently and rid your body of stored fat. Add these liberally to your food to help with weight loss:

Hot peppers and *chiles* help metabolize fat. The secret is in the capsaicin, an antioxidant that puts the heat in hot peppers. Hot peppers contribute to a decrease in insulin resistance and have anti-inflammatory effects (insulin resistance and inflammation are both involved in metabolic syndrome). Sprinkle a little crushed red pepper on vegetables and meat.

Piperine (in black pepper) decreases inflammation, has antioxidant properties, and can suppress cell damage. Cayenne pepper, mustard, and horseradish have similar effects. Grind fresh black pepper onto your meals. Dab fresh horseradish onto meats and use mustard and cayenne to flavor meats, vegetables, and legumes.

Curcumin, the active ingredient in turmeric, aids fat metabolism, lowers blood sugar, and increases insulin and leptin sensitivity. Reducing inflammation is another benefit of curcumin's antioxidant properties. It also acts as a stimulant, spurring weight loss with increased energy. Sprinkle turmeric onto any food and into soups and stews.

Garlic is another stimulant and also lowers blood pressure, helps metabolize fat, increases insulin sensitivity, and lowers oxidative stress. Use the flat of a knife to crush garlic cloves, releasing them from their papery skins. Mince and enjoy raw in salads or lightly steam or sauté for use in the savory food choices in my diet.

Cinnamon, with its distinctive scent and flavor from cinnamaldehyde, increases insulin sensitivity and can lower blood sugar if you're insulin resistant. Because cinnamon can improve insulin function and reduce inflammation, it's considered antidiabetic and a metabolic syndrome preventive. Given its ability to lower cholesterol, cinnamon is a metabolism-friendly spice. Sprinkle it on yogurt, fruit, and meats.

Gingerroot has been used for centuries for its medicinal effects. To aid weight loss, use fresh ginger as a stimulant to raise your metabolic rate. Ginger has anti-inflammatory effects, and has also been shown to lower cholesterol. Diabetics may find ginger helpful with blood sugar levels because it lowers both glucose and weight. Buy fresh gingerroot for a sweet-hot flavor explosion, mincing and sautéing it with garlic to add to vegetables, legumes, and meat. Dice raw and sprinkle on fruit, or boil sliced gingerroot in water and enjoy as a tea.

Cardamom is a plant native to southern India with a unique vanilla-like flavor. The cardamom seeds are what promote healthy metabolism and detoxification. By steeping the seeds and sipping cardamom tea, you'll relieve gas, indigestion, nausea, gallbladder issues, and intestinal irritation.

Ask Dr. Arem: Does Adding Turmeric to Food
Really Reduce Inflammation?

Q. Can I just buy organic turmeric and add it to my food to get its beneficial effects?

A. Absolutely. Inflammation is an inevitable outcome as your body metabolizes nutrients, and you want to use all safe methods possible for reducing it. Adding turmeric to your food is a safe, delicious way to fight inflammation. Bonus: turmeric tastes excellent on the lean meats and beans included in the Protein Boost Diet. Add it to omelets, too.

BENEFITS OF RESVERATROL

The Mediterranean diet includes a little alcohol in the form of red wine because resveratrol, a plant polyphenol that comes from grapes, activates proteins called "sirtuins" in your body that are helpful for weight loss. Rather than add toxins to your body by drinking a lot of alcohol (which breaks down into sugar and causes inflammation), take a capsule of resveratrol instead. It decreases fat buildup and slows the process by which sugar turns to fat. It also protects against the adverse cardiovascular and physical effects of eating too many calories. If you have metabolic syndrome, resveratrol can lower blood pressure, blood sugar, triglycerides, cholesterol, and free fatty acids, and also improve insulin levels. See the "Other Supplements" chart for dosing.

CALCIUM AND WEIGHT

In addition to its overall contribution to good health, calcium paves a path toward healthy weight. Studied widely for its beneficial properties, calcium is well-known for its role in increasing bone mass and muscle strength and in preventing osteoporosis. Animal research on calcium's effects on weight showed that a higher calcium intake prevented fat mass accumulation and accelerated fat loss. The combination of calcium and branched-chain amino acids (BCAAs) increases lean body mass. In a human clinical study, the group that consumed the most calcium lost nearly 10 percent of their body weight. Waist circumference and waist-to-hip ratio also drop with more calcium intake. Studies show that adequate calcium intake resulted in more than 4.4 pounds of lost weight in a year.

Research is also suggesting that not taking enough calcium can make you gain more fat, and that calcium deficiency leads to an increased appetite for calcium-rich food. In one study, supplementing with calcium and vitamin D significantly decreased spontaneous fat intake at a buffet-style lunch. The conclusion? Enough calcium can help you stay away from the wrong foods. Calcium has also been found to increase fasting leptin levels, which keeps you feeling fuller longer.

In combination with vitamin D, calcium can increase weight loss, as seen in a two-year study on humans. Obese people often have vitamin D deficiencies, and lack of vitamin D may contribute to weight gain and obesity. Research has also shown that women past menopause who took calcium along with vitamin D had less abdominal fat over a four-year period. Because the Protein Boost Diet is dairy product-restrictive, I recommend you supplement with calcium and vitamin D daily (see the "Other Supplements" chart).

YOUR HORMONE-HEALING, WEIGHT-LOSS SUPPLEMENT REGIMEN

"Do I really need all these supplements?" my patients ask. There's no doubt that to reset your metabolism to burn calories you need enough micronutrients and antioxidants to clear a path to weight loss. Supplements help you achieve this by revving up metabolism to promote mitochondrial activity to burn fat. Most people think they get enough nutrients from food, but due to the lag between harvest and plate, by the time you eat most produce its nutrient and antioxidant value has diminished significantly. Processing depletes food micronutrients, too.

Think of supplements as routine maintenance for your metabolism-boosting mitochondria. While you're losing weight and also when you're maintaining, take a well-rounded antioxidant blend, which should include the specifics shown in the chart. If you're a thyroid patient, I don't recommend a mix containing calcium or iron because these minerals interfere with thyroid hormone absorption. Even if you are not a thyroid patient, I suggest that you select a calcium-free antioxidant mix, and take your calcium supplement separately in a well-defined amount to avoid calcium excess. If you're on thyroid medication, take calcium supplements four hours after taking thyroid hormone. Read more about why these supplements are vital in "Essential Antioxidants/Micronutrients to Reshape Hormones for Weight Loss" (page 179).

MY FAVORITE VITAMIN-ANTIOXIDANT-MICRONUTRIENT REGIMEN*

Please do not be intimidated by this long list of micronutrients. Once you find a good-quality multivitamin that contains the right amount of the vitamins, antioxidants, and micronutrients below, you can get your antioxidants in 1 to 3 tablets (as directed) per day. Keep your daily routine simple. Get your antioxidant mix—remember, *without* calcium or iron if you are on thyroid medication—during breakfast, and take your calcium and vitamin D mix with lunch and dinner.

What to Take	Recommended Daily Dose
Vitamin A	2,500 IU natural, plant-derived beta-carotene
B vitamins:	
Thiamine	10–25 mg
Riboflavin	10–25 mg
Niacin	15–20 mg
Vitamin B_6	50 mg
Biotin (vitamin B_7)	300 mcg
Folate	400 mcg
Vitamin B_{12}	25–75 mcg
Vitamin C	500 mg
Pantothenic acid	20–40 mg
Vitamin D_3	1,000 to 2,000 IU; some people require as much as 5,000 IU daily
Vitamin E	200 IU
Alpha lipoic acid (ALA)	40–80 mg
Quercetin	40–60 mg
Turmeric	100–200 mg
Lycopene	2–10 mg
Coenzyme Q-10	10–50 mg
L-glutathione	40–60 mg
Para-aminobenzoic acid (PABA)	20–40 mg
Selenium	100 mcg
Zinc	15 mg
Copper	100–500 mcg

Manganese	2.5–5 mg
Molybdenum	25–50 mcg
Chromium	Chromium picolinate: 100–200 mcg or Niacin-bound chromium: 200–400 mcg
Iodine	150–400 mcg (a mixture of iodide and iodine)
Vanadium	25–50 mcg

*Can be found in commercially available multivitamin/antioxidant mixes as 1 to 3 capsules a day, such as *ThyroLife Optima.*

OTHER SUPPLEMENTS

What to Take	Recommended Daily Dose
Calcium	1,000 mg
Magnesium	200–400 mg (magnesium citrate)
Omega-3s	1,000 mg (600 mg EPA + 400 mg DHA)
Probiotic	20–50 billion CFU (colon forming units)
Relora* (optional)	250 mg, 2–3 times per day; enhance metabolism, reduce cravings, improve sleep
Resveratrol (optional)	100 mg
L-theanine (optional)	200 mg; take in the evening to enhance relaxation
Melatonin (optional)	1–3 mg; take at bedtime to improve sleep
GABA (optional)	250–500 mg; take in the evening for stress relief

*Found in natural supplement mixes such as Body Slim Mediterranean (also includes *Garcinia cambogia*, raspberry ketones, and yerba maté).

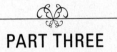

PART THREE

STEP-BY-STEP
WEIGHT-LOSS PROGRAM

CHAPTER NINE

DIET TOOLBOX

This is the place you'll find the tools you need to get ready to start my program. I've included all kinds of goodies, including a tracking chart to monitor progress and keep you motivated, a list of tests you might need if you suspect you have a thyroid or other disorder described in the book, and a few to-do lists so that you're well prepared to begin.

EIGHT STEPS TO A SUCCESSFUL LAUNCH

A beginning swimmer can't dive into the roiling Pacific safely or successfully. Neither can you dive into this program without preparation. Regardless of your fitness level or goals, you need to establish several routines to help your body prepare for the major changes it's about to undergo. This process takes just a couple of weeks, and you can begin these eight steps while you're being tested for any disorders (see "Tests You May Need" in this chapter). As soon as the following steps become routine, begin Phase 1. Note the first two items below focus on sleeping well and on schedule, which naturally feeds into meal timing. Sleep has an extreme impact on your weight hormones.

1. *Synchronize your clocks with meal timing.* Review Chapter 5 to understand why syncing your central circadian clock (your light/dark timepiece) and cellular clock (the one built into cells that expects nutrients on a regular sched-

ule) is fundamental to losing weight. On my diet, to ensure best clock alignment, you'll eat on a schedule during the day and not eat late at night (remember those fat mice who ate in the middle of the night?). Timing your meals to move in the same rhythm as your sleep schedule is fairly straightforward, but can vary among individuals. Most people on normal workday schedules can use the eating schedule I have laid out for you (see "Eat on a Schedule" in Chapter 10). But remember that Holly the teacher and Wanda the FedEx night worker in Chapter 5 had vastly different timetables based on their jobs, yet both committed to an eating schedule with good results.

2. *Address any sleep disturbances or shortages* using the recommendations in Chapter 5. Then begin a schedule of sleeping for eight to nine hours. Start by turning off all light-emitting, sound-emitting devices before 10:00 p.m., and snuggle in for a full eight-hour rest that will recharge your key weight-loss hormones—thyroid hormones, leptin, and growth hormone.

3. *Begin a relaxation technique.* Select one stress-reliever from Chapter 4 or choose your own and make space to practice, every day. You can meditate or practice breathing anytime and anywhere. Remember why you're doing this: stress and the way you perceive stress make you fat.

4. *Choose a start date and write it on your calendar.* Pick a date when you know you can dedicate your full attention to weight loss. I recommend a Saturday, a Sunday, or your day off.

5. *Plan to shop and cook.* The foods you'll be eating aren't difficult to prepare, but require that you shop, prep, and cook actual food. No more packaged convenience foods, which contain so many hormone-damaging ingredients. To get the best possible start, prep meals and snacks on the weekend for the week ahead. See "Eat-Smart Shopping Cart" later in this chapter for advice.

6. *Get acquainted with "My Favorite Foods" and portions.* Take a look at the foods you'll be eating every day by reviewing the Meal Plans and the Favorite Foods lists in

Chapter 10. All of the meals can be easily prepared. You don't actually need a recipe to enjoy eating this way, but if you're feeling adventurous, try some of my recipes, too.

7. *Schedule your 20/10 exercise.* Every other day you'll be doing the high-intensity interval training (HIIT; see "The Cardio 20" in Chapter 11) that's so effective for weight loss, ideally on a stationary bike. Plan what time of day you'll do this twenty-minute workout and locate an exercise bike you can use. Nothing fancy required—it could be a bike at your neighbor's house, at a health club, or at work; or you can purchase one or pick one up at a second-hand store (people with good intentions often leave them there). Your ten-minute strength training can be done at the same or another time of day. Choose some sets from the program and do just a few repetitions to get acquainted with the movements. For now, exercise three times a week; that will prepare you to work out every day.

8. *Identify the right antioxidant mix and start taking it consistently.* I recommend a complete, well-balanced mix of antioxidants and vitamins with weight-loss-promoting ingredients, such as ThyroLife Optima. If you prefer a basic supplement, check to ensure it has all the essential micronutrients described in Chapter 8. Don't forget your omega-3 supplement—it will boost your immune system and metabolism and suppress appetite.

TESTS YOU MAY NEED

To avoid weight-loss resistance, you want to address any hormone imbalance you have, such as an imbalance of thyroid hormones. Insulin resistance, growth hormone deficiency, food sensitivities, and toxins in your system are other factors. If you suspect you may have one or more of these, ask your doctor to test you. Here are the tests needed to determine if you have a hormonal imbalance or metabolic disorder.

You will not have to get all these tests. If you have been getting an annual physical, many of the blood tests have most likely already been taken care of.

METABOLIC AND INFLAMMATION TESTING

These blood tests reveal signs of inflammation in your system, often indicative of insulin resistance or metabolic syndrome. They're also helpful in detecting if prediabetes (a metabolic state that can lead to diabetes), diabetes, vitamin D deficiency, or liver dysfunction is a reason for your sluggish metabolism.

Fasting blood glucose and insulin levels
Two-hour glucose tolerance test (or fasting and two-hour postprandial blood glucose)
Fasting cholesterol and triglyceride levels
C-reactive protein
Homocysteine
Uric acid
25-hydroxyvitamin D
Liver function (AST, ALT, GGT)
Hemoglobin A_1 C
Plasminogen Activator Inhibitor-1 (PAI-1)

THYROID TESTING

These blood tests and ultrasound of the thyroid will reveal any thyroid imbalance and/or Hashimoto's thyroiditis (the autoimmune condition that causes low thyroid).

TSH
T4 (free)
Anti-TPO antibody
Thyroid ultrasound

GROWTH HORMONE (GH) TESTING

This blood test shows whether the activity or level of GH in your system is low. It helps determine if further GH testing is required.

Somatomedin-C (IgF-1)

HORMONE TESTS FOR POLYCYSTIC OVARY SYNDROME (PCOS)

These tests show if you have metabolic or hormonal changes indicating PCOS, and can assist your doctor in making a diagnosis of PCOS.

FSH, LH
Glucose tolerance test
Fasting insulin level
Insulin level fasting and two hours after a meal
Prolactin
Ultrasound of ovaries
Testosterone
SHBG
DHEA-sulfate

TESTS FOR MENOPAUSE

Your blood tests show your hormonal status—whether you're moving into menopause or you are menopausal. They also determine whether you have high or low male hormones during the periods before and after menopause.

FSH, LH
Estradiol
Progesterone
Testosterone
SHBG
DHEA-Sulfate

HEAVY METAL TOXICITY

This test reveals any accumulated amounts of heavy metals (mercury, cadmium, arsenic, lead, etc.) in your system.

Hair strand test

FOOD SENSITIVITIES

These tests can show if you have celiac disease or gluten sensitivity or other food sensitivities.

Celiac antibodies
IgG allergy test
IgE allergy test
ALCAT or Meridian Valley testing

ANTIOXIDANT DEFICIENCY

These tests reveal any deficiencies in antioxidants.

Blood tests for specific antioxidants (zinc, selenium, vitamin
    levels)
Spectra Cell

UPGRADE YOUR PANTRY

Go through your kitchen shelves, refrigerator, and freezer and rid your home of all the foods that can derail your best efforts. Give away cream and butter (loaded with saturated fat), margarines and shortenings (rich in trans fat), and junk snacks (cookies, chips, crackers, candy, ice cream, etc.). Also give away any other foods not included in my diet that may tempt you. Even low-calorie and no-calorie sweeteners can make you want to eat more sugar. You must treat your cravings seriously, like the addiction they are. Just as you wouldn't leave liquor on the shelves of an alcoholic's home, you must dispose of all foods that will tempt you to return to your former eating habits.

Once it's been cleared, restock your kitchen with the right tools, foods, and spices. Because grilling, steaming, and baking are the simplest healthy methods of cooking, quality pans are a good investment. Cast iron is ideal. Nonstick pans are practical for reducing the amount of oil, but use only nonstick pans that aren't scratched to avoid consuming toxicants from the nonstick surface. Get yourself a collapsible steamer basket to drop into a pot with a little boiling water. Lightly steamed vegetables are a treat.

For Phase 2, you'll need whole-grain flour to prepare bread, pizza crust, muffins, pancakes, and waffles. You may not find whole-grain flours in all grocery stores, though stores like Whole Foods Market carry them and Bob's Red Mill brand is available online. You can easily grind your own grains with a heavy-duty grain grinder, or get a blender powerful enough to grind whole grains (and use it to make your detox smoothies, too).

Stock your kitchen with these to make it more diet-friendly.

Oils: Olive, canola, peanut, sesame, safflower, soybean, and cottonseed oil—organic when possible. Remember, oil crops are sprayed with lots of pesticides with potentially damaging action on hormones.

Dairy: Low-fat yogurt, low-fat cottage cheese, fat-free cream cheese, fat-free mozzarella, reduced-fat feta, low-fat ricotta, and goat cheese

Dairy alternatives: Unsweetened soy and almond milks

Snacks: Unsalted nuts and edamame (soybeans), both rich in proteins and antioxidants

Sweets: Low-fructose fruits, nut butters

Sweet spices: Cardamom, ginger, nutmeg, cinnamon, allspice

Metabolism-boosting spices: Turmeric, cumin, ginger, red pepper, black pepper, cayenne, fennel seed, parsley, and garlic

EAT-SMART SHOPPING CART (SHOPPING TIPS)

Here's a secret: so-called convenience foods cost a lot more per serving than real whole foods that you cook yourself. Speaking of whole foods, if you're lucky enough to have a store that carries organics where you live, consider buying your hormone-free organic meats there. Most have excellent butchers who will even weigh and package your meats in individual portion sizes. Most also carry organic yogurt and cream cheese products in the low-, reduced-, and nonfat versions I recommend. Where these stores really shine is their bulk bins, filled with the dried lentils, beans, and quinoa you'll be enjoying, and the whole grains for Phase 2. Even if you choose canned versions of beans and lentils (already rehydrated), the cost for organic is comparable to that for most conventional versions. Organic produce is a little more expensive, but the cost savings from not buying junk snacks and prepared foods can easily offset the difference. Farmers' markets are the very best source for locally grown, no-pesticide or reduced-pesticide produce. Many also carry responsibly raised meats and eggs.

My Favorite Foods list has many items in each category, and on the Meal Plans you'll quickly see that some foods are eaten more often than others—protein being an obvious example. You want to be well-stocked with meats, fish and seafood, legumes, veggies, whole grains, fruits, and nuts. Meats can easily be frozen in portion sizes, and water-packed canned tuna and salmon are excellent choices. Ideally, you'll purchase fresh fruits and vegetables at least once a week. If you don't have time or you prefer buying these foods in bulk (especially seasonal items), with a little prep you can easily freeze them for later. Freezing doesn't interfere with nutritional content.

WEEKLY SHOPPING LIST

Plan a week's meals in advance and make a comprehensive list, consulting the meal plans and recipes you'll be following. Include the ingredients for your twice-daily detox smoothies and raw fennel. Remember: never shop when you're hungry, and stick to the Favorite Foods lists. Here are a few other pointers.

> *Select fish low or medium in mercury* such as wild salmon, scallops, cod, tilapia, sardines, haddock, anchovies, herring, mackerel (North Atlantic, chub), whitefish, trout, snapper, halibut, fresh tuna.
>
> For *dairy products,* select low-fat or fat-free cottage cheese, yogurt, and cream cheese. Grated Parmesan cheese (a good source of metabolism-boosting amino acids) can be used sparingly in some recipes.
>
> *You can purchase canned vegetables,* but make sure to rinse them thoroughly to remove the sodium.
>
> *You can purchase frozen vegetables,* as long as they are packed without sauce or other ingredients.

Select only the low-fructose, low-sugar fruits listed in "My Favorite Foods."

To save money, buy items on sale or in bulk, grow your own produce, and shop at farmers' markets. Dried beans are very cheap. Once cooked, they can be refrigerated for half a week at least.

Select whole-grain cereals for Phase 2, according to the list of My Favorite Whole Grains in Chapter 10. Avoid flavored oatmeals, as their sugar content is high.

For Phase 2 whole-grain products, choose only items on which the label clearly indicates "brown rice," "whole oats," or "whole wheat." Quinoa is the ideal gluten-free complete protein. There's nothing wrong with instant brown rice. Alternatives for brown rice in Phase 2 could be buckwheat, rye, or bulgur.

For pastas (such as spaghetti and lasagna), select whole wheat.

Breads are notoriously misleading when you're searching for whole-grain versions. Don't be fooled by "whole wheat" and labels that say "contains whole grains." The remaining flours are refined and not a healthful choice. Look for Ezekiel Breads (made by Foods for Life and sold at Whole Foods Market and other healthy food stores), made with sprouted whole grains. The best idea is to make your own bread, and my favorites are Protein Boost Diet Crusty Rolls, Quinoa Pizza Dough or Flatbread, and Protein Boost Diet Quinoa Sandwich Bread (in the Recipes section); all contain a mix of quinoa and whole grains.

Absolutely no commercially baked goods. Cookies, pies, and cakes are loaded with trans fat and sugar.

Avoid cocoa butter, palm oil, and tropical oils, which are found in many processed foods and are high in fats.

Don't buy packaged goods with "partially hydrogenated" or "hydrogenated" oils on the label, such as margarine, shortening, or foods made with them.

Avoid any foods or drinks containing sugar in its many disguises, among them: corn sugar, high fructose corn syrup (HFCS), sucrose, glucose, dextrose, maltose, turbinated sugar, fructose, and molasses.

WEIGH IN AND MEASURE

What's your BMI and how overweight are you? Read about this in Chapter 1. Here we're going to focus on the most important calculation: an estimate of your target body weight, which allows you to estimate the weight you need to lose. Using this chart, look for your height and then go to a BMI of 24 to see the target weight you're aiming for to be close to an acceptable range. If you are five feet, five inches, for example, you should weigh about 144 pounds or a little less. To determine how much weight you need to lose, subtract the target BMI weight from your current weight.

Weight-Loss Goal = Current Weight – Target Weight

On my diet you'll lose two to three pounds a week; try not to aim higher than that. Your goal needs to be achievable, not extreme. Forty to fifty pounds of weight loss in twenty weeks is achievable, so don't be afraid to set your sights high! Once you set your goal, push yourself to stick with my program, which will get you there.

	Normal		Overweight					Obese					Morbidly Obese*		
BMI	19	24	25	26	27	28	29	30	31	32	33	34	35	40	50
Height	Weight in Pounds														
4'10"	91	115	119	124	129	134	138	143	148	153	158	162	167	191	239
4'11"	94	119	124	128	133	138	143	148	153	158	163	168	173	198	247
5'0"	97	123	128	133	138	143	148	153	158	163	168	174	179	204	255
5'1"	100	127	132	137	143	148	153	158	164	169	174	180	185	211	264
5'2"	104	131	136	142	147	153	158	164	169	175	180	186	191	218	273
5'3"	107	135	141	146	152	158	163	169	175	180	186	191	197	225	282
5'4"	110	140	145	151	157	163	169	174	180	186	192	197	204	232	291
5'5"	114	144	150	156	162	168	174	180	186	192	198	204	210	240	300
5'6"	118	148	155	161	167	173	179	186	192	198	204	210	216	247	309
5'7"	121	153	159	166	172	178	185	191	198	204	211	217	223	255	319
5'8"	125	158	164	171	177	184	190	197	203	210	216	223	230	262	328
5'9"	128	162	169	176	182	189	196	203	209	216	223	230	236	270	338
5'10"	132	167	174	181	188	195	202	209	216	222	229	236	243	278	348
5'11"	136	172	179	186	193	200	208	215	222	229	236	243	250	286	358
6'0"	140	177	184	191	199	206	213	221	228	235	242	250	258	294	368

6'1"	144	182	189	197	204	212	219	227	235	242	250	257	265	302	378
6'2"	148	186	194	202	210	218	225	233	241	249	256	264	272	311	389
6'3"	152	192	200	208	216	224	232	240	248	256	264	272	279	319	399

* People within this range have significantly higher health risks.

Source: NIH/National Heart, Lung, and Blood Institute (NHLBI), *Evidence Report of Clinical Guidelines on the Identification, Evaluation, and Treatment of Overweight and Obesity in Adults,* NIH Publication No. 98-4083, September 1998.

MEASURE YOUR PROGRESS

Weigh yourself once a week, first thing in the morning on an empty stomach, after urination, and record your results on this chart. Measure your waist circumference (see "Are You Overweight or Obese?" in Chapter 1) once a month. Tracking your progress from start to finish with numerical values is a confidence builder—otherwise it's easy to look in the mirror after one or two weeks and feel discouraged. Record hip circumference as well, so you can see how your body begins to sculpt. Research tells us that people who weigh themselves weekly are more successful at losing weight. Monitoring your weight regularly can also help you see if you've gained some pounds so you can reverse the trend before you gain more. There's also a sleep column—aim for eight to nine hours a night.

Week	Weight (lbs.)	BMI	Waist Circumference (in.)	Hip Circumference (in.)	Waist/Hip Ratio	Avg. hrs. of sleep/night
1						
2						
3						
4						
5						
6						
7						
8						
9						
10						
11						
12						

(continued on next page)

Week	Weight (lbs.)	BMI	Waist Circumference (in.)	Hip Circumference (in.)	Waist/Hip Ratio	Avg. hrs. of sleep/night
13						
14						
15						
16						
17						
18						
19						
20						
21						
22						
23						
24						
25						
26						
27						
28						
29						
30						
31						
32						
33						
34						
35						
36						
37						
38						
39						
40						

TEN TIPS FOR LONG-TERM SUCCESS

Since you want my program to be effective in the long term, first engage mentally. Define your goals and motivation, and how you plan to honor your commitment to the plan. You also need to establish a well-defined program to track your progress. Here are ten recommendations to help you stay on track.

1. *Establish and maintain a contract with yourself.* Weight loss is foremost about better health and disease prevention. Recognizing the health issues at the outset will help you stick with the program in the long term. Focusing solely on your appearance can deter your progress by making you want to take shortcuts, which will only hurt your metabolism again. Condition your mind to view weight-gain-promoting factors as trouble, and your brain will stay in charge of your body and adhere to your goal. Write down your motivations such as self-esteem, body image, being fit for a job, keeping a relationship, or overcoming depression and make them a focus of daily life. Hang a photo of yourself when you were much slimmer on the wall or fridge. Have an unflattering picture of yourself taken and carry it in your wallet to look at every time you crave fattening foods. Wear a bracelet on your dominant hand that symbolizes the contract you've made with yourself and will remind you of your commitment.

2. *Carpe diem.* Focus on today. Make it a rule. With any behavior we want to change, we tend to convince ourselves that tomorrow we'll do it, but not today. How many times have you said, "I'll start my diet tomorrow," or "I'll eat this now and diet tomorrow"? Don't be tempted to take a break, eat bad foods, and restart tomorrow. Empower yourself to create an inner strength that will keep you in charge at all times. Follow my meal plans and honor your commitment to the 20/10 exercise program, sleep, and stress relief.

3. *Establish a weight-friendly social environment.* It's extremely important to surround yourself with people who

will commit to the diet with you and support you along the way. I've seen proof of it again and again in my patients. Losing weight is a challenging process, and to be successful you'll need encouragement from people who hold you accountable. Get everyone on your support team—partner, spouse, family member, friend, coworker, or any group of people with whom you're in regular contact. There's proof to support this idea. A six-month follow-up of the DIRECT spouse study, which analyzed the influence of spouses' attendance in the weight-loss program, showed that men on a diet program whose wives attended support sessions lost nearly one and a half times more weight than men whose wives didn't participate. Don't underestimate the importance of family and social circle in helping you stay with the program.

4. *Find a weight-loss partner.* Find one particular friend who will be your ally during your weight-loss program. He or she will ideally go through the program with you, and you'll hold each other accountable. You and your weight-loss buddy will follow up with each other on a weekly basis.

5. *Keep a diet and exercise diary.* Establish a notebook or electronic device you can carry with you everywhere to record the basics: *everything* you eat, how much you sleep, and when you exercise. The diary's main purpose is to track deviations from the program (not that you would have any) so you can address them where you've slipped and fix them immediately. If you slide, record where, how, the circumstances, and the reason. Your diary should give you encouragement.

6. *Prepare to address setbacks.* What causes your biggest setbacks? Is it the temptation to eat the wrong foods at the wrong times, or do you have trouble sleeping enough? Establish go-to activities to keep you from returning to those vices. For example, if you tend to snack out of boredom or as a result of bad moods, find an activity you like that elevates mood. It will keep your mind off food, and as you feel better your cravings for unhealthy snacks will

subside. Eating foods loaded with sugar and fats was most likely a major source of pleasure for you and by substituting favorite activities, you'll cut back on recreational eating. View sugars and fats as poisons. If you have an urge, remind yourself that it's temporary and likely to go away in half an hour. Or send cravings packing with a moment of breath meditation (see "To Release Stress, Focus and Relax" in Chapter 4). Imagine yourself on a sunny beach . . . with your new body. Call your weight-loss buddy. Look at the picture in your wallet and at your bracelet. Remind yourself that you're on a mission and you will succeed. Then go shopping for the foods that will keep you whole and full.

7. *Go for optimum weight loss with an optimistic mind.* Don't let negative thinking override motivation. After having lost some weight, you may notice you reach a plateau and stop losing even though you continue the diet. It's an almost universal occurrence, but don't be discouraged. The plateau period is short-lived—a few days to (rarely) a few weeks. This plateau is normal: your body senses that you've changed and is resisting weight loss. Think about how you're moving in the right direction, about how you'll continue to lose weight and be healthy. Have faith in yourself and be vigilant about doing the 20/10 workout. Miraculous changes are occurring inside.

8. *Pay close attention to sleep and stress.* Don't let stress or sleep problems interfere with hormonal balance. Schedule sleep and stress relief.

9. *Follow up with your doctor.* Your body is undergoing many changes while you're losing weight. Follow up with your doctor to monitor any medical conditions or hormone imbalances.

10. *When you grocery shop, stick to the list you've made from "My Favorite Foods."* When you get home, prep the foods you'll eat that week. And don't bring home any foods that can cause you to break your diet.

WEEKLY MEETING WITH YOUR WEIGHT-LOSS BUDDY

I'll be honest: my diet requires you to make a big lifestyle change. Get consistent feedback to track your progress, manage behavior, and give you encouragement. Each week, talk to your weight-loss buddy to discuss how to counter any deviations from the plan that occurred during the previous week. Then create individualized approaches for follow-up. It's fine to meet in person, but talking via phone, text, or e-mail works, too. Bring your diet diary and focus on one person's entire evaluation first before moving on to the next person. The follow-up has four sections.

1. *Deviations:* Small deviations like eating a piece of candy are just as important to mention as skipping exercise one day. Take every wrong turn into account.

2. *Reasons:* Talk through the behaviors that caused you to deviate. Discuss all possible factors: cravings, sleepiness, skipping meals, forgetting to pack your lunch/snack, temptation when eating out, lack of motivation. Share ideas to fix these.

3. *Action plan:* The most important part of your follow-up is an action plan to train you and your partner how not to deviate again. Anticipate your reasons for deviation and decide how you'll handle a similar situation in the future.

4. *Feedback:* It feels good to share gripes about temptations and deviations, but it feels even better to share accomplishments. Follow up on your action plans from the previous week. You may need to re-create an action plan for that behavior if the first one didn't work.

BECOME A CONFIDENT COOK

The best way to ensure that your food is fresh and pure is to shop for it and cook it yourself. You must start cooking regularly to stay on my plan. The food combination guidelines for each meal in Chapter 10 align with my diet's weight-loss benefits. Follow the meal plans, and you'll learn quickly the serving sizes and specific food options for each meal. Soon you won't have to look at the charts. To become an expert healthy cook, use "My Favorite Foods" list to create your own favorite meals according to the fundamentals of the diet. You don't actually need a recipe. Enjoy using spices to enhance the protein selections—get confident and creative! Here are some suggestions.

- When you establish favorite meals, print or write them on sheets of paper to create your own cookbook. Perhaps you'll find a certain breakfast combination suits your time constraints and palate. Write it down.

- Check recipes for your favorite dishes and replace ingredients that aren't included in "My Favorite Foods" list with items that are.

- If you're busy, cook basics like beans and whole grains once or twice a week and package them in portion-sized servings.

- Grilling, baking, broiling, braising, poaching, and roasting are the best ways to cook meats and fish. Avoid frying anything. Remove skin from poultry before cooking and trim visible fat from meats. If a recipe calls for ground meat, select ground turkey breast because it's the leanest. No breaded poultry, fish, or meat. Cook extra portions of meat for the following couple of days.

- For vegetables, steaming, blanching, boiling, and lightly stir-frying or sautéing are options. Overcooking vegetables will deplete their vitamins and raise their simple sugar content.

- Pack lunch to take to work. Assemble prepared meat, vegetables, and precooked beans or lentils in a container. Microwave on-site. Take a serving of fruit from the list for dessert and your healthy snack.

- I recommend you lose your sugar tooth altogether. "Sweet" spices such as cardamom, cinnamon, ginger, nutmeg, and allspice add sweetness to meats or fish and whole grains. Sprinkle cinnamon and unsweetened cocoa into coffee (instead of adding sugar) for even better metabolism and antioxidants.

- Portion foods for snacks so you won't eat too much. Even though you'll have only healthy snacks, too many nuts give you excess calories from fat. Convenient packaging also ensures that you can grab the snacks on the go, rather than succumbing to vending machine snacks.

- Make your own salad dressing. One part olive oil and one part either balsamic, apple cider, or flavored vinegar make an ideal dressing. Or use lemon or lime juice for the acid component. Add black pepper and other spices to taste.

- During Phase 2, make your own whole-grain breads—from grinding the grains to baking—and make pizza with Quinoa Pizza Dough or Flatbread (in the Recipes section). Whole-grain barley is a very good addition to soups.

- Keep foods wholesome and enjoy leftovers. No juicing your fruits—juices and caloric drinks have little satiating effect compared with solid food. Eat fresh fillets of fish or meat and don't overcook vegetables. Refried beans hold their nutritional value, and you may enjoy this variation because you'll be eating lots of beans at lunchtime (not at dinner). Look for vegetarian refried beans to avoid lard, or make your own.

- Cook meals with your weight-loss buddy.

Once you put effort into cooking something, you'll be more inclined to eat it. Challenge yourself to turn healthy foods into delicious dishes, and you'll see the reward in the mirror.

YOU CANNOT CHEAT THE PROGRAM: COMMON PITFALLS

Eating foods that support peak hormone function is central to upgrading your metabolism. As you adjust to the lifestyle, avoid these common impediments to weight loss.

Skipping meals, including snacks: A top priority is keeping your eating schedule steady to forestall cravings. Skipping any meal or your afternoon snack can push hunger out of control when you eat next.

Not focusing on eating, not waiting to feel full: Eat mindfully at a slow, steady pace to train your body's tempo. Not only does this aid digestion, it gives your stomach time to signal your brain that you're full. Eating proteins and fiber first will make hormones and GI chemicals give you a sense of fullness as quickly as ten minutes after you start, but it can take up to an hour for you to realize you feel full. For this reason, absolutely no mindless eating in front of the TV or computer, where it's easy to overeat without knowing it. Stop eating before you feel full to let the signals catch up.

Eating everything you're served: It's actually ideal to eat at home, eating food you've prepared yourself, for the first couple of weeks so you're very clear about food selections, portions, and the eating schedule. But life is to enjoy. When you do eat out or at a friend's house, no one's going to scold you for not eating everything on your plate. Choose wisely from what your host or the restaurant offers (see "Eating Out: Enjoy the Company, Not the Fattening Foods" in this chapter), staying as close as possible to the food combination guidelines of my diet. You should know what your protein portions are for every meal of the day, and obviously, if you're in Phase 1, you're off grains. So many people are, these days, that nobody will notice.

Drinking beverages loaded with calories: Soft drinks, energy drinks, sweetened tea, and sugared beverages of any kind are not a part of your diet. Neither is any fruit juice, which is simply fructose without the fiber of the whole fruit to help you feel full. All of these load your body with calories without even signaling your brain that you've consumed as many calories as a satisfying snack. Alcohol has a lot of calories too, which can come back to haunt you (see "Ask Dr. Arem: What About a Glass of Wine?" in Chapter 10).

Being seduced by flavorings and food additives: Many additives and flavorings have a detrimental effect on your metabolism and brain signaling. Monosodium glutamate can even potentially damage your sense of satiety (fullness) in the hypothalamus. Avoid additives by quitting all packaged and fast foods, and instead follow my meal plans with their whole foods and health-boosting spices. You'll also save money by not buying metabolism-damaging junk.

Forgetting to detox and to take antioxidants: You can follow my diet to the letter, but without a smooth detoxification system your metabolism will not adjust to its new pace. Drinking the Sensational Detox Smoothie (at the beginning of Chapter 8) and taking antioxidants, vitamins, and probiotics will help eliminate waste buildup as your body rapidly changes its metabolism. Also, remember to monitor calcium intake, especially now that you're cutting down on dairy. Taking adequate calcium with meals will help your metabolism and is a major factor in successful weight loss.

Eating processed foods or "diet" foods: The food industry makes enormous profits by selling food-like substances that may look/ smell/feel/taste appealing, but contain junk ingredients and little or no nutrition. No one is looking out for your health but you (and me), so turn to "My Favorite Foods" list. Then start using them to prepare your meals. Take what you learn from this book to create meals that sustain your cells and metabolism in a way "diet" foods never will.

Consuming alcohol regularly or excessively: You simply can't ignore the calories and sugar in alcoholic drinks. Liquor itself intoxicates your metabolic function as it pollutes your fat-clearing liver, and most mixers are loaded with sugar. Wine has a lot of sugar, too. If you want to drink alcohol (but I don't recommend it), limit yourself strictly. Choose red wine over white, as it has less sugar and you'll at least benefit from the resveratrol it contains (see "Benefits of Resveratrol" in Chapter 8). If you're addicted to drinking daily, work on your addiction first so that alcohol doesn't weaken your willpower.

Failing at consistency: My diet is a lifestyle, not a miracle cure or crash diet. Although it may take some time to adjust to, settling in and sticking to the program will be easier than deprivation dieting because you'll be eating foods that make you feel full, exercising efficiently daily, sleeping better, and feeling vibrant with more energy as your metabolism speeds its burn rate.

EATING OUT: ENJOY THE COMPANY, NOT THE FATTENING FOODS

I don't discourage you from eating out while you're following my diet, but be aware that it's easy to relapse into poor eating habits. For this reason and to ensure you have a sense of portion size and recommended foods, eat at home for at least a couple of weeks after starting the diet. When you eat out, make sure you're not hungry when you leave home—have your afternoon snack—and never skip a meal before going out (or ever). Here are some additional reminders.

- Instead of high-calorie drinks, order club soda with lime.
- Ignore the bread and butter.
- Order olive oil or balsamic vinaigrette salad dressing on the side—no high-calorie, high-saturated-fat dressings.
- Hold the mayo.
- Your entrée should include baked or grilled fish, chicken, veal, or lean meat. Decline sauces.
- Carbs can be brown or wild rice, which can often be substituted for potatoes. Mind your portion.
- Avoid altogether: white rice, potatoes, flour tortillas, bread, and croutons.
- Choose dinner restaurants that have a good selection of vegetables rich in protein and fiber, preferably grilled or steamed. For lunch, choose a restaurant that serves lentils or beans and baked, grilled, or blackened turkey, chicken, or fish.
- Definitely no desserts. Fruit for dessert at lunch is okay.
- Eat vegetables instead of foods rich in carbohydrates.

CHAPTER TEN

THE PROTEIN BOOST DIET

What, When, and How to Eat

My diet consists of two phases, and during both you'll be eating a broad variety of proteins to give your metabolism the well-rounded support it needs to get rid of fat and create lean muscle. The basic food combinations and serving amounts have been designed so you'll be consuming roughly 1,200 to 1,500 calories daily in both phases. The high-nutrient selections of vegetables, fruits, good fats, and the best carbs ensure that you—and your body—should never be hungry on this meal plan.

In this chapter, you'll find detailed meal plans for Phases 1 and 2 as well as DIY suggestions for building your own meals that conform to the diet. My Favorite Foods lists are here, too. You'll refer to them frequently as you get to know which food combinations create the well-balanced meals that constitute a perfect diet for your metabolism and your lean body to come. Did I mention the formula for making your own recipes? That's here, too. This food is real and satisfying. You'll never feel that you're on a diet, and in fact you might wonder how you'll eat everything I suggest for breakfast. The breakfasts might seem large compared with grabbing a slice of toast and coffee . . . and therein lies the magic. Enjoy this healthy way of eating, be satisfied, and be trim.

TEN FUNDAMENTALS OF THE PROTEIN BOOST DIET

1. Slightly low-calorie diet (roughly 1,200 to 1,500 calories per day). Adjust caloric intake according to BMR.

2. High-protein diet, with highest protein intake at dinner (for leptin and growth hormone's fat-burning effects at night) and a wide variety of protein sources throughout the day to ensure a balanced amino acid profile. This energizes your mitochondria to produce heat rather than storing energy for conversion into fat. Beans and lentils at lunchtime and lean meats and fish at dinnertime provide a generous amount of the branched-chain amino acids that have this powerful effect.

3. Synchronize central circadian and cellular clocks with meal timing: eat four to five meals (breakfast, optional midmorning snack, lunch, afternoon snack, dinner) at designated times.

4. No food three hours before bedtime to avoid spiking blood sugar and insulin levels.

5. Low-glycemic diet, with lowest-glycemic meals at dinner to keep insulin low. You'll avoid grains, legumes, and fruits at dinner and enjoy more good carbs at lunch and breakfast in the form of legumes, whole grains, quinoa, and low-fructose, high-fiber fruits.

6. High-fiber foods at every meal (daily total fiber roughly 35 to 40 grams).

7. Low in saturated fat, with more unsaturated fat (15 to 25 percent) daily.

8. Eat protein-rich and fiber-rich foods first at every meal. Fruits at the end of breakfast and lunch (as a dessert).

9. No added sugars and minimal fructose, in the form of low-fructose, moderately low–sugar fruits for breakfast and lunch only, at the end of the meal. And again, no fruit at dinner, to keep blood sugar low.

10. Detox smoothie and raw fennel to keep your body running cleanly for the first week of the diet and then ad lib.

Let's take a look at the two phases of your new diet.

Phase 1 is the first six weeks. This high-protein, grain-free approach will reverse the hormone imbalances that encouraged your extra fat. It's during Phase 1 that you'll be mending your metabolism, reshaping the hormones that control it so it runs in peak form. These first six weeks are also designed to detox your body and mind, eradicate cravings and sugar addictions, and teach you discipline with the food selections for every meal and snack. You could view Phase 1 as a six-week course in learning the very best foods to mix at breakfast, lunch, and dinner to energize your metabolism. My meal plans are simple and delicious, making these six weeks as delectable as they are educational. Once you start eating these highly nutritious foods in the correct order, in the right combinations, and on schedule, you can expect to lose an average of two to three pounds per week—or between twelve and eighteen pounds total during Phase 1.

With its elimination of grain, this initial phase can be challenging, but its purpose is to make the transition quick and effective. Knocking out the most difficult stage in the beginning will also make the program easier in the future. No matter how much weight you're trying to lose, Phase 1 should last six weeks. By eliminating grains, you will detox from the negative effects of any sensitivities to grains. Many of my patients also notice an overall improvement in well-being. Eliminating grains for six weeks also helps you overcome your addiction to sweets and carbohydrates and smooths your body's adjustment to low-glycemic foods.

For strong carb addictions, quitting cold turkey can be difficult initially, but it's the only way to eradicate cravings. For many of my patients, quitting grains was easier than they thought, thanks to the generous amounts of satisfying proteins at mealtime. Keep in mind that while you're eliminating grains, you're not eliminating all carbohydrates. The generous legume servings at lunch (lentil, chickpea, and other bean recipes) will help keep you full and satisfied. Addiction to sweets and carbohydrates is comparable to a drug addiction. It's natural to have intense cravings initially, but if you diligently follow the no-grains rule, you'll begin to want them less and less until the cravings diminish altogether. At that point, you'll reinstate healthful grains in a more structured, balanced way. My diet is actually easy compared with many others, because I designed it to make you feel better. Every aspect is conceived from scientific research, and there's no other diet I know of that takes into account the components of the food that affect your hormones.

Phase 2 continues everything you've learned in Phase 1, plus you'll start eating selected grains. That's because your metabolism now has the power to burn calories faster. You'll continue to consume a slightly reduced number of calories, but you can now substitute whole grains for other forms of carbohydrates. Stay with the whole grains included in "My Favorite Foods" list, leaving refined carbohydrates off your plate. Even in Phase 2, I discourage you from eating grain-derived foods at dinner. If you do, stick to quinoa (ideal) or brown rice in small amounts, and no more than twice weekly to minimize high sugar and insulin levels at night. I also highly recommend that for lunch you stick with beans or quinoa rather than whole grains. If you elect to eat whole grains for lunch, limit them to twice a week. My patients average a loss of two pounds per week during Phase 2. Don't underestimate these numbers. You're reshaping the health of your metabolism and resculpting your body. It's powerful and it works.

Every twelve weeks after beginning Phase 2, you'll spend two weeks following the Phase 1 diet. In this way, you'll ease any food sensitivities and periodically put the brakes on carb cravings before your body pushes you to eat more of them. You might notice you feel best when you don't eat grains at all, except for the quinoa (not actually a grain, after all). That's an indication of gluten sensitivity. If you choose to remain on a grain-free diet, continue with Phase 1 to eat gluten-free for life. You'll still be able to enjoy quinoa and use quinoa flour for the breads, pizza, and pasta in the recipe section.

Avoid packaged foods and snacks because they're virtually always rich in sugar, are processed, and contain chemicals. A few baby car-

Ask Dr. Arem: Dark Chocolate

Q. What's your position on dark chocolate?

A. Dark chocolate contains antioxidants and is the preferred form of chocolate in general for drinks or desserts. However, it's still high in sugar and should be minimized, if used at all, while you are following the Protein Boost Diet.

rots with hummus made from chickpeas or fava beans offer you the best carb/protein combo for a healthy midmorning or midafternoon snack. A cucumber with two boiled egg whites is an excellent alternative. Snacks that are high in fiber and protein and low in sugar—if you are lucky enough to find them—are okay.

SAY NO TO GHRELIN:
EAT ON A SCHEDULE, EAT IN THE CORRECT ORDER

When you train your dog, you dictate when he sits, walks, goes potty, and eats until the routine becomes second nature and he drools when it's dinnertime. You're training your body in much the same way to eat at the best times for hormone balance. Once you start, your body will come to expect food at the same time each day. That's a good thing because anticipating—and controlling—the hunger hormone ghrelin is one of the first steps to curbing your appetite. Ghrelin is produced in higher amounts at mealtimes and when your stomach is empty, making meal timing effective in quelling a creeping ghrelin level. High levels of ghrelin tell your brain and body to gain weight and preserve fat. Here's how to stop ghrelin before it prompts cravings.

EAT ON A SCHEDULE

Once you get used to eating at these ideal times, you'll be far less likely to crave food at odd hours. Sticking to the schedule will also help you with portion control.

Breakfast between 6:00 and 8:00 a.m.
Optional very light late-morning snack (only if you get hungry),
  one hour before lunch
Lunch between 11:00 a.m. and 12:30 p.m. (before hunger
  hormone ghrelin starts creeping up)
Midafternoon snack between 3:00 and 4:00 p.m.
Dinner between 5:00 and 7:00 p.m.

EAT FOODS IN CORRECT SEQUENCE THROUGHOUT THE DAY

Hormone levels that rhythmically rise and fall daily affect how your body handles nutrients, so the components in my meals differ as well. Breakfast and lunch are when you need the most carbs. They power activity and your pancreas is trained to deliver peak insulin early in the day to process them. This is why you eat grains and fruit early in the day and legumes and fruit at lunch. Later in the day, as you wind down, you need fewer carbs and more protein instead for better hormone balance. The object is to regain control of the hormones that are currently controlling the way you look and feel. Follow the meal plans and you'll do fine.

Ask Dr. Arem: What About a Glass of Wine?

Q. Can I drink a little wine after work on this diet?

A. For Phase 1, I don't recommend any alcohol, not even wine. The purpose of this phase is to lower the glycemic index and the glycemic load of your meals, particularly in the evening, and to consume the right amount of calories for optimal weight loss. For Phase 2, if your goal is to continue to lose fat, I also would be conservative with any alcoholic consumption, especially before dinner because the sugar content and alcohol effect can enhance your appetite. In Phase 2, one or two drinks can be allowed on occasion with dinner. Some of my patients, after achieving their desired weight, are able to have a drink after work and keep the weight off, but these people are rigorous followers of the diet guidelines and the 20/10 exercise program.

MY FAVORITE FOODS

(All gluten-free when fresh, unless otherwise specified)

My Favorite Vegetables	
Category 1: Higher protein	Category 2: Lower protein
Brussels sprouts	Cucumber
Broccoli	Cabbage
Cauliflower	Mustard greens
Mushrooms (cremini)	Collard greens
Asparagus	Radish
Tofu	Celery
Okra	Garlic
Yellow summer squash	Kohlrabi
Bamboo shoots	Arugula
Chives	Endive
Zucchini	Lettuce (all varieties)
Watercress	Bok choy
Sprouts*	Radicchio
Artichoke*	Banana peppers
Kale*	Parsley
Turnips*	Eggplant
Beets*	Spinach
Yams*	Turnip greens*
Snow peas*	Onions*
Scallions (green onions)*	Fennel*
Seaweed*	Shallots*
Butternut squash*	Leeks*
	String (green) beans*
	Bell peppers and chiles*
	Carrots*

*Less often at dinner because they're higher in fructose or carbs.

My Favorite Legumes	
10 Best Picks for Legumes (best amino acid profile for weight loss)	Alternatives
Soybeans	Pinto beans
Lentils	Black-eyed peas
Black beans	Pink beans
Kidney beans	Red beans
Mung beans	Green peas
Navy beans	Adzuki beans
Chickpeas	White beans
Fava beans	
Lima beans	
Flageolet beans	

My Favorite Fruits	
Category 1: Best Picks	Category 2: Alternatives (richer in fructose or carbs; to be eaten in smaller servings)
Cranberries	Grapefruit
Blackberries	Kiwi
Raspberries	Pear
Strawberries	Blueberries
Boysenberries	Apple
Honeydew melon	Apricot
Star fruit	Elderberries
Nectarines	
Peaches	
Cantaloupe	
Mulberries	
Pumpkin	
Plum	
Papaya	
Lemon	
Lime	
Avocado*	
Olives*	
Yellow tomatoes**	
Red tomatoes**	
Tomatillos**	

* Source of fat

** Can be eaten at dinner

My Favorite Whole Grains (Phase 2 Only)		
Four Best Picks	Alternatives (eat less often due to lower fiber or high carb content)	Others
Quinoa	Teff	Corn bran
Brown rice	Couscous*	Cornflakes
Amaranth	Rye*	Oat flakes*
Bulgur*	Barley*	Oatmeal*
	Buckwheat*	Oat bran*
	Whole-grain pasta*	Wheat bran*
		Rice bran*
		Wheat germ*

*Contains gluten

My Favorite Meats, Fish, and Seafood			
Meat/Poultry	Fish	Seafood	Game Meat
Turkey	Tilapia	Scallops	Venison
Chicken	Halibut	Shrimp	Duck
Beef liver	Catfish	Crab	Quail
Beef round	Flounder	Lobster	Cornish game hen
Beef sirloin	Mahimahi	Squid (calamari)	Rabbit
Beef tenderloin	Atlantic cod	Octopus	Pheasant breast
Veal	Wild salmon	Clams	Ostrich
Flank steak	Trout	Mussels	Squab
Lamb chops	Haddock	Oysters	
Pork tenderloin	Anchovies	Other mollusks	Turkey sausage*
Goat	Bass		
	Sole		
	Pollack		
	Perch		
	Yellowtail		
	Smelt		
	Pike		
	Turbot		
	Tuna,* canned in water		
	Salmon,* canned in water		
	Tuna,* fresh		
	Herring*		
	Mackerel*		
	Grouper*		

*Eat less often because of high mercury content or high calorie count

My Favorite Nuts and Seeds (Unsalted)
Almond butter (fresh, no salt)*
Almonds
Brazil nuts
Chia seeds
Flaxseed
Hazelnuts
Mustard seeds
Peanut butter (fresh, no salt)*
Peanuts
Pecans
Pine nuts
Pumpkin seeds
Sesame seeds
Sunflower seeds
Walnuts

*Some commercial products contain gluten. Nut butters made of ground nuts only are gluten-free.

My Favorite Dairy Products (with no added sugar or sugar substitutes)
Egg whites
Fat-free cottage cheese, plain
Fat-free cream cheese
Fat-free Greek-style yogurt, plain
Fat-free yogurt, plain
Goat cheese*
Low-fat cottage cheese, plain
Low-fat cream cheese
Low-fat or nonfat mozzarella*
Low-fat ricotta cheese*
Low-fat yogurt, plain
Parmesan cheese*
Reduced-fat feta cheese*

*Higher in fat and calories. See Meal Plans for serving sizes.

My Favorite Milks (with no added sugar or sugar substitutes)
Almond milk
Soy milk

My Favorite Spices and Condiments	
Black pepper	Balsamic vinegar
Caraway	Canola oil
Cardamom, cinnamon	Cider vinegar
Coriander	Cottonseed oil
Cumin	Extra virgin olive oil
Fennel seeds	Peanut oil
Garlic	Red and green salsas*
Ginger	Red wine vinegar
Mustard	Safflower oil
Nutmeg	Sesame oil
Oregano	Soybean oil
Paprika	Tahini
Spanish saffron	White vinegar
Thyme	
Turmeric	

* Some commercial products may contain gluten.

THE BIG PICTURE ON MEALS

You'll note my meal plans include two sources of protein for breakfast and lunch and two or three sources for dinner. For example, egg whites plus low-fat cottage cheese for breakfast; beans or lentils plus poultry or fish for lunch; and lean meat—though mostly fish (five times a week)—plus optional cheese protein and two or three Category 1 vegetables for dinner. You can see it's a high-protein diet with the highest protein content at dinner for optimal fat-burning leptin and growth hormone activity. Your daily choices will supply your body with a wide variety of different proteins providing a diverse amino acid profile that optimizes mitochondrial function and calorie burning. See "Protein and Its Aminos Help You Feel Full and Burn More Calories" in Chapter 7.

The meals have other highlights.

- *Each meal includes fiber:* light vegetables like cucumber and fruit for breakfast, beans or quinoa (and vegetables) and fruit for lunch plus a salad, and vegetables from Categories 1 and 2 for dinner.
- *There are good fats in every meal,* with very little saturated fat.
- *Low-glycemic eating* at every meal.
- *Lowest-glycemic-index foods eaten at night* keep your blood sugar nice and low while you sleep so you store less fat.
- *Fruits are for breakfast and lunch only,* carefully selected on the basis of fructose, sugar, and carbohydrate content. They're eaten last so you get your sugar last. All are rich in fiber.
- *No beans for dinner* because they're rich in carbs that raise blood sugar.

MEAL PLANS

Select foods from "My Favorite Foods" above. Combine one portion from each category listed below for each meal. For any meal you can also use two items from the same category as long as you reduce the portion of each item by half. Add "free" condiments (low-calorie sauces, dressings, spices, etc.) as needed. For vegetables, feel free to exceed the suggested portions in the chart. I do not recommend deli meats because many chemicals—including high fructose corn syrup—are used in their preparation. The cheese protein source at dinner is optional. You may reduce or eliminate it if you wish to reduce caloric intake.

Ask Dr. Arem: Should I Weigh My Protein?

Q. How do I know how much 4 ounces of protein is? Should I weigh it? And is that raw or cooked?

A. The weights listed are raw food items, unless otherwise specified. I recommend you purchase a food scale to use until you're clear on the quantities you should eat. Usually you can easily see how many ounces of protein you're purchasing by looking at the net weight on the label. If a package of four chicken breasts is sold with a net weight of 28 ounces, each piece is about 7 ounces. Typically, a chicken breast or a frozen fish fillet is 7 to 8 ounces, making the recommended serving of 4 ounces slightly larger than half a chicken breast.

PHASE 1

Protein choices include turkey and salmon, a perfect way to use cooked leftovers.

BREAKFAST, PHASE 1

- Drink your Sensational Detox Smoothie (Chapter 8) and eat the raw fennel for at least the first week.
- Choose one from each category: Protein #1, Protein #2, Fiber, Fat, and Carbs.

Sample breakfast: 2 egg whites plus 1 whole egg (Protein #1), ½ cup low-fat or non-fat yogurt (Protein #2), 1½ cups cucumber (Fiber), 2 tablespoons avocado (Fats), and 1 cup blackberries (Carbs)

Protein Source #1 (egg white, poultry, fish, and meat)	Protein Source #2 (low-fat dairy, legumes)	Vegetables	Good Fats	Fruits
4 egg whites	½ cup fat-free Greek-style yogurt, plain	1½–2 cups cucumber	⅛ avocado	1 cup Category 1 favorite fruit
2 egg whites + 1 whole egg	½ cup low-fat or fat-free yogurt, plain	1 cup fennel	¼ cup tofu	½–¾ cup Category 2 favorite fruit
2–3 oz turkey	½ cup low-fat or fat-free cottage cheese	2 cups celery	1 tbsp flaxseed, ground	
		1 cup mushrooms		
	¼ cup reduced-fat feta cheese	3 cups spinach	3 walnut halves	
		2 cups radicchio		
2–3 oz smoked or canned salmon	½ oz goat cheese	1 cup zucchini	7 almonds	
	2 tbsp low-fat cream cheese	1 cup cauliflower	¾ tbsp sunflower seeds	
¼ can water-packed tuna	¼ cup low-fat ricotta cheese			
	1 cup soy or almond milk	½ cup broccoli	¾ tbsp sesame seeds	
2–3 oz scallops	2 tbsp cooked beans + ⅓ cup low-fat cottage cheese	1 cup radishes	1 tsp olive oil	
		1 cup asparagus	1 tsp vegetable oil	
2–3 oz shrimp	⅓ cup cooked beans	⅓ cup artichoke (hearts or baby)	1 tsp coconut oil	
2 egg whites + 1 oz turkey, salmon or scallops or ⅛ can water-packed tuna		¾ cup eggplant	4 kalamata olives	
		⅓ cup onion	1½ tsp almond butter	
		¾ cup seaweed	1½ tsp peanut butter	
		¾ cup peppers		

- Add and mix reduced portions of above proteins and vegetables.
- Feel free to add extra pepper, onions, broccoli, mushrooms, and spinach to your omelet.

OPTIONAL MIDMORNING SNACK, PHASE 1

Enjoy one of these snacks if you have cravings late in the morning.

Option 1	½ cup baby carrots + 2 tbsp hummus
Option 2	½ cup baby carrots + 6 almonds
Option 3	½ cup baby carrots + 6 hazelnuts
Option 4	¼ cup berries + 6 almonds

LUNCH, PHASE 1

Choose one from each category. Note that lunch has two protein sources from meat, fish, or cheese, and legumes or quinoa.

Sample lunch: 4 oz fish (Protein #1), 1 cup lentils (Protein #2), 1 cup broccoli (Fiber), ⅛ avocado (Fat), and 1 cup blackberries (Carbs)

Protein Source #1 (egg white, poultry, fish, meat, and cheese)	Protein Source #2 (legumes and quinoa)	Vegetables	Good Fats	Fruits
2–3 oz chicken or any other meat from the Favorite Foods	1 cup cooked lentils or beans (excluding chickpeas, adzuki beans)	1 cup Category 2 vegetables	⅛ avocado	1 cup Category 1 favorite fruit
2–4 oz turkey, light	¾ cup cooked quinoa, chickpeas, adzuki beans	⅓–½ cup Category 1 vegetables	¼ cup tofu	½–¾ cup Category 2 favorite fruit
⅓ cup reduced-fat feta cheese				
1 oz goat cheese				
½ cup low-fat ricotta cheese				
2–4 oz fish*	2 slices Protein Boost Diet Quinoa Sandwich Bread (see Recipes)		1 tsp olive oil	
3–4 oz shellfish			1 tsp vegetable oil	
2–3 oz canned water-packed salmon			1 tsp coconut oil	
½–¾ cup shredded nonfat mozzarella			4 kalamata olives	
½–¾ can water-packed tuna				
3 egg whites + 2 cups any Category 1 vegetable				
3 egg whites + ¼ cup water-packed tuna or salmon				

*For fresh salmon, 2–3 oz

AFTERNOON SNACK, PHASE 1

Option 1	10 almonds
Option 2	8 hazelnuts
Option 3	5 walnut halves
Option 4	10 peanuts (no salt)
Option 5	1 cup raw broccoli
Option 6	1 cup cucumber + 2 tbsp hummus
Option 7	1 cup raw brussels sprouts
Option 8	½ cup baby carrots + 2 tbsp hummus

DINNER, PHASE 1

Choose one from each category.

Protein Source #1 (poultry, seafood, and meat)	Protein Source #2 (cheeses) (Optional)	Protein Source #3 / Fiber Source #1 (Category 1 vegetables or quinoa)	Vegetables	Good Fats
5–8 oz turkey or other lean meats	½–¾ oz goat cheese	2 cups Category 1 vegetables (excluding tofu)	1–2 cups Category 1 vegetables (excluding tofu)	⅛ avocado
4–6 oz chicken or lean meat	3 tbsp reduced-fat feta			¼ cup tofu
6–8 oz fish*	¼ cup low-fat or fat-free mozzarella	½ cup cooked quinoa**		1 tsp olive oil
6–8 oz shellfish	3 tbsp grated Parmesan		2–4 cups Category 2 vegetables	1 tsp coconut oil
¾–1 cup tofu				1 tsp vegetable oil
4–6 oz game meat				4 kalamata olives

* For fresh salmon, 4–5 oz

** No more than twice weekly

PHASE 2

In this second phase, you'll continue eating exactly the same protein, fiber, fat, and fruit combinations. The only difference is that now you can eat some grains or grain-derived foods, which are good sources of protein and fiber. Since they also provide carbs, portions of whole-grain foods may replace other sources of carbs such as legumes and fruits. Protein choices include turkey and salmon, a perfect way to use cooked leftovers (not deli types, although canned salmon is fine).

BREAKFAST, PHASE 2

- Choose one from each category: Protein #1, Protein #2, Fiber, Fats, and Carbs (grains and fruits).

Protein Source #1 (egg white, poultry, fish, and meat)	Protein Source #2 (low-fat dairy, legumes)	Vegetables	Good Fats	Grains and Quinoa	Fruits
4 egg whites	½ cup fat-free Greek-style yogurt	1½–2 cups cucumber	⅛ avocado	1 packet instant oatmeal, plain	¼ cup Category 1 favorite fruits
2 egg whites + 1 whole egg	½ cup low-fat or fat-free yogurt, plain	1 cup fennel	¼ cup tofu	1 slice whole-grain bread	
				1 slice Protein Boost Diet Quinoa Sandwich Bread (see Recipes)	
2–3 oz turkey	½ cup low-fat or fat-free cottage cheese	1–2 cups celery	1 tbsp flaxseed, ground	1 cup cereal*	
	¼ cup reduced-fat feta cheese	1 cup mushrooms			
		3 cups spinach	3 walnut halves		
		2 cups radicchio			
2–3 oz smoked or canned salmon	½ oz goat cheese	1 cup zucchini	7 almonds		
	2 tbsp low-fat cream cheese	1 cup cauliflower	¾ tbsp sunflower seeds		
¼ can water-packed tuna	¼ cup low-fat ricotta cheese				
	1 cup soy or almond milk	½ cup broccoli	¾ tbsp sesame seeds	1 cup oat bran	

2–3 oz scallops	2 tbsp cooked beans + ⅓ cup low-fat cottage cheese	1 cup radishes 1 cup asparagus	1 tsp olive oil 1 tsp vegetable oil		¼ cup Category 1 favorite fruits
2–3 oz shrimp	⅓ cup cooked beans	⅓ cup artichoke	1 tsp coconut oil		
2 egg whites + 1 oz turkey, salmon, or scallops, or ⅛ can water-packed tuna		¾ cup eggplant	4 kalamata olives		
		⅓ cup onion	1½ tsp almond butter		
		¾ cup seaweed ¾ cup peppers	1½ tsp peanut butter		

*Recommended cereals: TOTAL Whole Grain, Special K Low-Carb Lifestyle Protein Plus, All-Bran Complete Wheat Flakes, and Smart Start Strong Heart Original Antioxidants

- Add and mix reduced portions of above proteins and vegetables.
- Feel free to add extra pepper, onions, broccoli, mushrooms, and spinach to your omelet.

MIDMORNING SNACK, PHASE 2

Enjoy one of these midmorning snacks if you have late-morning cravings.

Option 1	½ cup baby carrots + 2 tbsp hummus
Option 2	½ cup baby carrots + 6 almonds
Option 3	½ cup baby carrots + 6 hazelnuts
Option 4	¼ cup berries + 6 almonds

LUNCH, PHASE 2

Choose one from each category. Note that your lunch has two protein sources.

Protein Source #1 (egg white, poultry, fish, meat, and cheese)	Protein Source #2 (legumes, grains, and quinoa)***	Vegetables	Good Fats	Fruits
2–3 oz chicken or any other meat from Favorite Foods	1 cup cooked lentils or beans (excluding chickpeas and adzuki beans)	1 cup Category 2 vegetables	⅛ avocado	1 cup Category 2 fruit
2–4 oz turkey, light ½ cup reduced-fat feta cheese 1 oz goat cheese ½ cup low-fat ricotta cheese	½–¾ cup cooked quinoa, chickpeas, or adzuki beans	⅓–½ cup Category 1 vegetables	¼ cup tofu	½–¾ cup Category 2 fruit
2–4 oz fish* 3–4 oz shellfish 2–3 oz water-packed canned salmon	Pizza with Quinoa Pizza Dough (see Recipes; toppings to be chosen from other food categories)		1 tsp olive oil 1 tsp vegetable oil	
½–¾ cup shredded nonfat mozzarella	2 slices Protein Boost Diet Quinoa Sandwich Bread (see Recipes)		1 tsp coconut oil	
	2 slices whole-grain bread**		4 kalamata olives	
	½–¾ cup whole grains (brown rice, multigrain pasta, etc.)			
½–¾ can water-packed tuna				
3 egg whites + 2 cups any Category 1 vegetables				
3 egg whites + ¼ can water-packed tuna or salmon				

* For fresh salmon, 2–3 oz

** See "Shopping Lists" in Chapter 9 for discussion of whole-grain breads.

*** If you choose to eat grains, reduce fruit portion by half to minimize sugar load. Also limit to twice weekly.

AFTERNOON SNACK, PHASE 2

Option 1	10 almonds
Option 2	8 hazelnuts
Option 3	5 walnut halves
Option 4	10 peanuts (no salt)
Option 5	1 cup raw broccoli
Option 6	1 cup cucumber + 2 tbsp hummus
Option 7	1 cup raw brussels sprouts
Option 8	½ cup baby carrots + 2 tbsp hummus

DINNER, PHASE 2

Choose one from each category.

Protein Source #1 (poultry, seafood, and meat)	Protein Source #2 (cheese) (Optional)	Protein Source #3 (Category 1 vegetables and grains)**	Vegetables	Good Fats
5–8 oz turkey, or other lean meats	½–¾ oz goat cheese	2 cups Category 1 vegetables (excluding tofu)	1–2 cups Category 1 vegetables (excluding tofu)	⅛ avocado
4–6 oz chicken or lean meat	3 tbsp reduced-fat feta	½ cup cooked quinoa, brown rice, bulgur, teff, couscous, or amaranth	2–4 cups Category 2 vegetable	¼ cup tofu
6–8 oz fish*	¼ cup low-fat or fat-free mozzarella			1 tsp olive oil
6–8 oz shellfish	3 tbsp grated Parmesan			1 tsp coconut oil
				1 tsp vegetable oil
¾–1 cups tofu				4 kalamata olives
4–6 oz game meat		½ cup cooked whole grain pasta		

*For fresh salmon, 4–5 oz

**Grains to be included no more than two times weekly.

CREATE YOUR OWN PHASE 1 AND 2 MENUS

The goal is roughly 1,200 to 1,500 calories per day and to follow these flexible guidelines for each meal. Adjust your portions according to your frame and physical activity. For example, reduce portions if you are less active or small-framed; the best way to accomplish this is to reduce the fruit portion at lunch, and reduce or eliminate the cheese component at dinnertime. If you have a larger frame and/or are physically very active, you can slightly increase the meat or fish protein source at lunch and dinnertime.

BREAKFAST, PHASE 1

Roughly 250 to 300 calories

- **4 egg whites** or substitute 2–3 oz lean meat (such as salmon or turkey), 3 oz seafood, or ¼ can water-packed tuna
- ½ **cup low-fat cottage cheese** or substitute ½ cup fat-free Greek-style yogurt, ⅓ cup cooked beans, 1 cup soy or almond milk, ¼ cup cheese (reduced-fat feta or low-fat ricotta), ½ oz goat cheese, or 2 tbsp low-fat cream cheese
- 1½ **cups cucumber** or substitute same amount of any Category 1 or 2 vegetables
- ⅛ **avocado** or substitute ¼ cup tofu, 1 tbsp ground flaxseed, 3 walnut halves, 7 almonds, 1 tsp oil, ½ tsp almond butter or peanut butter, or 4 olives
- **1 cup berries** or substitute papaya or ½ cup of Category 2 fruits

BREAKFAST, PHASE 2

Same as Phase 1, but you can add the same amount of grains listed in Breakfast Meal Plans and a reduced fruit portion (restrict to Category 1 fruits).

LUNCH, PHASE 1

Roughly 400 to 500 calories

- **2–3 oz turkey** or substitute 3 egg whites plus 2 cups Category 1 or 2 vegetables, ⅓ cup reduced-fat feta cheese, ½ cup low-fat ricotta cheese, 1 oz goat cheese, 2–4 oz fish or seafood, or 2–3 oz any other meat from the Favorite Foods list.
- **¾–1 cup cooked beans or lentils** or substitute ¾ cup cooked quinoa, or 1 portion Quinoa Pizza or Quinoa Flatbread
- **1 cup cucumbers** or substitute any Category 2 vegetable, or ⅓–½ cup Category 1 vegetable
- **⅛ avocado** or substitute 1 tsp oil (vegetable, olive, or coconut), 4 kalamata olives, or ¼ cup tofu
- **1 cup Category 1 fruit** or substitute ½–¾ cup Category 2 fruit

LUNCH, PHASE 2

Same as Phase 1, but you can substitute quinoa for the same amount of grains listed in Lunch Meal Plans. Also, if you select grains, reduce fruit portion by half.

DINNER, PHASE 1

Roughly 400 to 500 calories

- **6–8 oz fish or shellfish** or substitute ¾ cup tofu, 4–6 oz chicken or veal, 4–6 oz game, or 5–8 oz turkey
- **¼ cup low-fat or fat-free mozzarella** or substitute 3 tbsp reduced-fat feta or ½ oz goat cheese
- **1 cup each of three or four different Category 1 vegetables** or substitute 2 cups Category 1 vegetables + 2–4 cups Category 2 vegetables, or 2 cups Category 1 vegetables + ½ cup quinoa
- **1 tsp oil (vegetable, coconut, or olive)** or substitute ⅛ avocado, ¼ cup tofu (but not if tofu was chosen as main protein), or 4 kalamata olives

DINNER, PHASE 2

Same as Phase 1, but you can substitute quinoa for the same amount of grains listed in dinner meal plans. Limit substitution to twice a week.

THE PROTEIN BOOST DIET FOR LIFE

Once you reach your ideal body weight, you'll feel energetic and very good about yourself. To maintain your new body and metabolism, just continue eating the Phase 2 food choices (increase food portions judiciously to keep a constant healthy weight) and continue to follow all other program components—stress reduction, sleep, the 20/10 workout. And remember, if you've ever been overweight at any point in your life, you're susceptible to gaining that weight back. Stay within the rules of the eating plan for the rest of your life, so you can stay as trim, healthy, and youthful as possible. One last thing: keep your antioxidant system up to gear at all times by taking your daily comprehensive mix of antioxidants (see Chapter 8).

CHAPTER ELEVEN

THE 20/10 EXERCISE PROGRAM

My 20/10 program is a brand-new protocol for exercising as efficiently as possible, making every move count toward your svelte new profile while boosting brainpower, too. If—like me—you dislike spending a lot of time working out, you'll share my excitement at the new research showing it's possible to achieve maximum exercise benefits in minimal time.

Take twenty minutes of cardio-focused high-intensity interval training plus ten minutes of strength training, add a little stretching to the mix, and you get the half-hour mind-body workout you've been waiting for. Who knew effective exercise didn't require long, hard hours of sweaty strain? Knowledge is power. You've got it right here.

Remember, every time you exercise you're charging up your cells' power plants, the mitochondria, and strengthening your metabolism so it burns calories at a faster rate even when you're sitting. Exercise is vital to keeping you youthful, trim, smart, and happy, and it also actually increases new cell growth in your brain, having the same effect on cell generation as an antidepressant. Animal research demonstrates up to a triple increase in brain cell generation in the hippocampus, the brain structure that regulates mood. Exercise also improves your immune system by enhancing the circulation of immune-related cells through your bloodstream.

The 20/10 workout is built on a formula that requires spending less time mindlessly exercising and spending more energy focusing on performance. This in turn accelerates your energy level because you're pushing your mitochondria to work better even when you're not exercising—the well-functioning metabolism we've been aiming for. I created the 20/10 program, and I designed it specifically to be easily folded into the busiest life. As you'll see later in this chapter, it can even be adapted for travel.

Many people still erroneously think weight is a simple matter of calories eaten and calories burned—that less food plus an increase in exercise equals weight loss. The reality is a bit more complex. Studies show that exercise alone results in minimal weight loss when compared with watching your food intake alone, the latter resulting in nearly twice as much weight loss. But here's the kicker: combining the two increases initial weight loss by a massive 20 percent compared with diet alone. Follow my diet and other recommendations for hormone balancing and do about half an hour of exercise daily to give yourself the very best chance of getting control of your weight. Many studies show that exercise plays a significant role in weight maintenance, even more important once you start shedding pounds.

Three aspects of my workout keep the switch on your metabolism set to high calorie burning.

- *People who exercise in intense spurts (high-intensity interval training or HIIT)* have about a 15 percent higher resting metabolic rate (meaning they burn 15 percent more calories when doing nothing) than sedentary counterparts of the same age, gender, and muscle mass. That means this workout triggers your body to burn more calories even at rest. Muscle also produces hormones including myokines and recently discovered irisin that make white fat turn into metabolism-accelerating brown fat. Exercise causes your muscles to release these hormones, which in turn increase the activity of mitochondria, making your body burn more fat.

- *Strength training* builds lean muscle mass, the main contributor to a resting metabolic rate.

- *Relaxation techniques* (see Chapter 4) help you cope with stress and its counterpart, compulsive eating, reining in your emotional brain and its authority over hormone balance. We also know that practicing relaxation techniques regularly relieves anger, tension, and confusion.

Many of us gained weight because we didn't make eating well a priority and our lives were too busy for us to exercise. That's why I kept the 20/10 workout simple and easy to complete in half an hour. What's most important is that you stay with the program and begin to enjoy its rich benefits, physical and mental. Both the high-intensity cardio (the 20) and strength training (the 10) incorporate focused intensity to achieve maximum weight-loss results in a short-ened time. Plus, your energy and mood will zoom upward.

Start the 20/10 workout and stick with it. As you build more lean muscle alongside your improved metabolism, exercising will become exponentially easier. And one day you'll wonder how you ever lived without it.

EFFECTS OF EXERCISE ON APPETITE

One question I hear from my patients a lot is this: "But Dr. Arem, won't exercising give me more of an appetite?" The answer is no. Physical activity has actually been shown to modulate appetite for the better, helping your body recognize that it's eaten enough in the previous meal and feel more easily satisfied during your next meal. When you're active, your body is better able to detect how much you need to eat and adjust its intake at subsequent meals. On the other hand, sitting a lot can easily lead to trouble controlling hunger. Eating a large lunch, for example, causes your body to "want" a similarly large calorie load at the next meal. Recently, scientists have been researching the effects of physical exercise on appetite, and they've seen exercise produce better short-term and long-term appetite control.

THE CARDIO 20: HIGH-INTENSITY INTERVAL TRAINING (HIIT)

For decades, scientists thought extended periods of cardio—long hours on the treadmill or jogging—were key to losing weight. However, the most recent research shows that high-intensity interval training (HIIT) is effective for fat reduction, especially in people who are overweight, and it's an incredible time-saver. HIIT is a workout made up of short bursts of fast-as-you-can cardio exercise, such as pedaling a stationary bike, followed by lower-intensity exercise or rest before you push through the next interval.

Your goal is the all-important enhancement of your resting metabolic rate, sign of a highly functioning metabolism, so your body continues to burn calories while you're at your desk or relaxing. The point of exercising is not fatigue after burning calories, but rather to boost calorie burn even after you stop exercising. Studies show that HIIT makes you burn more calories and leads to increased production of the thyroid hormone thyroxine (T4), which itself speeds up your metabolism.

At the hormone level you benefit tremendously from HIIT. Look at the evidence.

FAT-BLASTING CATECHOLAMINES

Levels of catecholamines (adrenaline and noradrenaline—aka epinephrine and norepinephrine—hormones released by your adrenal glands and the autonomic nervous system) rise immediately after high-intensity exercise, acting on fat cells to make them break down fat and release it into the bloodstream for further breakdown. Catecholamines have the ability to break down both subcutaneous fat and fat found in muscles. What's even more exciting is that research shows that HIIT has the potential to make you burn more fat around your waist and in your abdomen as well.

SUGAR-FLUSHING CORTISOL

To keep blood sugar from falling below normal during HIIT, cortisol rises briefly, triggering the sugar stores in your liver to break down and be released into the bloodstream as an immediate form of energy for muscles to perform adequately.

MUSCLE-BUILDING GROWTH HORMONE

HIIT also kicks up levels of growth hormone (GH), encouraging your body to burn extra fat and build lean muscle. In people sprinting on a treadmill for just thirty seconds of short-burst HIIT, levels of GH were higher than in those training for endurance (longer periods of exercise). Remarkably, GH concentration was ten times higher in the high-intensity group even one hour after cooling down. During exercise, GH prevents blood sugar from falling below normal, keeping sugar available for the muscles to use. Essential GH also helps break down fat in fat cells. In general, higher GH levels have an overall metabolism-boosting effect, enhancing insulin sensitivity and consequently minimizing fat accumulation.

QUICK FAT-BURNING RESPONSE TO HORMONES

Fat burning occurs quickly during HIIT, peaking for untrained women at twenty minutes (ten minutes for trained athletic women). In other words, you reach the summit of fat burn at twenty minutes or less—and that's the end of your HIIT cardio period. Also important: when compared with people doing slower, steady aerobic exercise, people who did HIIT lost more fat. The decrease in fat occurs whether you have a lot of abdominal fat or not. That means regardless of how much extra fat you're trying to shed, HIIT will help you do it.

DAMPED-DOWN INSULIN

Remember, high insulin means fat accumulation. Look at these numbers, based on data from a collection of studies. Within just three months after HIIT was added to their workout, participants' insulin sensitivity increased anywhere from 19 to 58 percent, a staggering improvement in the ability of their bodies to use insulin and keep levels low.

These remarkable results tell the story of HIIT's effectiveness.

- *Nearly 50 percent belly fat loss in just eight weeks:* A study of type 2 diabetic men found that those who exercised with HIIT for just eight weeks decreased their abdominal fat by nearly 50 percent. The relationship of HIIT to weight loss seems to be that the more body fat you have, the greater the reduction in fat—a powerful result indeed when you consider that intermittent bursts of exertion during a twenty-minute workout are beneficial to all body types.
- *Your body starts using its energy stores (fat) more efficiently* within seven weeks after you start HIIT.
- *These workouts boost overall metabolic activity,* meaning you burn more calories regardless of your activity level when you're not exercising.
- *In as little as two weeks, your muscle oxidative capacity can significantly increase,* which means your muscles and mitochondria start burning more fat for energy.
- *The long-term response of your body* to exercising with HIIT includes better all-around fitness, skeletal muscle endurance, decreased fasting insulin and insulin resistance, and best of all, an increase in fat loss.

THE PERFECTING 10: STRENGTH TRAINING

Strength training, also called "resistance training," has been shown to significantly increase total calorie burn. In this portion of my 20/10 program, you'll be working your muscles against weight to build them up. You can accomplish this by working with weight machines, free weights, or rubber bands, or simply by pushing against your own weight, as you do during a push-up. As you increase the amount of muscle you have through strength training, your resting metabolic rate increases. The 10 portion of the 20/10 helps you create this lean muscle, which leads to the high-functioning metabolism that burns

Ask Dr. Arem: High-Intensity Exercise
to Stimulate Growth Hormone

Q. I've heard high-intensity interval training makes the pituitary gland generate more growth hormone, which you say breaks down fats and speeds up
metabolism. Is it true that doing your high-intensity workout every other
day can boost my growth hormone levels?

A. Amazingly, yes, it can. High-intensity interval training (HIIT) does stimulate growth hormone production, and it's growth hormone that helps your
body build muscle and stay youthful. Here's how it works: HIIT's short,
intense bursts of cardio, by stretching muscle, trigger the pituitary gland
to increase its production of growth hormone to strengthen the muscle.
HIIT also builds more calorie-burning mitochondria in your cells and thus
expands your ability to burn more fat in the long run. As you age, your
body produces less growth hormone, but with this type of exercise you
elevate growth hormone levels so you can reacquire—and maintain—the
metabolism of your glory days.

calories 24/7. This kind of training also strengthens your bones and
improves posture. You won't look like a bodybuilder using my program. Instead, you'll develop a stronger, leaner look—muscle instead
of fat, remember?

STRETCHING

Flexibility is essential when you're building muscle and working hard
at cardio. It can prevent soreness, increase your range of motion, and
minimize injury. It also helps you maintain proper form throughout your ten minutes of strength training, where form is everything.

Give yourself five minutes to stretch and warm up your body
before your workout. Move through the five stretches below, holding
each for 30 seconds on both sides, and never bouncing.

You can learn lots of other stretches from yoga instructors, stretch
exercise classes, or a personal trainer.

Take a couple of five-minute stretch breaks daily to keep muscles loose and posture perfect. You'll be amazed at how well stretching relieves the stiffness you might feel after sitting at a computer
all day.

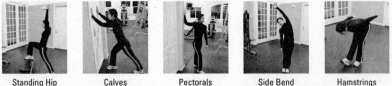

| Standing Hip Flexors | Calves | Pectorals | Side Bend | Hamstrings |

Ten to fifteen minutes of yoga is a perfect trifecta of strength, stretching, and relaxation. Some of my patients who choose yoga as their relaxation technique (see Chapter 4) incorporate its powerful poses into both stretching and strength training. Yoga looks fluid and easy when done by people with great strength . . . and yoga is how they usually got so strong.

Tamara, a 37-year-old lawyer at a large law firm in downtown Los Angeles, had neither the time nor the energy to lose the 100 pounds she'd gained between working full-time and raising her two children. She told me she hadn't had any drastic weight gain until she started having children. She said she'd been very self-conscious and determined to lose a lot of weight while she was in college and law school. At one point, Tamara was thinner than average at size 2. But once she got pregnant with her son, she gained thirty pounds, and she held on to twenty of it after having him. Five years later she gained fifty pounds when she became pregnant with her second son. After delivery, she gained even more. "I would have lost some of that weight, but my son was so sick we spent most of our time at the hospital for one month, and we ate fast food there because there was nowhere else to eat. I just couldn't leave him," she explained. "Not only did I not lose the baby weight; I gained. I thought, 'Well, when the baby gets better I'll work on losing it,' but I've never been able to."

Tamara originally became my patient because she had a history of Hashimoto's thyroiditis (an autoimmune attack on the thyroid gland) and wanted to make sure she was getting the best treatment. She also understood she needed to lose 100 pounds. "At my age, it's not that I'm so vain, but I'm acutely aware of how other people perceive me and that's definitely affected my career in the last few years," said Tamara. "I deliberately don't take certain cases where I know I'll have to be in front of a jury because I think it would be very difficult. Their perception of you is everything, and I don't want to put myself in that position because I think it could harm my client.

This is terrible on so many levels, plus it's changed my career path and that's huge for me."

Tamara knew she had to start taking her weight issue seriously. A few weeks before seeing me, she'd started exercising for an hour, two or three days a week. She told me she'd stopped exercising because she felt exhausted and hungry, and the next day, her appetite would rage out of control. "I'd get some fast food on the way to pick up my kids, and of course then I'd feel guilty and ride my stationary bike for an hour. I don't have time to work out like I did when I was thirty. So I stopped."

Tamara listened carefully as I explained the benefits of high-intensity interval training. I recommended that she use her stationary bike and follow my 20/10 program. She knew changing her diet was imperative and started eating according to my hormone-friendly program.

When Tamara returned for her six-month follow-up, she weighed 196 pounds, down from 250 when we first met. She smiled and said, "I still have fifty pounds to go, but just watch me lose it in the next few months! Over the past couple of months, I've lost three pounds a week. I *love* this half-hour workout, which I can get done before I leave for work. Plus, I've lost five inches off my waist already."

THE 20/10 WORKOUT

The 20/10 workout includes the three important types of exercise: aerobic/cardio, strength training, and stretching. I designed it so you can cover it all in minimal time. In addition, because you can adjust frequency, speed, and intensity according to your capabilities, you can start and continue to follow the 20/10 program regardless of your fitness level.

The 20/10 has two major parts—twenty minutes of aerobic plus ten minutes of strength training—and you'll want to stretch (see "Stretching" in this chapter, above) before starting them.

- High-intensity 20: do this every other day—20 minutes of high-intensity interval training (HIIT, routines described below)

- Low-intensity 20: do this every day in between—20 minutes of walking, biking, or other regular aerobic exercises
- Perfecting 10: do this every day—10 minutes of strength training (routines described below)

Most likely you'll need to get back into the swing of an exercising routine, and by that I mean sticking with a half-hour workout each day. Don't push too hard as you begin in anticipation of seeing fast results, but don't baby yourself, either. Know that the health risks of *not exercising* are highest of all. You can do this, and the results will be spectacular. Don't fall into the trap of giving yourself a break on your workout after you lose weight. The only outcome you can expect is regaining it. Adult women who lost 10 percent of their initial body weight and engaged in exercise for thirty to forty minutes a day were able to keep the weight off for two years, the duration of the study. Multiple studies show that people who don't exercise after losing weight soon gain it back.

Once you get in the habit of doing the 20/10, you'll realize how much better you feel with regular exercise. This is because working out increases feel-good endorphins and elevates mood, decreasing stress and any depression or anxiety you feel.

THE HIGH-INTENSITY 20

The most vital part of your workout routine, whether you're losing or maintaining weight, is the cardio portion. During these twenty minutes, you'll raise your heart rate in 30-second bursts as vigorously as your body can handle. A stationary bike offers the best means of safely accomplishing high-intensity interval training, and you don't need fancy equipment. Some bikes have adjustments that make the resistance stronger (making pedaling harder), and this is a useful feature. You can start with the easiest pedaling and soon you'll be adjusting upward.

Consult your physician, as with any other health advice, before starting if you're over 40 and/or have a heart condition. Begin your 30-second bursts by pedaling as fast as you can. The exercise intensity that leads to the highest rate of fat burn is about 60 to 70 percent of maximum oxygen consumption by your body or about 70 to

80 percent of your maximum heart rate. Put simply: push yourself during the 30-second fast-as-you-can bursts, pedaling hard enough so you can't speak.

As you move into your second or third week, gradually increase the resistance on the bike. Counting revolutions is one way to track your progress. Once you've reached a plateau, up your challenge by increasing the resistance. Progression varies from person to person, but after a few weeks (or even sooner) you should feel that you can handle a higher level of exertion. You don't have to keep a record of how you progress with the HIIT, but it can give you exciting proof of your improvement. Note when you started the 20/10, and monitor your progress.

Follow this formula for an effective high-intensity interval training (HIIT) workout using a stationary bike.

Warm up with 2 minutes of stretches
Pedal as fast as you can for 30 seconds
Relaxed pedaling for 4 minutes
Pedal as fast as you can for 30 seconds
Relaxed pedaling for 4 minutes
Pedal as fast as you can for 30 seconds
Relaxed pedaling for 4 minutes
Pedal as fast as you can for 30 seconds
Relaxed pedaling for 4 minutes

If you have the option to increase intensity on your stationary bike, try this slightly different plan using a higher resistance.

Warm up, cycling at a moderate pace for 5 minutes. Then do six segments of
    Pedaling at a higher resistance and fast pace for 30 seconds
    Pedaling at moderate resistance and speed for 2 minutes

Are you obese or very frail? Try this lower-intensity interval workout. Most of my extremely overweight patients, along with those who are frail, are able to begin HIIT with a lower-intensity program like this.

Warm up, walking at a brisk pace for 5 minutes
Set a timer for 20 minutes and press the start button
Power-walk or jog lightly for 15 seconds (use a watch with a
    sweep-second hand to monitor time)
Walk briskly for 1 minute
Repeat for 20 minutes

Many businesses are investing in employee health by offering on-site fitness centers and a wellness staff (such as registered dietitians and fitness professionals). The power of wellness is evident in the pay-off: by reducing health risks through corporate wellness programs, one study revealed savings of $311,755 over one year, with returns typically seen in reduced health care expenses, increased productivity, and reduced employee turnover due to job satisfaction. Some forward-thinking employers offer discounted memberships to local gyms and health clubs. If your employer does, snap up the offer. You can easily follow my program there on the latest stationary bike or in a pool.

You can apply the same HIIT formula to swimming, going as hard as you can during your 30-second intervals followed by easy swimming until your next 30-second burst. Water is fifteen times more resistant than air, but it's easy on your joints if you have arthritis. Swimming is also good for pregnant women.

I don't recommend running or biking outdoors for HIIT because with running, you'll be slamming your knee joints, and the risk of injury is high. With biking, it's difficult to watch for traffic and pedal flat-out. Still, I have a couple of high-performing patients who are able to do their HIIT outside on a bike successfully. You'll find out what works for you.

THE PERFECTING 10

This scientifically based series of strength training moves is designed to slim your waistline, build nice, lean, calorie-burning muscle, and tone your entire body. I designed it with the help of an exercise specialist. Each day you'll focus on a specific muscle group, performing five exercises carefully selected to address problem areas. Because abdominal fat is essential to eliminate, you'll focus on your core three times a week.

Remember: always stretch first.

Follow this 10-minute formula for the most efficient strength training workout.

1. Start with the Day 1 exercise set. For each of the five moves, do 30 seconds of continuous repetition (about 12 to 15 reps) with 30 seconds of rest in between exercises.

2. Repeat Step 1, going though each of the five exercises again, switching from the right side to the left side if applicable.

3. In the days that follow, move to the Day 2 through 7 exercises, performing them using the same routine. Return to the Day 1 moves after a week and continue.

4. As you become stronger, increase to 45 seconds of continuous repetitions (about 15 to 20 reps) with 15 seconds of rest in between exercises.

5. Add free weights when you're ready for more resistance.

Over seven days, you'll work on a different part of your body, sculpting it to perfection. The only equipment needed is a resistance band for a few of the exercises. The most important part of toning your core muscles—your abdominals (or abs)—is learning to breathe. Breathe by expanding your chest outward and keeping your core tight, drawing air in through your nose and exhaling through pursed lips during the exertion portion of your move. Mastering this method of breathing helps tighten your core while you walk, stand, do yoga, or do other exercises. It's essential to breathe right and keep your core muscles tight through each move.

Use a mirror to check your form—good form means good muscle control, and it's everything!

This strength training will also address problem areas such as flabby arms or a protruding belly. The reason for rotating the focus is that muscles need time to recover. The seven daily sets are designed so you'll be working your abs at least three times a week. Go ahead and add abdominal exercises every day as long as your core isn't sore. Because you're slimming and toning your core muscles during this phase, the core exercises consist of light movements with higher repetitions.

Don't try to "max out" on any exercise. It's important that you gradually increase resistance to match your growing muscles. Initial ambition to push the limit can backfire if you make your body too sore to continue your daily workout.

For all exercises one set equals 30 seconds. Some patients like to set a timer while others look at a clock with a second hand.

DAY 1: FRONT OF BODY (INCLUDING YOUR BELLY)

1. CRUNCHES

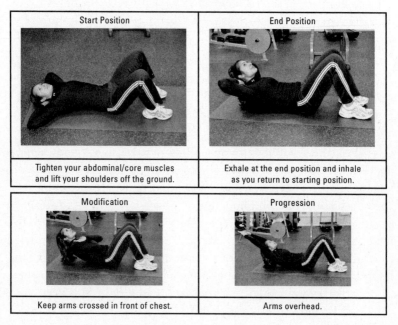

Start Position	End Position
Tighten your abdominal/core muscles and lift your shoulders off the ground.	Exhale at the end position and inhale as you return to starting position.
Modification	Progression
Keep arms crossed in front of chest.	Arms overhead.

COMMON ERROR

- Lifting head only, which works the neck muscles instead of the abdominals

2. LEG RAISES

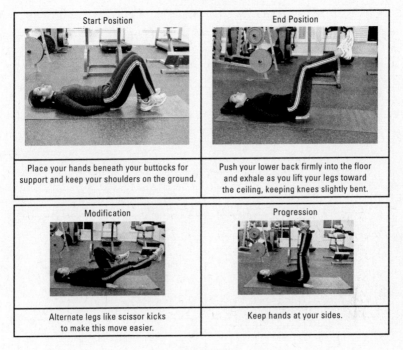

Start Position	End Position
Place your hands beneath your buttocks for support and keep your shoulders on the ground.	Push your lower back firmly into the floor and exhale as you lift your legs toward the ceiling, keeping knees slightly bent.

Modification	Progression
Alternate legs like scissor kicks to make this move easier.	Keep hands at your sides.

COMMON ERRORS

- Allowing lower back to arch
- Allowing feet to extend out too far

3. PUSH-UPS

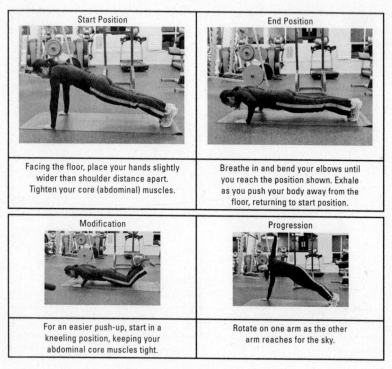

Start Position	End Position
Facing the floor, place your hands slightly wider than shoulder distance apart. Tighten your core (abdominal) muscles.	Breathe in and bend your elbows until you reach the position shown. Exhale as you push your body away from the floor, returning to start position.
Modification	Progression
For an easier push-up, start in a kneeling position, keeping your abdominal core muscles tight.	Rotate on one arm as the other arm reaches for the sky.

COMMON ERRORS

- Not engaging the core area
- Shrugging shoulders
- Allowing abdomen to sag

4. RESISTANCE BAND SHOULDER PRESS

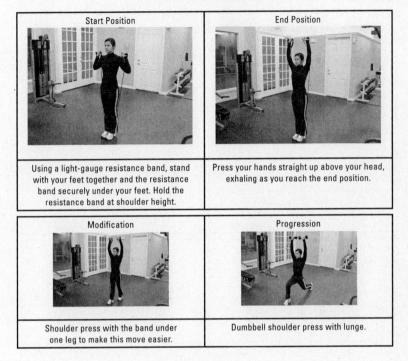

Start Position	End Position
Using a light-gauge resistance band, stand with your feet together and the resistance band securely under your feet. Hold the resistance band at shoulder height.	Press your hands straight up above your head, exhaling as you reach the end position.

Modification	Progression
Shoulder press with the band under one leg to make this move easier.	Dumbbell shoulder press with lunge.

COMMON ERRORS

- Arching lower back, a result of engaging core muscles
- Not maintaining good posture

5. RESISTANCE BAND CHEST PRESS

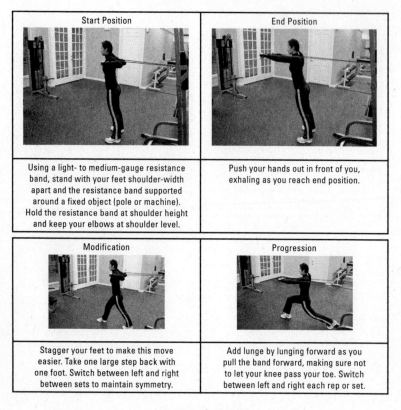

Start Position	End Position
Using a light- to medium-gauge resistance band, stand with your feet shoulder-width apart and the resistance band supported around a fixed object (pole or machine). Hold the resistance band at shoulder height and keep your elbows at shoulder level.	Push your hands out in front of you, exhaling as you reach end position.
Modification	Progression
Stagger your feet to make this move easier. Take one large step back with one foot. Switch between left and right between sets to maintain symmetry.	Add lunge by lunging forward as you pull the band forward, making sure not to let your knee pass your toe. Switch between left and right each rep or set.

COMMON ERRORS

- Dropping elbows
- Shrugging shoulders

DAY 2: CORE (INCLUDING HIPS AND THIGHS)

1. QUADRUPED

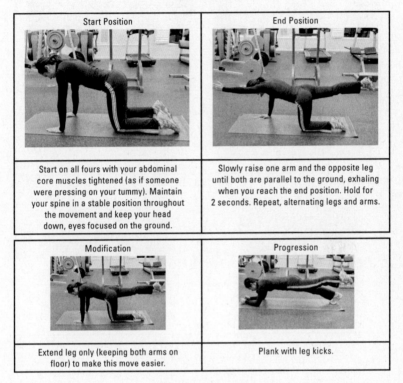

Start Position	End Position
Start on all fours with your abdominal core muscles tightened (as if someone were pressing on your tummy). Maintain your spine in a stable position throughout the movement and keep your head down, eyes focused on the ground.	Slowly raise one arm and the opposite leg until both are parallel to the ground, exhaling when you reach the end position. Hold for 2 seconds. Repeat, alternating legs and arms.

Modification	Progression
Extend leg only (keeping both arms on floor) to make this move easier.	Plank with leg kicks.

COMMON ERRORS

- Arching lower back and not bracing core (abdominals) throughout
- Head looking forward instead of down throughout movement

2. SIDE PLANK

Start Position	End Position
Lie on your side with your forearm directly under your shoulder, weight on your forearm. Tighten your abdominal/core muscles, as if someone were pressing on your tummy.	Lift your torso until your body makes a straight line. Exhale as you lift your body to the end position. Hold for 2 seconds and return to start position, breathing in. Repeat this lift-and-hold 7 times. Then repeat on the other side.
Modification	Progression
Kneeling: When you lift your torso, keep your knees together so your body makes a straight line from head to knees. Slightly bend your knees for balance.	Arm overhead: In the end position, lift your free arm straight above your head, keeping it close to your ear.

COMMON ERRORS

- Forearm not directly under shoulder
- Not tightening abdominals, causing balance problems

3. PLIÉ SQUATS

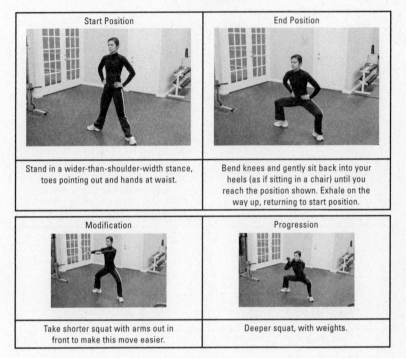

Start Position	End Position
Stand in a wider-than-shoulder-width stance, toes pointing out and hands at waist.	Bend knees and gently sit back into your heels (as if sitting in a chair) until you reach the position shown. Exhale on the way up, returning to start position.
Modification	**Progression**
Take shorter squat with arms out in front to make this move easier.	Deeper squat, with weights.

COMMON ERROR

- Knees going past toes

4. SIDE LUNGES

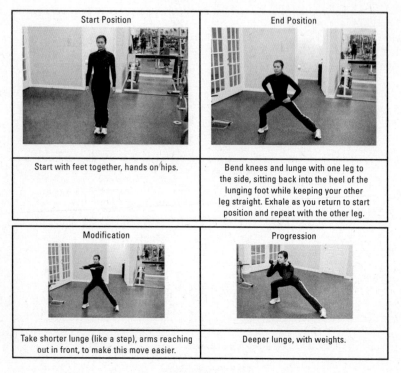

Start Position	End Position
Start with feet together, hands on hips.	Bend knees and lunge with one leg to the side, sitting back into the heel of the lunging foot while keeping your other leg straight. Exhale as you return to start position and repeat with the other leg.

Modification	Progression
Take shorter lunge (like a step), arms reaching out in front, to make this move easier.	Deeper lunge, with weights.

COMMON ERROR

- Starting out with a range of motion that is too deep (build range of motion gradually)

5. SIDE STEP-UPS

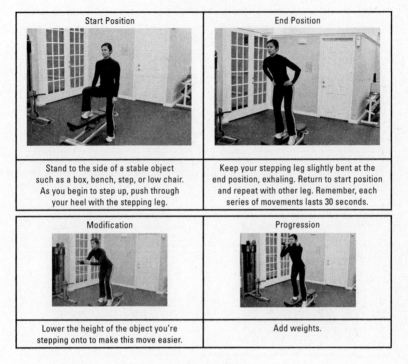

Start Position	End Position
Stand to the side of a stable object such as a box, bench, step, or low chair. As you begin to step up, push through your heel with the stepping leg.	Keep your stepping leg slightly bent at the end position, exhaling. Return to start position and repeat with other leg. Remember, each series of movements lasts 30 seconds.
Modification	Progression
Lower the height of the object you're stepping onto to make this move easier.	Add weights.

COMMON ERRORS

- Locking knee at the end position
- Raising heel off the stable object
- Starting with a stable object that is too high (gradually build to higher objects)

DAY 3: BACK OF BODY

1. COBRA

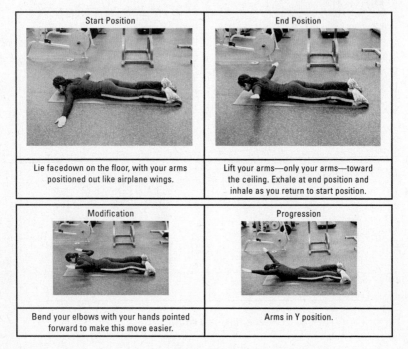

Start Position	End Position
Lie facedown on the floor, with your arms positioned out like airplane wings.	Lift your arms—only your arms—toward the ceiling. Exhale at end position and inhale as you return to start position.
Modification	Progression
Bend your elbows with your hands pointed forward to make this move easier.	Arms in Y position.

COMMON ERRORS

- Looking up (keep eyes focused on the floor)
- Shrugging shoulders

2. MARCHING BRIDGE

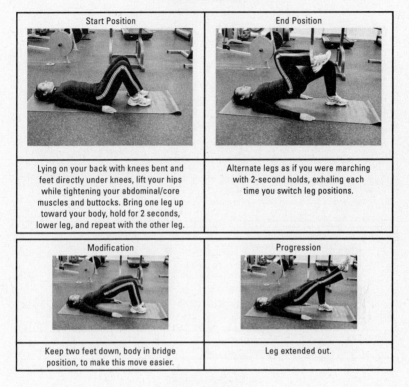

Start Position	End Position
Lying on your back with knees bent and feet directly under knees, lift your hips while tightening your abdominal/core muscles and buttocks. Bring one leg up toward your body, hold for 2 seconds, lower leg, and repeat with the other leg.	Alternate legs as if you were marching with 2-second holds, exhaling each time you switch leg positions.

Modification	Progression
Keep two feet down, body in bridge position, to make this move easier.	Leg extended out.

COMMON ERROR

- Positioning feet too far out, not under the knees

3. RESISTANCE BAND ROW

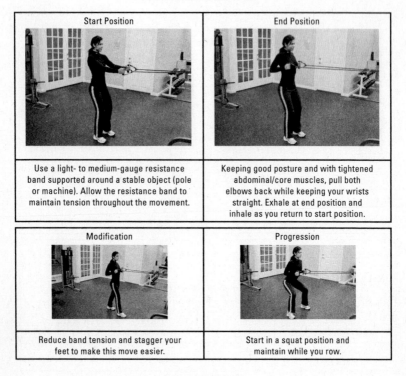

Start Position	End Position
Use a light- to medium-gauge resistance band supported around a stable object (pole or machine). Allow the resistance band to maintain tension throughout the movement.	Keeping good posture and with tightened abdominal/core muscles, pull both elbows back while keeping your wrists straight. Exhale at end position and inhale as you return to start position.

Modification	Progression
Reduce band tension and stagger your feet to make this move easier.	Start in a squat position and maintain while you row.

COMMON ERRORS

- Shrugging shoulders
- Not maintaining good posture

4. RESISTANCE BAND REVERSE FLY

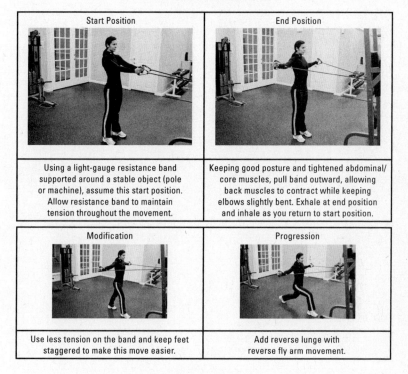

Start Position	End Position
Using a light-gauge resistance band supported around a stable object (pole or machine), assume this start position. Allow resistance band to maintain tension throughout the movement.	Keeping good posture and tightened abdominal/core muscles, pull band outward, allowing back muscles to contract while keeping elbows slightly bent. Exhale at end position and inhale as you return to start position.

Modification	Progression
Use less tension on the band and keep feet staggered to make this move easier.	Add reverse lunge with reverse fly arm movement.

COMMON ERRORS

- Shrugging shoulders
- Not maintaining good posture

5. WALL SHOULDER PRESS

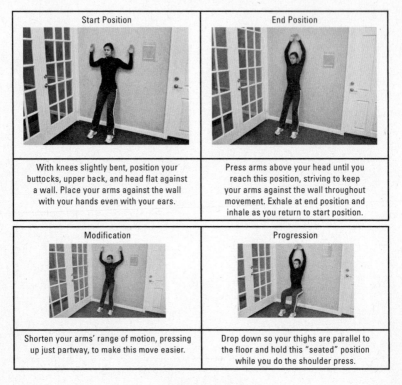

Start Position	End Position
With knees slightly bent, position your buttocks, upper back, and head flat against a wall. Place your arms against the wall with your hands even with your ears.	Press arms above your head until you reach this position, striving to keep your arms against the wall throughout movement. Exhale at end position and inhale as you return to start position.

Modification	Progression
Shorten your arms' range of motion, pressing up just partway, to make this move easier.	Drop down so your thighs are parallel to the floor and hold this "seated" position while you do the shoulder press.

COMMON ERRORS

- Arching lower back excessively
- Allowing head to come off the wall
- Trying to press arms too high (go slowly and work through any shoulder pain)

DAY 4: LEGS

1. FORWARD LUNGE WITH ROTATION

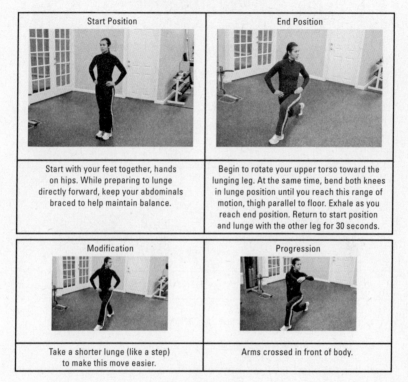

Start Position	End Position
Start with your feet together, hands on hips. While preparing to lunge directly forward, keep your abdominals braced to help maintain balance.	Begin to rotate your upper torso toward the lunging leg. At the same time, bend both knees in lunge position until you reach this range of motion, thigh parallel to floor. Exhale as you reach end position. Return to start position and lunge with the other leg for 30 seconds.

Modification	Progression
Take a shorter lunge (like a step) to make this move easier.	Arms crossed in front of body.

COMMON ERRORS

- Starting out with a range of motion that is too deep (gradually build range of motion)
- Allowing the knee of the lunging leg to move beyond toe

2. SQUAT

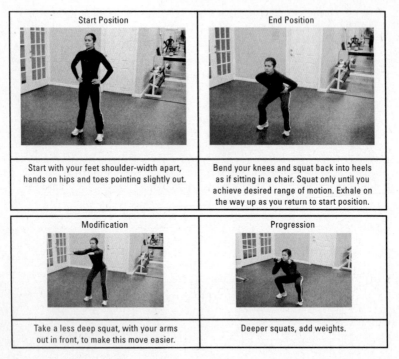

Start Position	End Position
Start with your feet shoulder-width apart, hands on hips and toes pointing slightly out.	Bend your knees and squat back into heels as if sitting in a chair. Squat only until you achieve desired range of motion. Exhale on the way up as you return to start position.

Modification	Progression
Take a less deep squat, with your arms out in front, to make this move easier.	Deeper squats, add weights.

COMMON ERRORS

- Knees moving beyond toes
- Starting out with a range of motion that is too deep (gradually build range of motion)

3. REVERSE LUNGE

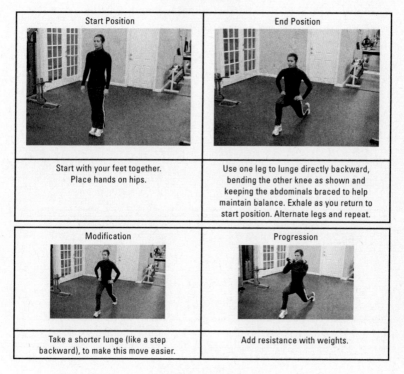

Start Position	End Position
Start with your feet together. Place hands on hips.	Use one leg to lunge directly backward, bending the other knee as shown and keeping the abdominals braced to help maintain balance. Exhale as you return to start position. Alternate legs and repeat.
Modification	Progression
Take a shorter lunge (like a step backward), to make this move easier.	Add resistance with weights.

COMMON ERRORS

- Starting out with a range of motion that is too deep (gradually build range of motion)
- Allowing the knee of the front leg to move over toe

4. STEP-UPS

Start Position	End Position
With hands on hips, stand in front of a stable object such as a box, bench, step, or chair. As you step up, push through the heel of the stepping leg.	Keep your leg slightly bent at the end position, exhaling. Repeat, alternating legs.

Modification	Progression
Lowering the height of the stable object makes this move easier.	Add resistance with weights.

COMMON ERRORS

- Raising stepping heel off stable object (keep it planted)
- Locking knee at the end position
- Starting with a stable object that is too high (gradually build to higher objects)

5. LEANING TOE TOUCHES

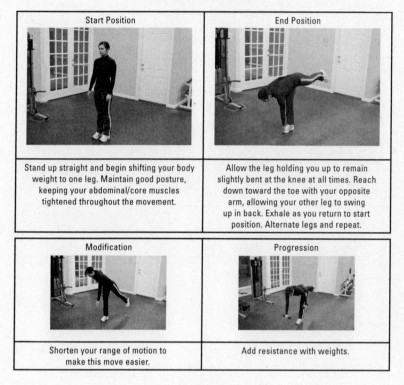

Start Position	End Position
Stand up straight and begin shifting your body weight to one leg. Maintain good posture, keeping your abdominal/core muscles tightened throughout the movement.	Allow the leg holding you up to remain slightly bent at the knee at all times. Reach down toward the toe with your opposite arm, allowing your other leg to swing up in back. Exhale as you return to start position. Alternate legs and repeat.
Modification	Progression
Shorten your range of motion to make this move easier.	Add resistance with weights.

COMMON ERRORS

- Rounding lower and upper back muscles, losing good posture
- Locking the knee of the balancing leg

DAY 5: CORE (ABDOMINALS AND LOWER BACK)

1. OBLIQUE CRUNCHES

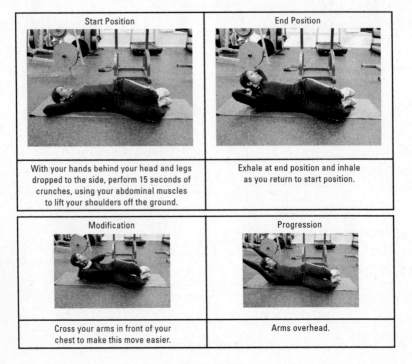

Start Position	End Position
With your hands behind your head and legs dropped to the side, perform 15 seconds of crunches, using your abdominal muscles to lift your shoulders off the ground.	Exhale at end position and inhale as you return to start position.
Modification	Progression
Cross your arms in front of your chest to make this move easier.	Arms overhead.

COMMON ERROR

- Lifting head only, which works the neck muscles instead of the abdominals

2. LEG RAISES (SEE DAY 1, EXERCISE 2)

3. BACKSTROKE

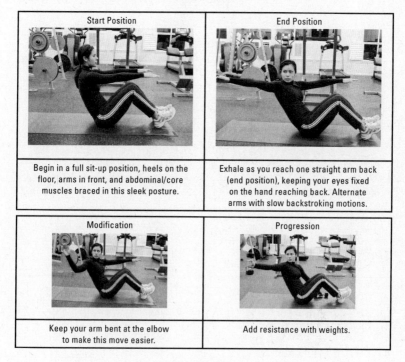

Start Position	End Position
Begin in a full sit-up position, heels on the floor, arms in front, and abdominal/core muscles braced in this sleek posture.	Exhale as you reach one straight arm back (end position), keeping your eyes fixed on the hand reaching back. Alternate arms with slow backstroking motions.

Modification	Progression
Keep your arm bent at the elbow to make this move easier.	Add resistance with weights.

COMMON ERRORS

- Not maintaining good posture
- Not keeping eyes on the hand reaching back

4. QUADRUPED (SEE DAY 2, EXERCISE 1)

5. COBRA (SEE DAY 3, EXERCISE 1)

DAY 6: ARMS

1. PLANK

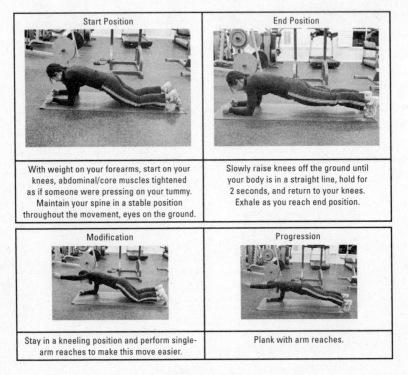

Start Position	End Position
With weight on your forearms, start on your knees, abdominal/core muscles tightened as if someone were pressing on your tummy. Maintain your spine in a stable position throughout the movement, eyes on the ground.	Slowly raise knees off the ground until your body is in a straight line, hold for 2 seconds, and return to your knees. Exhale as you reach end position.
Modification	Progression
Stay in a kneeling position and perform single-arm reaches to make this move easier.	Plank with arm reaches.

COMMON ERRORS

- Allowing lower back to sag, caused by not bracing your abdominals throughout the move
- Head looking forward (eyes should look at ground throughout movement)

2. RESISTANCE BAND ROW (SEE DAY 3, EXERCISE 3)

3. CLOSE HAND PUSH-UP

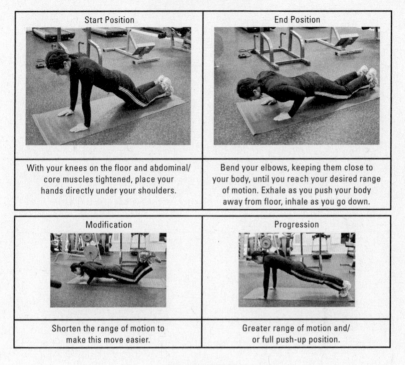

Start Position	End Position
With your knees on the floor and abdominal/core muscles tightened, place your hands directly under your shoulders.	Bend your elbows, keeping them close to your body, until you reach your desired range of motion. Exhale as you push your body away from floor, inhale as you go down.

Modification	Progression
Shorten the range of motion to make this move easier.	Greater range of motion and/or full push-up position.

COMMON ERRORS

- Not engaging the core area
- Shrugging shoulders
- Allowing elbows to drift away from body

4. RESISTANCE BAND BICEPS CURLS

Start Position	End Position
Using a light- to medium-gauge resistance band, stand with your feet hip-width apart, the resistance band placed firmly under your feet. Hold the resistance band at hip height. Engage your abdominal/core muscles and stand straight, looking forward.	Curl your arms from the elbows until your hands reach shoulder height. Exhale as you reach this end position. Inhale as you lower your hands and repeat. Maintain tension on the resistance band throughout the movement.

Modification	Progression
Position band under just one foot to make this move easier.	Add a lunge and add weights.

COMMON ERROR

- Not maintaining good posture

5. DIPS

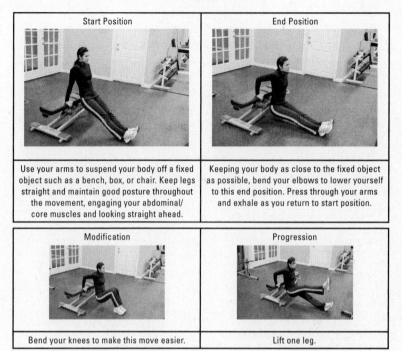

Start Position	End Position
Use your arms to suspend your body off a fixed object such as a bench, box, or chair. Keep legs straight and maintain good posture throughout the movement, engaging your abdominal/core muscles and looking straight ahead.	Keeping your body as close to the fixed object as possible, bend your elbows to lower yourself to this end position. Press through your arms and exhale as you return to start position.

Modification	Progression
Bend your knees to make this move easier.	Lift one leg.

COMMON ERRORS

- Not maintaining good posture
- Shrugging shoulders

DAY 7: CORE AND GLUTEUS

1. RESISTANCE BAND SIDE WALKING

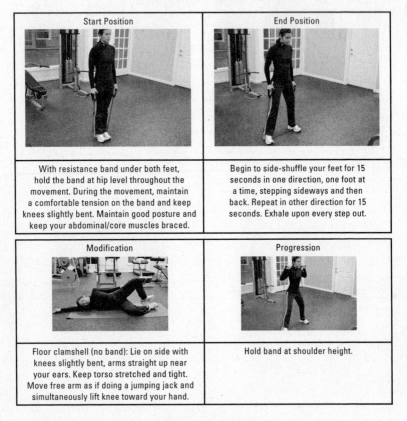

Start Position	End Position
With resistance band under both feet, hold the band at hip level throughout the movement. During the movement, maintain a comfortable tension on the band and keep knees slightly bent. Maintain good posture and keep your abdominal/core muscles braced.	Begin to side-shuffle your feet for 15 seconds in one direction, one foot at a time, stepping sideways and then back. Repeat in other direction for 15 seconds. Exhale upon every step out.

Modification	Progression
Floor clamshell (no band): Lie on side with knees slightly bent, arms straight up near your ears. Keep torso stretched and tight. Move free arm as if doing a jumping jack and simultaneously lift knee toward your hand.	Hold band at shoulder height.

COMMON ERRORS

- Not maintaining good posture
- Locking the knees during the movement

2. MARCHING BRIDGE (SEE DAY 3, EXERCISE 2)

3. KNEELING PLANK WITH KICKS

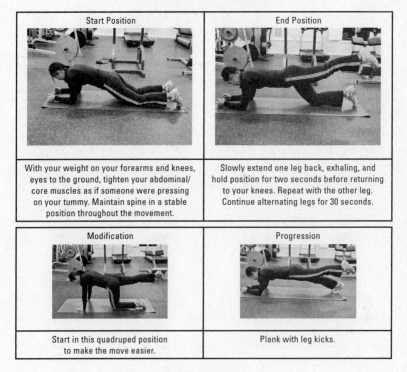

Start Position	End Position
With your weight on your forearms and knees, eyes to the ground, tighten your abdominal/core muscles as if someone were pressing on your tummy. Maintain spine in a stable position throughout the movement.	Slowly extend one leg back, exhaling, and hold position for two seconds before returning to your knees. Repeat with the other leg. Continue alternating legs for 30 seconds.

Modification	Progression
Start in this quadruped position to make the move easier.	Plank with leg kicks.

COMMON ERRORS

- Allowing lower back to sag, due to not tightening abdominal/core muscles throughout the move
- Head looking forward (keep eyes on the ground throughout movement)

4. CURTSY LUNGE

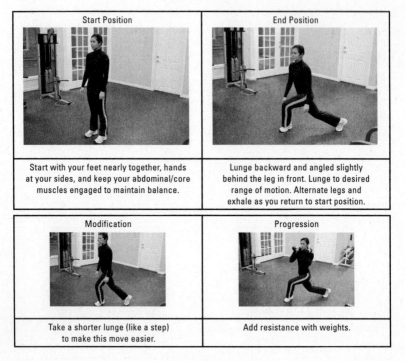

Start Position	End Position
Start with your feet nearly together, hands at your sides, and keep your abdominal/core muscles engaged to maintain balance.	Lunge backward and angled slightly behind the leg in front. Lunge to desired range of motion. Alternate legs and exhale as you return to start position.

Modification	Progression
Take a shorter lunge (like a step) to make this move easier.	Add resistance with weights.

COMMON ERROR

- Starting out with a range of motion that is too deep (build range of motion gradually)

5. SQUAT FEET TOGETHER

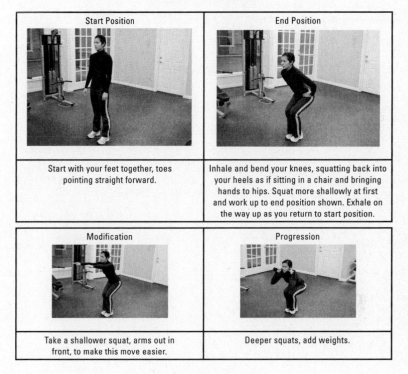

Start Position	End Position
Start with your feet together, toes pointing straight forward.	Inhale and bend your knees, squatting back into your heels as if sitting in a chair and bringing hands to hips. Squat more shallowly at first and work up to end position shown. Exhale on the way up as you return to start position.
Modification	Progression
Take a shallower squat, arms out in front, to make this move easier.	Deeper squats, add weights.

COMMON ERRORS

- Knees going past toes
- Starting out with a range of motion that is too deep (build range of motion gradually)

Ask Dr. Arem: Substitutions on Some 20/10 Workout Days

Q. I tend to get bored quickly doing the same exercise program day in and day out. I already like the seven-day rotation of strength exercises in your 20/10, but would it be okay to substitute other exercise on some days?

A. By all means, go for it! Switching out your 20/10 for sports or classes is a fine idea. Fitness classes offered at local health clubs usually last about an hour, and playing an entire game can take even longer. Here are some suggestions for substitute days that will give you both cardio and strength training.

- Fitness classes (kickboxing, boot camp)
- Team sports (soccer, basketball, kickball, ultimate Frisbee)
- Racket sports (tennis, racquetball, badminton)
- Combative sports with higher intensity (tae kwon do, extreme martial arts, fencing, kendo)
- Dancing (salsa, jazz, hip-hop, pole)

A gentle reminder: for all the reasons discussed at the beginning of this chapter, you need to stay with my structured 20/10 workout when you're not exploring other exercise options. I prescribe weight-dampening, metabolism-boosting high-intensity interval training and strength training because all the evidence shows they work.

EXERCISE WHEN YOU TRAVEL: THE MINI WORKOUT

I designed my 20/10 workout to fit easily into your schedule, and you can even use a variation of it—the Mini Workout—on the road when traveling for business or pleasure. The Mini Workout is a shortened version of the 20/10 program for a total of twenty minutes rather than thirty. Because you'll be quickly switching exercises, the travel adaptation works best with minimal equipment. However, some of my patients love their resistance bands, so go ahead and pack them if you want.

MINI WORKOUT

Alternate 1 minute of high-intensity cardio with 30 seconds of a strength exercise.

- For the 1-minute cardio portion: as hard as you can, run in place, jog in place with high knees, do jumping jacks, hop around on both feet, or dance intensely.
- Break and breathe for 15 to 30 seconds.
- For the 30-second strength training: choose any exercises from the seven-day list, excluding planks. Be mindful of your form.
- Break and breathe for 15 to 30 seconds.
- Keep alternating until you've worked out for 20 minutes.

YOU'RE A LEAN, MEAN CALORIE-BURNING MACHINE! ACTIVE ADDITIONS (NOT REPLACEMENTS) FOR STAYING TRIM AND FIT

Once you've accelerated your resting metabolic rate, you'll burn more calories no matter what you do. But this is no time to relax. Instead, become even more active by replacing sedentary hours with physical activity. I'm proud of your success so far—practicing your relaxation technique and sticking with the 20/10 workout. It may seem like a lot more exercise than you've ever done, but don't stop now. And remember, whatever you incorporate into your life is in addition to—not a substitute for—your daily half-hour 20/10 workout. You still need that half hour every day to achieve and maintain your calorie-burning metabolism. Ponder these ideas, develop your own, and integrate them into your day.

Walk at least part of the way instead of driving or taking public transportation. One of my patients started walking for her groceries instead of driving to the store. She buys two bags of provisions per trip (yes, she makes trips more often, but she's worked it into her routine) and carries the bags home, using them as a strength training exercise for her arms. Research shows weight loss is minimal with slow-paced walking alone, but any walking is better than sitting in the driver's seat or on the train or bus.

Get on your bike, not in your car. A sixteen-year study of women showed that more time spent bicycling correlated with significantly lower weight gain. Even women who biked five minutes a day or less experienced less weight gain. The study argues that bike riding could be the answer to controlling weight gain by replacing time spent in a car, calling it an almost unconscious form of exercise as you focus on the trip's destination rather than the exercise itself. A study done on nearly 1,000 adult men found that men who walked or biked to work for more than thirty minutes daily had a lower BMI and a smaller waist circumference (by 1 cm) compared with men who didn't walk or bicycle to work.

Taking stairs instead of the elevator is common advice, but it's solid. So why not do that every once in a while? I've even heard of stair-walking groups of employees who use the stairs to their best advantage during breaks.

Instead of meeting friends for a weekly happy hour and appetizers, suggest a sport every other week or plan a group walk to a park for a picnic.

Get off the train or bus early and walk. Disembark a couple of stops ahead of your destination and walk the rest of the way.

Play with your kids instead of watching a movie. Get outside and stroll in your neighborhood, kick a soccer ball around, throw a baseball, or walk to the park. This is especially good for your postprandial metabolism.

RECIPES

For your meals to be compliant with the guidelines of the Protein Boost Diet, you will be provided with suggested additions to the following recipes— indicated as "serving suggestion." Feel free to substitute other choices for the serving suggestion by consulting the meal plan charts in Chapter 10.

BREAKFAST, PHASE 1

Egg whites and seafood such as smoked salmon or tuna are the primary Phase 1 breakfast proteins, with low-fat cottage cheese, yogurt, and beans your secondary protein. Fat in this phase is primarily from olive oil, avocado, or nuts and seeds. (Don't worry if your total meal fat ratio is slightly higher if you choose a protein with more fat, such as salmon, as opposed to a lower-fat protein like egg whites; it will not adversely affect the diet as these are healthy fats in small quantities.) The fiber source will be low-carbohydrate, high-fiber vegetables like spinach and broccoli. Fruits like berries, kiwi, and grapefruit provide carbohydrates to complete your 250 to 300 average calories. Check the charts in the Meal Plans in Chapter 10 for quantities.

Recipes for ingredients in *italics* can be found elsewhere in this section.

SMOKED SALMON WITH CAPERS AND ASPARAGUS
(MAKES 1 SERVING)

½ teaspoon capers, rinsed and soaked in cold water for 15 minutes
3 ounces smoked salmon
2 teaspoons minced shallots
¼ to ½ lime
8 medium spears asparagus, steamed (about 1 cup)

Drain and finely chop the capers. Arrange the salmon on a serving plate and sprinkle the capers and shallots on top. Squeeze lime juice over the salmon to taste and serve with the asparagus on the side.

Each serving: 131 calories, 19 g protein, 7 g carbohydrates, 3 g fiber (net carbs: 4 g), 2 g sugar, 4 g fat (1 g saturated fat), 20 mg cholesterol, 1,546 mg* sodium

Serving suggestion: Protein #2: ½ cup nonfat yogurt; Fat: 3 walnut halves; Carbohydrate: 1 cup grapefruit sections

Each serving, with suggestions: 306 calories, 28 g protein, 29 g carbohydrates, 5 g fiber (net carbs: 24 g), 23 g sugar, 9 g fat (2 g saturated fat), 27 mg cholesterol, 1,833 mg* sodium

* Sodium content varies widely by brand of smoked fish, so check the label if you are concerned about sodium intake.

TOFU WITH SPINACH (MAKES 1 SERVING)

A nonstick skillet or nonstick grill pan works best, but you can also cook the tofu in an enameled cast-iron skillet.

¼ cup (2 ounces) firm tofu, drained and patted dry
¼ teaspoon olive or grapeseed oil
3 cups fresh spinach
1 tablespoon balsamic vinegar
Kosher salt and ground black pepper

1. Wrap the tofu in a paper towel and gently press to remove as much excess moisture as possible. Brush a medium nonstick skillet with the oil and cook the tofu undisturbed until it begins to brown along the edges, about 5 minutes. Flip the tofu and cook until the other side is lightly golden, about 4 minutes.

2. Add the spinach and cook until just wilted, about 1 minute. Add the balsamic vinegar and cook until the liquid in the pan is reduced by half, about 1 minute. Remove from the heat and season with salt and pepper. Serve hot.

Variation: To make ginger-soy marinated tofu, marinate the tofu in 1 tablespoon low-sodium soy sauce and ½ teaspoon ground ginger for 10 minutes before cooking. Drain the tofu, pat dry with paper towels, and cook as directed, but omit the balsamic vinegar.

Each serving: 78 calories, 8 g protein, 5 g carbohydrates, 3 g fiber (net carbs: 2 g), 1 g sugar, 4 g fat (1 g saturated fat), 0 mg cholesterol, 79 mg sodium

Serving suggestion: Protein #1: 3 ounces smoked turkey breast; Protein #2: ½ cup low-fat yogurt; Carbohydrate: 1 cup strawberries

Each serving, including suggestions: 300 calories, 30 g protein, 28 g carbohydrates, 6 g fiber (net carbs: 22 g), 19 g sugar, 7 g fat (2 g saturated fat), 44 mg cholesterol, 1,010 mg sodium

MEXICAN SCRAMBLE (MAKES 1 SERVING)

If you use store-bought salsa, check the label to make sure it does not contain added sugar or carbohydrate-rich ingredients like corn.

This recipe has little added fat, so using a nonstick skillet is essential to keep the eggs from sticking.

>   4 egg whites or ½ cup pasteurized egg whites
>   2 tablespoons cooked black beans, drained and rinsed if canned
>   ¼ teaspoon olive or grapeseed oil
>   ½ garlic clove, minced
>   Kosher salt and ground black pepper
>   ⅓ cup low-fat cottage cheese
>   2 tablespoons *Fresh Tomato Salsa* or store-bought salsa
>   ⅛ avocado, sliced or diced
>   2 teaspoons chopped fresh cilantro

In a small bowl, whisk the egg whites. Stir in the black beans. Brush a small nonstick skillet with the oil and cook the garlic for 30 seconds. Add the egg mixture and cook, stirring occasionally with a heat-resistant silicone spatula, until the eggs are set, about 2 minutes. Season with salt and pepper. Serve topped with the cottage cheese, salsa, avocado, and cilantro.

Each serving: 227 calories, 28 g protein, 14 g carbohydrates, 4 g fiber (net carbs: 10 g), 3 g sugar, 7 g fat (2 g saturated fat), 6 mg cholesterol, 720 mg sodium

Serving suggestion: Fiber: 1 cup raw or lightly steamed string (green) beans; Carbohydrate: ½ kiwi

Each serving, with suggestions: 284 calories, 31 g protein, 28 g carbohydrates, 9 g fiber (net carbs: 19 g), 8 g sugar, 7 g fat (2 g saturated fat), 6 mg cholesterol, 728 mg sodium

ZUCCHINI FRITTATA (MAKES 1 SERVING)

This recipe has little added fat, so using a nonstick skillet is essential to keep the eggs from sticking to the pan.

>   1 teaspoon olive or grapeseed oil
>   1 tablespoon minced shallot or onion
>   ½ garlic clove, minced
>   1 small zucchini, shaved into thin strips with a vegetable peeler (about 1 cup)
>   4 egg whites or ½ cup pasteurized egg whites
>   Kosher salt
>   ½ teaspoon fresh thyme leaves or a generous pinch of dried thyme
>   Ground black pepper

1. Brush a medium nonstick skillet with the oil and cook the shallot and garlic until softened, about 1 minute. Add the zucchini and cook, stirring occasionally, until tender, 2 to 3 minutes.

2. In a small bowl, whisk the egg whites with a generous pinch of salt and the thyme. Add to the zucchini, mixing well. Cook undisturbed over low heat until the frittata is set, about 2 minutes. Flip the frittata and cook 1 minute more. Season with salt and pepper and serve hot.

Variations: This is also great with chopped fresh oregano or rosemary instead of thyme.

Use ½ cup chopped broccoli instead of the zucchini.

Each serving: 124 calories, 16 g protein, 5 g carbohydrates, 2 g fiber (net carbs: 3 g), 3 g sugar, 5 g fat (1 g saturated fat), 0 mg cholesterol, 226 mg sodium

Serving suggestion: Protein #2: ½ cup nonfat yogurt; Carbohydrate: 1 cup blackberries

Each serving, with suggestions: 254 calories, 24 g protein, 29 g carbohydrates, 9 g fiber (net carbs: 20 g), 20 g sugar, 6 g fat (1 g saturated fat), 2 mg cholesterol, 322 mg sodium

SPINACH OMELET (MAKES 1 SERVING)

This recipe has little added fat, so using a nonstick skillet is essential to keep the eggs from sticking.

> ¾ teaspoon olive or grapeseed oil
> 2 teaspoons minced shallots or onions
> 1 garlic clove, minced
> 3 cups fresh spinach
> 4 egg whites or ½ cup pasteurized egg whites
> Kosher salt
> 1 kalamata or other cured black olive, pitted and minced
> Ground black pepper
> 2 teaspoons chopped fresh parsley
> 2 teaspoons grated Parmesan cheese

1. Brush a medium nonstick skillet with the oil and cook the shallots and garlic, stirring occasionally, until softened, 2 to 3 minutes. Add the spinach and cook another 2 minutes or until wilted.

2. In a small bowl, whisk the egg whites with a generous pinch of salt. Pour the egg whites over the vegetables and scatter the olive on top. Cook until the eggs are set, 3 to 4 minutes. Season with salt and pepper and serve sprinkled with the parsley and Parmesan.

(continued on next page)

Variation: Use ½ cup chopped broccoli or ¾ cup chopped bell pepper instead of the spinach.

Each serving: 141 calories, 19 g protein, 7 g carbohydrates, 2 g fiber (net carbs: 5 g), 1 g sugar, 5 g fat (1 g saturated fat), 3 mg cholesterol, 383 mg sodium

Serving suggestion: Protein #2: ½ cup low-fat cottage cheese; Carbohydrate: 1 cup mixed berries

Each serving, with suggestions: 319 calories, 35 g protein, 28 g carbohydrates, 7 g fiber (net carbs: 21 g), 12 g sugar, 8 g fat (2 g saturated fat), 12 mg cholesterol, 842 mg sodium

---

POACHED EGGS (MAKES 1 SERVING)

This is a supereasy version of poached eggs; you don't even need to swirl the water as you add the eggs. The key is to use a small (5- to 6-inch-diameter) saucepan to keep the egg whites from spreading too much.

> 1 whole egg
> 2 egg whites or ¼ cup pasteurized egg whites
> Kosher salt
> 2 tablespoons white or cider vinegar
> Ground black pepper

Crack the egg and egg whites into small cup. Bring 2 cups water to a low boil in a small saucepan and add ¼ teaspoon salt and the vinegar. Immediately slide the eggs gently into the water, reduce the heat to a simmer, and cook until the whites are firm but the yolk is still runny, 2 to 3 minutes. Remove the eggs with a slotted spoon and drain any excess water. Season with salt and pepper and serve immediately.

Each serving: 95 calories, 13 g protein, 1 g carbohydrates, 0 g fiber (net carbs: 1 g), 1 g sugar, 5 g fat (1 g saturated fat), 164 mg cholesterol, 326 mg sodium

Serving suggestion: Protein #2: ½ cup fat-free cottage cheese; Fat: 7 almonds; Fiber: 3 cups cooked spinach; Carbohydrate: ½ cup sliced kiwi

Each serving, with suggestions: 308 calories, 34 g protein, 26 g carbohydrates, 6 g fiber (net carbs: 20 g), 15 g sugar, 9 g fat (2 g saturated fat), 164 mg cholesterol, 999 mg sodium

BREAKFAST, PHASE 2

In this phase, your calories will stay in the same 250-to-300 range on average, but you will increase your carbohydrates slightly with a whole-grain fiber source (see the chart in the Meal Plans in Chapter 10).

WHOLE-GRAIN FRENCH TOAST (MAKES 1 SERVING)

If you prefer sweet French toast, add a pinch of stevia to the egg mixture.

  1 whole egg
  2 egg whites or ¼ cup pasteurized egg whites
  1 tablespoon low-fat milk
  1 slice whole-grain bread or *Protein Boost Diet Quinoa Sandwich Bread*
  1 teaspoon olive or grapeseed oil

1. In a shallow, wide bowl, whisk the egg, egg whites, and milk. Add the bread and allow to soak in the egg mixture for 5 minutes, gently flipping it once.

2. Brush a small nonstick skillet with the oil. Drain excess batter from the bread and place the bread in the skillet. Cook undisturbed until the bottom of the bread begins to brown, about 3 minutes. Flip and cook until golden, about 3 minutes. Serve hot.

Each serving: 199 calories, 16 g protein, 13 g carbohydrates, 2 g fiber (net carbs: 11 g), 3 g sugar, 10 g fat (2 g saturated fat), 164 mg cholesterol, 321 mg sodium

Serving suggestion: Protein #2: ½ cup fat-free yogurt; Fiber: 1 cup sliced fennel; Carbohydrate: ¼ cup strawberries

Each serving, with suggestions: 306 calories, 24 g protein, 32 g carbohydrates, 5 g fiber (net carbs: 27 g), 14 g sugar, 10 g fat (2 g saturated fat), 166 mg cholesterol, 461 mg sodium

EGGS BENEDICT WITH SPINACH (MAKES 1 SERVING)

1 teaspoon olive or grapeseed oil
1 garlic clove, minced
3 cups fresh spinach
Kosher salt
1 slice whole-grain bread or *Protein Boost Diet Quinoa Sandwich Bread*, toasted
1 whole egg plus 2 egg whites, poached (see *Poached Eggs*) and kept warm
Ground black pepper
½ cup nonfat cottage cheese, at room temperature
2 teaspoons chopped fresh parsley

1. Brush a small nonstick skillet with the oil and cook the garlic for 30 seconds. Add the spinach and a pinch of salt and cook, stirring occasionally, until wilted, 1 to 2 minutes.

2. Place the toast on a serving plate and top with the spinach and poached eggs. Season with salt and pepper, top with the cottage cheese and parsley, and serve.

Each serving: 295 calories, 32 g protein, 23 g carbohydrates, 5 g fiber (net carbs: 18 g), 8 g sugar, 10 g fat (2 g saturated fat), 169 mg cholesterol, 804 mg sodium

Serving suggestion: Carbohydrate: ¼ cup blackberries

Each serving, with suggestions: 311 calories, 32 g protein, 26 g carbohydrates, 7 g fiber (net carbs: 19 g), 10 g sugar, 10 g fat (2 g saturated fat), 169 mg cholesterol, 805 mg sodium

LUNCH, PHASE 1

At lunch, much of your protein and fiber source will come from fiber-rich legumes such as lentils, chickpeas, and other beans, as well as quinoa. Your meat source will primarily be lean meats and seafood, though you can substitute low-fat cheeses as an option. Your vegetable fiber source will be a variety of Category 1 and 2 vegetables, with fruit continuing to serve as an additional carbohydrate source. Total calories should range from 400 to 500.

The grain and bean salads keep well for a week, so each recipe makes six servings; for a quick lunch, serve with canned tuna or salmon, roast turkey breast, or chicken. Perishable salads, like the Niçoise, serve four. All can be easily halved or doubled. You can cook large quantities of dried beans ahead and freeze them in recipe- or individual-size portions in resealable plastic bags.

MEDITERRANEAN LENTIL SALAD (MAKES 6 SERVINGS)

Be careful not to overcook the lentils so they will retain their shape.

2 cups dried green or brown lentils, sorted and rinsed
2 tablespoons olive or grapeseed oil
¼ cup lemon juice, plus more as needed
½ cup chopped fresh parsley (1 small bunch)
Kosher salt and ground black pepper
1 cup diced cucumber (1 medium cucumber)
1 cup diced tomato (1 medium tomato)
1 cup diced red onion (1 medium onion)
1 cup diced green bell pepper (1 medium pepper)

1. In a medium pot, combine the lentils with enough water to cover by 3 inches. Bring to a boil, reduce the heat to low, and simmer until just tender, 15 to 17 minutes. Drain the lentils and set them aside to cool.

2. In a large bowl, whisk together the oil, lemon juice, parsley, ¾ teaspoon salt, and ½ teaspoon pepper. Add the cucumber, tomato, onion, and bell pepper. Gently stir in the lentils, being careful not to break them apart. Season with additional salt, pepper, and lemon juice to taste. Serve at room temperature or chilled.

Each serving: 290 calories, 17 g protein, 44 g carbohydrates, 21 g fiber (net carbs: 23 g), 4 g sugar, 5 g fat (1 g saturated fat), 0 mg cholesterol, 203 mg sodium

(*continued on next page*)

Serving suggestion: Protein #1: 3 ounces boneless, skinless chicken breast, or ⅓ cup
(1½ ounces) reduced-fat feta, crumbled on the salad; Fiber: 1 cup grilled radicchio (the
salad has half your vegetables); Carbohydrate: ¾ cup grapefruit sections

Each serving, with suggestions: 461 calories, 40 g protein, 65 g carbohydrates, 24 g fiber
(net carbs: 41 g), 20 g sugar, 6 g fat (1 g saturated fat), 42 mg cholesterol, 259 mg sodium

---

PICNIC CHICKPEA SALAD (MAKES 6 SERVINGS)

To quick-soak chickpeas, in a pot, cover them with water by 2 inches and
bring to a boil for 2 minutes. Remove from the heat, cover, and set aside
for 1 hour. The cooking time later will vary depending on the size and age
of the chickpeas.

> Scant 2 cups dried chickpeas, soaked overnight in 6 cups water or
>   quick-soaked
> 1 tablespoon plus 2 teaspoons olive or grapeseed oil
> ¼ cup lemon juice, plus more as needed
> 1 tablespoon capers, drained and minced
> 2 garlic cloves, minced
> ½ cup chopped fresh parsley (1 small bunch)
> 2 tablespoons chopped fresh mint
> 4 kalamata or other cured black olives, pitted and chopped
> Kosher salt and ground black pepper
> ¾ cup thinly sliced red onion (¾ medium onion, quartered and sliced)
> 1 cup diced red or yellow bell pepper (1 medium pepper)
> 2 cups diced cucumber (1 large cucumber)
> 1 cup diced tomato (1 medium tomato)

1. Drain the chickpeas. Transfer them to a medium pot and add enough
fresh water to cover them by 3 inches. Bring to a boil, reduce the heat to
low, and simmer until tender, 1 to 1½ hours, adding additional water if the
chickpeas appear dry. Drain the chickpeas and set them aside to cool.

2. In a large bowl, whisk together the oil, lemon juice, capers, garlic, parsley, mint, olives, ¾ teaspoon salt, and ½ teaspoon pepper. Add the chickpeas, onion, and bell pepper, then gently fold in the cucumber and tomato.
Season with additional salt, pepper, and lemon juice to taste. Serve at room
temperature or chilled.

Variation: For a southwestern-style salad, use ¼ cup chopped fresh cilantro
and 2 tablespoons minced jalapeño chile instead of the mint.

Each serving: 290 calories, 13 g protein, 44 g carbohydrates, 12 g fiber (net carbs: 32 g),
9 g sugar, 8 g fat (1 g saturated fat), 0 mg cholesterol, 267 mg sodium

Serving suggestion: Protein #1: 3 ounces turkey breast; Fiber: ½ cup cooked kohlrabi (the salad has half your vegetables); Carbohydrate: ½ cup sliced apple

Each serving, with suggestions: 426 calories, 29 g protein, 59 g carbohydrates, 17 g fiber (net carbs: 42 g), 20 g sugar, 10 g fat (1 g saturated fat), 37 mg cholesterol, 966 mg sodium

---

SPICED QUINOA WITH YAMS (MAKES 6 SERVINGS)

Some brands of quinoa are not prewashed. If yours has a powdery residue, rinse it well in a fine-mesh strainer under cold running water until the water runs clear, then drain thoroughly, or the quinoa will have a bitter flavor. Toasting the quinoa lends a fantastic nuttiness to this dish, but it's also great untoasted.

 2¼ cups quinoa
 ½ cup diced red onion (1 small onion)
 2 tablespoons olive or grapeseed oil
 2 teaspoons ground cumin
 1½ teaspoons ground turmeric
 1 teaspoon paprika
 2 garlic cloves, minced
 2 cups peeled and diced yams, in ½-inch cubes (2 small yams)
 Kosher salt and ground black pepper
 3 tablespoons red wine vinegar
 ¼ cup chopped fresh parsley, plus more as needed
 2 tablespoons chopped fresh mint

1. If you like, toast the quinoa in a dry medium saucepan over high heat, stirring frequently, until the seeds begin to brown and smell nutty, 2 to 3 minutes (be careful not to let them burn).

2. Add 4½ cups water (if you toasted the quinoa, expect it to spit), bring to a boil, reduce the heat to low, cover, and simmer until the grains are tender, the little tails have unfurled, and the water is mostly absorbed, about 15 minutes. Remove from the heat and allow to steam, covered, for 5 minutes.

3. In a medium skillet, cook the onion in the oil, stirring occasionally, until softened, 3 to 4 minutes. Add the cumin, turmeric, paprika, and garlic and cook for 30 seconds. Add the yams, ¼ cup water, and a generous pinch of salt. Cover and cook until the yams are tender, about 10 minutes.

4. Remove from the heat and stir in the vinegar. Gently fold the onion-yam mixture and parsley into the quinoa. Season with salt and pepper. Sprinkle with the mint and more parsley, if you like, and serve warm or at room temperature. (*continued on next page*)

Variation: For a version to go with leftover holiday turkey, use ½ teaspoon ground cinnamon and ⅛ teaspoon ground cloves instead of the cumin, paprika, and mint.

Each serving: 326 calories, 10 g protein, 53 g carbohydrates, 7 g fiber (net carbs: 46 g), 1 g sugar, 8 g fat (1 g saturated fat), 0 mg cholesterol, 302 mg sodium

Serving suggestion: Protein #1: 4 ounces tilapia, baked; Carbohydrate: 1 cup blackberries

Each serving, with suggestions: 483 calories, 33 g protein, 67 g carbohydrates, 15 g fiber (net carbs: 52 g), 8 g sugar, 10 g fat (2 g saturated fat), 55 mg cholesterol, 343 mg sodium

---

QUINOA TABBOULEH (MAKES 6 SERVINGS)

Some brands of quinoa are not sold prewashed. If yours has a powdery residue, rinse it well or the quinoa will have a bitter flavor.

To shred the mint, first stack a few leaves. Roll up the leaves tightly, like a cigar. Cut across the roll with a sharp knife.

You can find jars of pickled vegetables (carrots, celery, and cauliflower; also called "giardiniera"), such as Mezzetta Italian Mix, at well-stocked grocery stores.

2¼ cups quinoa, rinsed if necessary
¼ cup pickled mixed vegetables, drained
2 tablespoons olive or grapeseed oil
⅓ cup lemon juice, plus more to taste
Kosher salt and ground black pepper
2½ cups chopped fresh curly parsley (about 3 large bunches)
¼ cup finely shredded mint leaves (about 1 bunch)
1½ cups diced tomatoes (2 medium tomatoes)
½ cup diced red onion (1 small onion)
2 cups diced cucumber (1 large cucumber)
1 jalapeño chile, seeded and minced (optional)

1. Combine the quinoa and 4½ cups water in a medium saucepan. Bring to a boil, reduce the heat to low, cover, and simmer until the grains are tender, the little tails have unfurled, and the water is mostly absorbed, about 15 minutes. Remove from the heat and allow to steam, covered, for 5 minutes.

2. Meanwhile, soak the pickled vegetables in water for 15 minutes. Drain and chop coarsely.

3. In a large bowl, whisk together the oil, lemon juice, ½ teaspoon salt, and ½ teaspoon pepper. Add the parsley, mint, tomatoes, red onion, cucumber,

pickled vegetables, and jalapeño, if using, then gently fold in the quinoa. Season with salt and pepper and additional lemon juice to taste. Serve at room temperature or chilled.

Variation: The backbone of tabbouleh is a fantastic amount of parsley, but otherwise the salad varies widely by region. Experiment with replacing some of the parsley with different fresh herbs like dill or cilantro.

Each serving: 290 calories, 10 g protein, 45 g carbohydrates, 6 g fiber (net carbs: 39 g), 3 g sugar, 8 g fat (1 g saturated fat), 0 mg cholesterol, 215 mg sodium

Serving suggestion: Protein #1: 3 ounces flounder, baked; Fiber: 2 cups spinach salad (the salad has half your vegetables); Carbohydrate: ¾ cup blackberries (the salad has ¼ your fruit)

Each serving, with suggestions: 450 calories, 33 g protein, 57 g carbohydrates, 13 g fiber (net carbs: 44 g), 8 g sugar, 11 g fat (2 g saturated fat), 58 mg cholesterol, 362 mg sodium

---

NIÇOISE SALAD (MAKES 4 SERVINGS)

Be sure to use flavorful cured black olives, rather than canned, here.

> 1 tablespoon olive or grapeseed oil
> 3 tablespoons lemon juice
> 4 kalamata or other cured black olives, pitted and chopped
> 1 bunch scallions (green onions), including 3 inches of green tops, finely chopped
> Kosher salt and ground black pepper
> Two 5-ounce cans water-packed tuna, drained (about 1 cup)
> 6 cups loosely packed baby salad greens
> 2 cups string (green) beans, trimmed and lightly steamed (about 12 ounces)
> ½ cup halved cherry tomatoes
> ½ cup thinly sliced red or yellow bell pepper (1 small pepper)
> Whites from 3 hard-boiled eggs, quartered

1. To make the dressing, whisk together the oil, lemon juice, olives, scallions, ¼ teaspoon salt, and ¼ teaspoon pepper in a small bowl.

2. In a medium bowl, toss the tuna with 1½ tablespoons of the dressing.

3. In a large bowl, lightly toss the salad greens with the remaining dressing and season with salt and pepper. Divide the salad greens among four serving plates. Top equally with the green beans, tomatoes, peppers, and egg whites. Arrange the tuna on top.

(continued on next page)

Variation: Try steamed asparagus or baby artichokes instead of string beans.

Each serving: 175 calories, 24 g protein, 10 g carbohydrates, 4 g fiber (net carbs: 6 g), 2 g sugar, 5 g fat (1 g saturated fat), 42 mg cholesterol, 352 mg sodium

Serving suggestion: Protein #2: 1 cup cooked chickpeas or fava beans; Carbohydrate: ¾ cup grapefruit sections

Each serving, with suggestions: 466 calories, 38 g protein, 63 g carbohydrates, 18 g fiber (net carbs: 45 g), 21 g sugar, 9 g fat (1 g saturated fat), 42 mg cholesterol, 362 mg sodium

BLACK BEAN AND TUNA SALAD WITH RADICCHIO
(MAKES 4 SERVINGS)

This salad is even better for lunch the next day.

If you're grilling, quarter a small head of radicchio and toss it on the grill until lightly charred.

    2 cups packed parsley leaves and stems (2 large bunches)
    1 tablespoon plus 1 teaspoon olive or grapeseed oil
    3 tablespoons lemon juice
    2 teaspoons red wine vinegar
    1 garlic clove, minced
    Kosher salt and ground black pepper
    2 medium heads radicchio, cored, leaves coarsely torn (7 to 8 cups)
    4 cups cooked black beans, drained and rinsed if canned
    2 celery stalks, thinly sliced
    12 ounces grilled albacore tuna, cubed, or three 5-ounce cans water-packed
        tuna, drained
    Lemon wedges, for serving

1. To make the dressing, pulse the parsley, oil, lemon juice, vinegar, garlic, ¼ teaspoon salt, and ¼ teaspoon pepper in a food processor until no large stems remain.

2. In a medium bowl, toss the radicchio with 2 tablespoons of the dressing and season with salt and pepper.

3. In another bowl, combine the beans and celery with the remaining dressing.

4. Arrange the radicchio on four serving plates, divide the beans among them, and top with the tuna. Serve with lemon wedges.

Each serving: 398 calories, 37 g protein, 48 g carbohydrates, 12 g fiber (net carbs: 36 g), 2 g sugar, 8 g fat (2 g saturated fat), 37 mg cholesterol, 326 mg sodium

Serving suggestion: Carbohydrate: ¾ cup sliced apple

Each serving, with suggestions: 441 calories, 37 g protein, 60 g carbohydrates, 15 g fiber (net carbs: 45 g), 11 g sugar, 8 g fat (2 g saturated fat), 37 mg cholesterol, 327 mg sodium

GREEK FAVA BEAN SOUP (MAKES 6 SERVINGS)

Make sure the favas you buy have been peeled.

If you reduce the serving size by half, you can serve the soup with 1 slice whole-grain or crusty bread, as is traditional in Greece.

½ cup diced onion (1 small onion)
2 tablespoons olive or grapeseed oil
3 garlic cloves, minced
Rounded 2 cups small dried fava beans, sorted and rinsed
2 teaspoons fresh thyme leaves or ¾ teaspoon dried thyme
1 bay leaf
Kosher salt and ground black pepper
3 tablespoons chopped fresh parsley
Lemon wedges, for serving

In a medium pot, cook the onion in the oil, stirring occasionally, until softened, 3 to 4 minutes. Add the garlic and cook for 30 seconds. Add the favas, thyme, bay leaf, ¾ teaspoon salt, and 6 cups water. Bring to a boil, reduce the heat to low, and simmer, stirring occasionally, until the beans are fall-apart tender, about 45 minutes. Add more water if the beans seem dry (the soup should be thick). Remove the bay leaf. Season with salt and pepper. Sprinkle with parsley and serve with the lemon wedges.

Variation: For a Moroccan-spiced variation, add ½ teaspoon caraway seeds, ½ teaspoon ground cumin, ½ teaspoon ground coriander, and ⅛ teaspoon cayenne pepper when you add the garlic.

Each serving: 261 calories, 17 g protein, 38 g carbohydrates, 17 g fiber (net carbs: 21 g), 4 g sugar, 6 g fat (1 g saturated fat), 0 mg cholesterol, 204 mg sodium

Serving suggestion: Protein #1: 4 ounces shelled mussels, steamed; Fiber: 1 cup *Mediterranean Salad*; Carbohydrate: ½ cup sliced pear

Each serving, with suggestions: 426 calories, 32 g protein, 59 g carbohydrates, 21 g fiber (net carbs: 38 g), 11 g sugar, 9 g fat (1 g saturated fat), 32 mg cholesterol, 534 mg sodium

LENTIL-VEAL RAGOUT (MAKES 6 SERVINGS)

This is a great Sunday stew with leftovers for the week. You can cook the ragout in a slow cooker if you prefer.

> 1 teaspoon ground turmeric
>
> ⅛ teaspoon cayenne pepper, or more to taste
>
> Kosher salt
>
> 1 pound boneless veal stew meat, trimmed of excess fat and cut into
>   ½-inch cubes
>
> ½ cup diced onion (1 small onion)
>
> 2 tablespoons olive or grapeseed oil
>
> 2 garlic cloves, minced
>
> 2 teaspoons dried oregano leaves or 1 teaspoon ground oregano
>
> One 14.5-ounce can low-sodium chicken broth
>
> 2 cups dried green or brown lentils, sorted and rinsed
>
> 1 bunch scallions (green onions), including 3 inches of green tops, sliced
>   crosswise
>
> Ground black pepper
>
> ¼ cup chopped fresh parsley

1. In a medium bowl or resealable plastic bag, mix together the turmeric, cayenne, and ½ teaspoon salt. Add the veal and toss to coat.

2. In a medium pot, cook the veal and onion in the oil, stirring occasionally, until the meat is lightly browned, 4 to 5 minutes.

3. Add the garlic and oregano and cook for 30 seconds. Add the broth and bring to a boil. Reduce the heat to low, cover, and simmer for 30 minutes. (If using a slow cooker, transfer the mixture to the cooker after it comes to a boil. Add the remaining ingredients and enough water to cover. Cook on low for 7 to 8 hours.)

4. Add the lentils, scallions, and enough water to cover by 1 inch. Simmer until the lentils and veal are tender, 20 to 25 minutes, adding more water if the lentils seem dry. (In the slow cooker, add water just to cover, and cook for 7 to 8 hours.)

5. Season with salt and pepper. Serve sprinkled with the parsley.

Variation: To make a curried version, cook 1 tablespoon curry powder with the garlic instead of the oregano.

Each serving: 428 calories, 44 g protein, 42 g carbohydrates, 21 g fiber (net carbs: 21 g), 2 g sugar, 9 g fat (2 g saturated fat), 110 mg cholesterol, 290 mg sodium

Serving suggestion: Fiber: 1 cup diced or sliced cucumber; Carbohydrate: ½ cup grilled apricots

Each serving, with suggestions: 481 calories, 46 g protein, 55 g carbohydrates, 23 g fiber (net carbs: 32 g), 11 g sugar, 9 g fat (2 g saturated fat), 110 mg cholesterol, 293 mg sodium

MEDITERRANEAN-STYLE TURKEY AND PINTO BEAN CHILI

(MAKES 6 SERVINGS)

Increase the amount of chili powder and cayenne depending on how hot you like your chili. You can also make this with diced leftover roast turkey breast instead (add during the last 10 minutes of cooking).

1 pound lean ground turkey breast

¾ cup diced onion (¾ medium onion)

2 tablespoons olive or grapeseed oil

3 garlic cloves, minced

2 tablespoons chili powder

¼ teaspoon cayenne pepper or chipotle powder, or to taste

1 teaspoon ground cumin

1 teaspoon ground coriander

2 teaspoons dried oregano leaves or ½ teaspoon ground oregano

2 teaspoons minced fresh rosemary or sage or ½ teaspoon ground rosemary
    or sage

3 tablespoons tomato paste

One 14.5-ounce can diced tomatoes

1 tablespoon cider vinegar

¾ cup diced red or yellow bell pepper (about ½ large pepper)

6 cups cooked pinto beans, drained and rinsed if canned

2 cups peeled and diced yams, in ½-inch cubes (2 small yams)

Kosher salt and ground black pepper

¼ cup chopped fresh parsley

1. In a medium pot, cook the turkey and onion in the oil, stirring occasionally to break up clumps, until the meat is lightly browned, 4 to 5 minutes. Stir in the garlic, chili powder, cayenne, cumin, coriander, oregano, and rosemary and cook for 30 seconds.

2. Stir in the tomato paste. Add 2½ cups water, the tomatoes and their juice, the vinegar, bell pepper, beans, yams, ¾ teaspoon salt, and ¾ teaspoon pepper. Bring to a boil, reduce the heat to low, and simmer for 45 minutes, stirring occasionally and adding more water if the chili seems dry.

3. Season with salt, pepper, and additional cayenne if desired. Serve sprinkled with the parsley.

(continued on next page)

Each serving: 464 calories, 31 g protein, 61 g carbohydrates, 15 g fiber (net carbs: 46 g), 6 g sugar, 12 g fat (3 g saturated fat), 54 mg cholesterol, 496 mg sodium

Serving suggestion: Carbohydrate: ½ cup diced cantaloupe (the chili has half your fruit)

Each serving, with suggestions: 490 calories, 32 g protein, 68 g carbohydrates (net carbs: 53 g), 15 g fiber, 12 g sugar, 12 g fat (3 g saturated fat), 54 mg cholesterol, 508 mg sodium

CHICKEN QUINOA (MAKES 4 SERVINGS)

Some brands of quinoa are not sold prewashed. If yours has a powdery residue, rinse it well or the quinoa will have a bitter flavor.

- ¾ pound bone-in chicken breasts, skin removed, cut into 4 pieces
- Kosher salt and ground black pepper
- ½ cup diced onion (1 small onion)
- 1 tablespoon plus 1 teaspoon olive or grapeseed oil
- 2 garlic cloves, minced
- 1 teaspoon ground turmeric
- Generous pinch of cayenne pepper
- 1 tablespoon tomato paste
- 1½ cups quinoa, rinsed if necessary
- ¼ cup chopped fresh parsley

1. Season the chicken with ¼ teaspoon salt and ¼ teaspoon pepper. In a medium skillet, cook the chicken and onion in the oil, stirring occasionally, until the chicken is lightly browned, 4 to 5 minutes.

2. Add the garlic, turmeric, and cayenne and cook for 30 seconds. Stir in the tomato paste. Add 3 cups water and stir well. Add the quinoa and bring to a boil. Reduce the heat to low, cover, and simmer until the grains are tender and the chicken is no longer pink, about 15 minutes.

3. Remove from the heat and allow to steam, covered, for 5 minutes. Season with salt and pepper and serve sprinkled with the parsley.

Variation: For a Mediterranean variation, add 1 teaspoon dried oregano with the garlic, and sprinkle with chopped fresh basil instead of (or in addition to) the parsley.

Each serving: 374 calories, 30 g protein, 42 g carbohydrates, 5 g fiber (net carbs: 37 g), 1 g sugar, 9 g fat (1 g saturated fat), 68 mg cholesterol, 356 mg sodium

Serving suggestion: Fiber: ½ cup grilled asparagus (about 4 medium spears); Carbohydrate: 1 cup blackberries with mint

Each serving, with suggestions: 449 calories, 33 g protein, 58 g carbohydrates, 14 g fiber (net carbs: 44 g), 14 g sugar, 10 g fat (1 g saturated fat), 68 mg cholesterol, 359 mg sodium

SHRIMP QUINOA RISOTTO (MAKES 4 SERVINGS)

Some brands of quinoa are not prewashed. If yours has a powdery residue, rinse it well or the quinoa will have a bitter flavor.

1 pound shrimp, peeled, deveined, and cut in half
1 tablespoon plus 1 teaspoon olive or grapeseed oil
½ cup diced onion (1 small onion)
1 garlic clove, minced
Generous pinch of saffron threads, crumbled (optional)
¼ cup white wine or water
1½ cups quinoa, rinsed if necessary
3 cups *Shrimp or Fish Broth*, warmed
Kosher salt and ground black pepper
2 tablespoons chopped parsley

1. In a large saucepan, cook the shrimp in the oil until the shrimp are almost opaque in the center, about 3 minutes. Remove with a slotted spoon and set aside on a plate.

2. Add the onion to the oil and cook until softened, 3 to 4 minutes. Add the garlic and saffron, if using, and cook for 30 seconds. Add the wine and scrape up any residue on the bottom of the pan with a cooking spoon. Add the quinoa and cook for 2 minutes, stirring constantly. Add ½ cup of the broth and stir until the broth is absorbed. Repeat, adding broth ½ cup at a time, until all of the broth has been used and the quinoa is tender. Add water if the quinoa is dry but not yet tender.

3. Season with salt and pepper. Divide the quinoa among four serving plates and arrange the shrimp on top. Serve sprinkled with the parsley.

Variation: Instead of shrimp, try mussels or a mix of your favorite fish.

Each serving: 386 calories, 33 g protein, 41 g carbohydrates, 5 g fiber (net carbs: 36 g), 1 g sugar, 9 g fat (1 g saturated fat), 221 mg cholesterol, 285 mg sodium

Serving suggestion: Fiber: 1 cup grilled fennel; Carbohydrate: 1 cup blackberries with grated orange zest (the colored part only of the skin)

Each serving, with suggestions: 482 calories, 36 g protein, 62 g carbohydrates, 16 g fiber (net carbs: 46 g), 8 g sugar, 10 g fat (1 g saturated fat), 221 mg cholesterol, 343 mg sodium

LUNCH, PHASE 2

In this phase, your lunch calories will remain between 400 and 500, but you can add whole grains like whole wheat pasta two days a week. At those meals, reduce your fruit portion by half.

EGG SANDWICHES WITH GREENS AND GUACAMOLE
(MAKES 4 SERVINGS)

If you use store-bought salsa, check the label to be sure it does not contain added sugar or carbohydrate-rich ingredients like corn.

This recipe has little added fat, so using a nonstick skillet is essential to keep the eggs from sticking.

½ avocado
½ teaspoon lemon or lime juice
½ teaspoon paprika
Kosher salt and ground black pepper
½ teaspoon olive or grapeseed oil
1 tablespoon minced shallot or onion
8 cups coarsely chopped mustard or collard greens,
     (about 2 bunches, stems removed)
3 whole eggs
4 egg whites or ½ cup pasteurized egg whites
8 slices *Protein Boost Diet Quinoa Sandwich Bread*, toasted
2 tablespoons *Fresh Tomato Salsa* or store-bought salsa
     (optional)

1. To make the guacamole, mash the avocado in a small bowl and add the lemon juice, paprika, and a generous pinch of salt and pepper. Cover and set aside.

2. Brush a medium nonstick skillet with ¼ teaspoon of the oil and cook the shallot, stirring occasionally, until softened, about 1 minute. Add the greens, cover, and cook until the leaves are wilted, 3 to 4 minutes. Season with salt and pepper and transfer to a bowl. Wipe out the skillet with paper towels to remove any excess water.

3. In a small bowl, whisk the eggs and egg whites with a pinch each of salt and pepper. Brush the skillet with the remaining ¼ teaspoon oil and cook the eggs over medium heat, undisturbed, until set, 1 to 2 minutes. Flip the eggs and cook 1 minute more.

4. Slice the omelet into quarters. Spread the guacamole on 4 slices of bread and top with the greens and omelet. Top each with the salsa, if using, and the second slice of bread.

Variations: Spice up the guacamole with minced jalapeño instead of paprika. Or make the sandwiches with turkey breast instead of eggs.

Use 12 cups coarsely chopped spinach or Swiss chard (with or without the stems) instead of the greens, if you prefer.

Each serving: 399 calories, 22 g protein, 59 g carbohydrates, 12 g fiber (net carbs: 47 g), 7 g sugar, 13 g fat (2 g saturated fat), 123 mg cholesterol, 691 mg sodium

Serving suggestion: Protein #2: 1 cup cooked brussels sprouts (the sandwich has the egg component of your protein); Fiber: 1 cup strawberries with ½ teaspoon aged balsamic vinegar

Each serving, with suggestions: 445 calories, 25 g protein, 69 g carbohydrates, 15 g fiber (net carbs: 54 g), 14 g sugar, 13 g fat (2 g saturated fat), 123 mg cholesterol, 692 mg sodium

PIZZA (MAKES 3 PIZZAS, 6 SERVINGS)

You can use a pizza pan if you prefer.

If you use store-bought tomato sauce, avoid those with added sugar or carbohydrate-rich ingredients like caramelized onions. Classico marinara with plum tomatoes and Mezzetta homemade style or tomato-basil marinara are good choices.

    1 recipe *Quinoa Pizza Dough*
    Quinoa flour, for rolling
    1 to 1½ cups *Homemade Tomato Sauce* or store-bought tomato sauce
    1½ cups shredded fat-free mozzarella cheese
    1 additional protein topping (see chart)
    2 to 3 vegetable toppings, plus free toppings (see chart)
    Kosher salt and ground black pepper

1. Place a pizza stone in the bottom of the oven. (If you don't have a pizza stone, flip a baking sheet upside down and place on the bottom rack in the oven.) Preheat the oven to 450°F.

2. Divide the dough into three pieces and form each into a loose ball. Sprinkle the work surface lightly with flour. Pat and roll each ball of dough into a 10- to 11-inch round, dusting the top very lightly with flour if needed. Transfer one round of dough to a lightly floured cutting board. Top with ⅓ to ½ cup tomato sauce, ½ cup mozzarella, and your choice of protein, vegetable, and free toppings. Season with salt and pepper.

(continued on next page)

Protein (per pizza; 2 servings)	Vegetables (See Vegetable chart on page 222)
4 ounces cooked calamari, shrimp, mussels, or clams	Grilled baby artichokes or canned artichoke hearts
4 ounces grilled fresh sardines, or water-packed tuna	Roasted eggplant, zucchini, or asparagus
3 ounces cooked lean ground turkey or veal	Sautéed red or yellow onions
2 ounces grilled chicken breast	Sautéed sliced cremini mushrooms or spinach
Vegetarian alternative: Add an extra ½ cup shredded fat-free mozzarella or ¼ cup grated Parmesan per pizza	Sliced red, yellow, or green bell peppers
	Free toppings: Capers, minced garlic, fresh herbs such as basil

3. Slide the dough directly onto the stone or baking sheet and bake until the crust is lightly golden brown on the bottom and around the edges, as little as 8 minutes if you are using a pizza stone to as long as 12 minutes if you are using a baking sheet. Watch closely the last few minutes so it doesn't burn. Carefully transfer the pizza to a wire rack to cool slightly before serving.

4. Repeat with the remaining 2 pizzas.

Each serving (approximately; will vary depending on toppings): 424 calories, 28 g protein, 55 g carbohydrates, 9 g fiber (net carbs: 46 g), 4 g sugar, 10 g fat (2 g saturated fat), 33 mg cholesterol, 710 mg sodium

Serving suggestion: Fiber: 1 cup diced cucumber and mint salad; Fruit: ½ cup diced apple (the pizza has half your vegetable serving; the tomato sauce is half your fruit)

Each serving, with suggestions: 468 calories, 29 g protein, 66 g carbohydrates, 11 g fiber (net carbs: 55 g), 11 g sugar, 10 g fat (2 g saturated fat), 33 mg cholesterol, 713 mg sodium

SPINACH AND MUSHROOM LASAGNA (MAKES 6 SERVINGS)

If you use store-bought tomato sauce, avoid those with added sugar or carbohydrate-rich ingredients like caramelized onions. Classico marinara with plum tomatoes and Mezzetta homemade style or tomato-basil marinara are good choices.

> 4 cups sliced cremini mushrooms (two 6- or 8-ounce packages)
> 2 cups sliced shiitake mushrooms (one 5-ounce package)
> 2 garlic cloves, minced
> 2 teaspoons fresh thyme leaves or ½ teaspoon dried thyme
> 1 tablespoon olive or grapeseed oil
> Kosher salt and ground black pepper
> Two 10-ounce packages frozen chopped spinach, thawed

2 cups low-fat cottage cheese
3 egg whites or 6 tablespoons pasteurized egg whites
¼ cup grated Parmesan cheese
Pinch of ground nutmeg
2½ cups *Homemade Tomato Sauce* or one 24-ounce jar tomato sauce
9 whole wheat lasagna noodles (about 8 ounces), uncooked
½ cup shredded fat-free mozzarella cheese

1. In a large skillet, cook the mushrooms, garlic, and thyme in the oil, stirring occasionally, until the mushrooms are softened, 8 to 10 minutes. Season with salt and pepper. Remove from the heat and set aside.

2. Preheat the oven to 350°F.

3. Squeeze the water out of the spinach. Stir together the spinach, cottage cheese, egg whites, Parmesan, and nutmeg in a medium bowl.

4. Spread ¼ cup of the tomato sauce on the bottom of a 9 by 13-inch baking pan. Arrange 3 lasagna noodles on top. Spread half of the spinach mixture over the noodles. Top with half of the mushroom mixture, then 1 cup sauce. Repeat, using 3 noodles, the remaining spinach mixture, the remaining mushrooms, and 1 cup sauce. End with the remaining noodles and sauce.

5. Cover the pan with aluminum foil. Bake the lasagna for 40 minutes.

6. Remove the foil, sprinkle the mozzarella on top, and return to the oven until the cheese is melted, about 15 minutes. Let rest for 10 minutes before cutting and serving.

Each serving: 375 calories, 29 g protein, 50 g carbohydrates, 11 g fiber (net carbs: 40 g), 7 g sugar, 7 g fat (2 g saturated fat), 11 mg cholesterol, 1,039 mg sodium

Serving suggestion: Fiber: 1 cup steamed string (green) beans with lemon juice (the tomato sauce is your fruit serving)

Each serving, with suggestions: 409 calories, 31 g protein, 58 g carbohydrates, 14 g fiber (net carbs: 44 g), 9 g sugar, 7 g fat (2 g saturated fat), 11 mg cholesterol, 1,046 mg sodium

MEDITERRANEAN BEAN MEDLEY (MAKES 6 SERVINGS)

This hearty, freezer-friendly stew is great with crumbled feta. The cooking time will vary depending on the size and age of the chickpeas and favas. Make sure the favas you buy have been peeled. For how to quick-soak chickpeas, see *Picnic Chickpea Salad*.

- ½ cup dried chickpeas, sorted and rinsed, soaked overnight in 2 cups water or quick-soaked, and drained
- ½ cup small dried fava beans, sorted and rinsed
- ½ cup dried green or brown lentils, sorted and rinsed
- ⅔ cup coarsely ground bulgur, pearled barley, or brown rice (not quick-cooking), rinsed
- 2 tablespoons tomato paste
- 1 tablespoon dried oregano or 1½ teaspoons ground oregano
- Kosher salt and ground black pepper
- 6 garlic cloves, minced
- ⅛ teaspoon cayenne pepper, or more to taste
- 2 teaspoons ground turmeric
- 1 tablespoon ground cumin
- 2 tablespoons olive or grapeseed oil
- ¼ cup lemon juice, plus more to taste
- ¼ cup chopped fresh parsley

1. Combine the chickpeas, favas, lentils, bulgur, tomato paste, oregano, and 8 cups water in a large pot. Bring to a boil, reduce the heat to low, cover, and simmer, stirring occasionally to prevent sticking, until the chickpeas are tender, 1 to 1½ hours. Add more water if the mixture appears dry. When the beans are tender, add 1 teaspoon salt and 1 teaspoon pepper.

2. In a small skillet, cook the garlic, cayenne, turmeric, and cumin in the oil for 30 seconds. Add to the beans and simmer for 5 minutes.

3. Remove from the heat and stir in the lemon juice. Season with salt, pepper, and more lemon juice, if desired. Serve sprinkled with the parsley.

Variation: For an Italian-style stew, decrease the water to 5 cups and add one 28-ounce can whole tomatoes (crush tomatoes with your hands). Omit the lemon juice and serve sprinkled with basil. The tomatoes will serve as your fruit.

Each serving: 287 calories, 13 g protein, 46 g carbohydrates, 14 g fiber, 4 g sugar, 6 g fat (1 g saturated fat), 0 mg cholesterol, 404 mg sodium

Serving suggestion: Protein Source #1: Crumble ⅓ cup (about 1½ ounces) reduced-fat feta on the beans. Fiber: 1 cup *Mediterranean Salad*; Carbohydrate: 1 cup diced cantaloupe

Each serving, with suggestions: 472 calories, 24 g protein, 64 g carbohydrates, 16 g fiber (net fiber: 48 g), 18 g sugar, 11 g fat (4 g saturated fat), 17 mg cholesterol, 913 mg sodium

WHOLE-GRAIN PASTA WITH VEGETABLES (MAKES 6 SERVINGS)

The cooking time will vary depending on the size and age of the chickpeas and favas.

Make sure the favas you buy have been peeled.

⅓ cup dried chickpeas, sorted and rinsed, soaked in 2 cups of water overnight or quick-soaked (see *Picnic Chickpea Salad*), and drained
⅓ cup small dried fava beans, sorted and rinsed
⅓ cup dried green or brown lentils, sorted and rinsed
2 tablespoons tomato paste
⅛ teaspoon cayenne pepper, or more to taste
1 teaspoon ground turmeric
½ cup diced onion (1 small onion)
¾ cup thinly sliced celery
Kosher salt and ground black pepper
6 garlic cloves, minced
2 teaspoons caraway seeds
2 teaspoons ground coriander
2 tablespoons olive or grapeseed oil
2 cups diced zucchini (1 medium zucchini)
6 cups fresh spinach, coarsely chopped
6 ounces whole-grain cut pasta, such as penne (about 2 cups)
¼ cup chopped fresh parsley

1. Combine the chickpeas, favas, lentils, tomato paste, cayenne, turmeric, onion, celery, and 6 cups water in a medium pot. Bring to a boil, reduce the heat to low, cover, and simmer, stirring occasionally, until the chickpeas are tender, 1 to 1½ hours. Add 1 teaspoon salt and 1 teaspoon pepper.

2. In a small skillet, cook the garlic, caraway, and coriander in 1 tablespoon of the oil for 30 seconds, then stir into the beans.

3. In another skillet, stir-fry the zucchini in the remaining 1 tablespoon oil until crisp-tender, about 5 minutes, and season with salt. Add the zucchini, spinach, and pasta to the beans; if the beans appear dry, add 1 cup water before adding the pasta. Bring to a simmer and cook, stirring occasionally

(continued on next page)

to prevent sticking, until the pasta is al dente, 5 to 6 minutes. Season with additional salt and pepper and serve sprinkled with the parsley.

Each serving: 300 calories, 14 g protein, 49 g carbohydrates, 14 g fiber, 5 g sugar, 7 g fat (1 g saturated fat), 0 mg cholesterol, 262 mg sodium

Serving suggestion: Protein Source #1: 3 ounces turkey or ½ can light tuna; Carbohydrate: ½ cup sliced peaches

Each serving, with suggestions: 422 calories, 30 g protein, 60 g carbohydrates, 15 g fiber (net fiber: 45 g), 16 g sugar, 8 g fat (1 g saturated fat), 37 mg cholesterol, 1,125 mg sodium

DINNER, PHASE 1

At dinner, your focus in this phase will be on eating lean protein, primarily seafood (see the charts in the Meal Plans in Chapter 10 for quantities of specific proteins). Aim for five nights of seafood per week, along with three to six servings of Category 1 and 2 vegetables. Your fat will come from good oils and avocados again, and you will also have a small amount of cheese protein (optional) to round out the meal. Two nights a week, you can substitute ½ cup cooked quinoa for a portion of your vegetables. Your total calorie intake will be between 400 and 500 calories.

In the lunch section, many of the recipes were fairly complete meals with side dish additions like fruit. At dinner, you will be choosing several vegetable sides to complete your meal, so many of the recipes here leave ¼ or ½ teaspoon olive oil to brush on your vegetables before grilling or roasting or to use in a salad dressing. Your cheese serving is another great way to vary dinners (add a few tablespoons of Parmesan to roasted brussels sprouts one night, goat cheese to a spinach salad the next). You can also easily design your own quick dinners by grilling or baking your favorite lean proteins and vegetables.

SEAFOOD

SEAFOOD CEVICHE (MAKES 4 SERVINGS)

To shred the cilantro, first stack a few leaves. Roll up the leaves tightly, like a cigar. Cut across the roll with a sharp knife.

Kosher salt

10 ounces large sea scallops, quartered, or bay scallops

10 ounces cleaned calamari, bodies sliced into ¼-inch-wide rings, tentacles left whole

10 ounces shrimp, peeled, deveined, and cut into thirds

1 small red onion, quartered and thinly sliced

¾ cup lime juice

½ avocado, cut into ¼-inch dice

¼ cup shredded fresh cilantro

Ground black pepper

(*continued on next page*)

1. Place a large bowl of ice water next to the sink. Bring a medium saucepan of water and ½ teaspoon salt to a boil. Add the scallops, calamari, and shrimp and simmer for 45 seconds. Drain, immediately transfer to the ice water to stop the cooking, then drain again.

2. Place the scallops, calamari, shrimp, and onion in a large shallow bowl and stir in the lime juice. Cover and refrigerate until the seafood is firm but still tender, 45 minutes to 1 hour, stirring occasionally.

3. Drain off the excess lime juice into a cup. Gently fold the avocado and cilantro into the seafood. Season with salt and pepper. Add back a few tablespoons of the lime juice, adding more if you prefer a tangier ceviche. Transfer to a serving bowl or divide among individual martini glasses and serve immediately.

Variation: Use whatever mix of seafood you prefer, for a total of about 2 pounds. If you use fish fillets, cut them into ½-inch cubes.

Each serving: 260 calories, 38 g protein, 11 g carbohydrates, 2 g fiber (net carbs: 9 g), 2 g sugar, 6 g fat (1 g saturated fat), 324 mg cholesterol, 308 mg sodium

Serving suggestion: Fiber #1 (+ Cheese Protein): 2 cups roasted broccoli and cauliflower, sprinkled with 3 tablespoons Parmesan; Fiber #2: 1 cup diced cucumber; 2 cups grilled radicchio drizzled with 1 teaspoon balsamic vinegar

Each serving, with suggestions: 414 calories, 50 g protein, 30 g carbohydrates, 8 g fiber (net carbs: 22 g), 8 g sugar, 11 g fat (3 g saturated fat), 337 mg cholesterol, 616 mg sodium

GRILLED SHRIMP WITH OREGANO AND LEMON
(MAKES 4 SERVINGS)

Instead of metal skewers, you can thread the shrimp on rosemary branches for more flavor (remove the leaves first).

¼ cup capers, rinsed and soaked in cold water for 15 minutes
3 tablespoons chopped fresh oregano, 1 teaspoon dried oregano leaves,
    or ¼ teaspoon ground oregano
1 garlic clove, minced
2 teaspoons olive or grapeseed oil
1 teaspoon finely grated lemon zest (only the colored part of the skin)
2 tablespoons lemon juice
Ground black pepper
2 pounds large shrimp, peeled and deveined, tails intact

1. To make the sauce, drain and chop the capers. Place them in a medium bowl and stir in the oregano, garlic, oil, lemon zest, and lemon juice. Season with pepper.

2. Heat a grill to medium-high. Thread the shrimp on metal skewers and grill until lightly charred and cooked through, 2 to 3 minutes per side.

3. Remove the shrimp from the skewers and transfer to a platter. Spoon the sauce on top and serve immediately.

Variation: To make tandoori-style shrimp, omit the caper-oregano sauce. Combine 2 teaspoons oil with 1 teaspoon finely grated gingerroot, ½ teaspoon ground cumin, ½ teaspoon ground coriander, ½ teaspoon ground turmeric, ½ teaspoon paprika, a pinch of cayenne pepper, and ¼ teaspoon salt. Toss the shrimp in the marinade before skewering.

Each serving: 218 calories, 43 g protein, 8 g carbohydrates, 2 g fiber (net carbs: 6 g), 0 g sugar, 3 g fat (0 g saturated fat), 334 mg cholesterol, 539 mg sodium

Serving suggestion: Fiber #1 (+ Cheese Protein): 2 cups garlic-roasted brussels sprouts with 3 tablespoons Parmesan; Fiber #2 (+ ½ Fat): Classic slaw with 2 to 2½ cups shredded cabbage, 1 tablespoon minced red onion, ½ teaspoon olive oil, and ½ teaspoon cider vinegar (or to taste)

Each serving, with suggestions: 422 calories, 57 g protein, 34 g carbohydrates, 13 g fiber (net carbs: 21 g), 10 g sugar, 10 g fat (4 g saturated fat), 337 mg cholesterol, 844 mg sodium

WEEKNIGHT BAKED FISH (MAKES 4 SERVINGS)

This is an easy technique for roasting any skinless white fish fillet for lunch or dinner (reduce the serving size at lunch).

Four 6- to 8-ounce skinless mahimahi, tilapia, halibut, sole, or flounder fillets
Kosher salt and ground black pepper
2 teaspoons olive or grapeseed oil
¼ cup chopped fresh parsley
4 lemon wedges, for serving

1. Preheat the oven to 375°F. Pat the fish dry with paper towels and season with salt and pepper. Brush a baking dish lightly with ½ teaspoon of the oil.

2. Place the fish in the baking dish in one layer and drizzle with the remaining oil. Bake the fish until it flakes, 8 to 12 minutes, depending on the thickness of the fillets. Sprinkle with the parsley and serve with the lemon wedges.

Variations: You can also cook the fish in a nonstick skillet. Brush a large skillet lightly with oil. Working in batches if necessary, place the fish in the skillet in a single layer. Drizzle with a little oil. Cook until the bottom is lightly golden. Flip the fish carefully and cook until firm to the touch.

Sprinkle the fish with ½ teaspoon smoked paprika before baking.

(continued on next page)

Top with chopped jalapeños and serve with limes instead of lemons.

In addition to parsley, you can sprinkle the fish with chopped chives, scallions (green onions), or your favorite fresh herbs.

Each serving: 213 calories, 42 g protein, 0 g carbohydrates, 0 g fiber, 0 g sugar, 4 g fat (1 g saturated fat), 165 mg cholesterol, 202 mg sodium

Serving suggestion: Fiber #1: 2 cups steamed asparagus with lemon (about 15 medium spears); Fiber #2 (+ Cheese Protein + ½ Fat): Endive salad with 2 cups endive, ¼ cup sliced yellow bell pepper, 4 radishes, ¾ ounce goat cheese, and 1½ teaspoons *Basic or Dijon Vinaigrette* (made with red wine vinegar)

Each serving, with suggestions: 407 calories, 56 g protein, 16 g carbohydrates, 10 g fiber (net carbs: 6 g), 7 g sugar, 14 g fat (6 g saturated fat), 188 mg cholesterol, 309 mg sodium

---

LEMONY ROAST SALMON OR SNAPPER (MAKES 4 SERVINGS)

Salmon cooking time varies, depending on thickness and desired doneness. If using whole snapper, have your fishmonger clean and bone it for you.

> One 1-pound skin-on salmon fillet, or one 1¼-pound snapper, boned, without head or tail
> Kosher salt and ground black pepper
> 1 teaspoon olive or grapeseed oil
> ½ teaspoon ground turmeric
> Generous pinch of cayenne pepper, or more to taste
> 12 thin slices lemon
> 12 thin slices red onion
> 2 tablespoons minced fresh chives

1. Preheat the oven to 375°F. Pat the salmon dry with paper towels and season with salt and pepper. Brush a baking dish lightly with the oil.

2. Place the salmon in the pan, skin side down. Mix together the turmeric, cayenne, and ¼ teaspoon salt and sprinkle over the salmon. Arrange the lemon and onion slices on top and bake the salmon until just turning opaque in the center, 18 to 22 minutes, or to preferred doneness. Serve sprinkled with the chives.

Variations: Omit the lemon and onion slices and top the salmon with fresh herbs, such as oregano or tarragon, and grated citrus zest (lemon or orange, only the colored part of the skin) before baking.

To make mustard-glazed salmon, whisk together 2 tablespoons Dijon mustard with 1 tablespoon each lemon juice and minced chives. Spread on the fillet before baking.

Each serving: 244 calories, 25 g protein, 0 g carbohydrates, 0 g fiber, 0 g sugar, 15 g fat (3 g saturated fat), 71 mg cholesterol, 69 mg sodium

Serving suggestion: Fiber #1 (+ Cheese Protein + ½ Fat): 2 cups sliced or diced zucchini cooked in ½ teaspoon olive oil with 3 tablespoons Parmesan; Fiber #2 (+ ¼ Fat): 2½ cups cooked kohlrabi and watercress

Each serving, with suggestions: 437 calories, 38 g protein, 21 g carbohydrates, 10 g fiber (net carbs: 11 g), 8 g sugar, 24 g fat (6 g saturated fat), 86 mg cholesterol, 391 mg sodium

POULTRY AND MEAT

CHICKEN VEGETABLE SOUP (MAKES 4 SERVINGS)

This recipe can be enjoyed at lunch if you add 4 cups cooked chickpeas to the broth when you add the greens. You can remove the chicken from the bones and shred it, if you prefer.

> ½ cup diced onion (1 small onion)
> 1 medium leek, white and light green parts, thoroughly rinsed and minced
> 2 celery stalks, minced
> 1 carrot, peeled and minced
> 1 tablespoon olive or grapeseed oil
> 1½ pounds bone-in chicken breasts, skin removed, cut into 8 pieces
> 4 cups diced zucchini (about 4 medium)
> Kosher salt
> 2 cups diced peeled turnips (about 3 medium)
> 2 cups coarsely chopped turnip greens (remove stems first) or 4 cups coarsely
>   chopped fresh spinach
> Kosher salt and ground black pepper

1. In a large pot, cook the onion, 1 tablespoon of the leek, 1 tablespoon of the celery, and 1 tablespoon of the carrot in the oil, stirring occasionally, until softened, 3 to 4 minutes.

2. Add the chicken and cook undisturbed until the chicken begins to brown, about 3 minutes. Flip the chicken pieces and cook until lightly brown on the other side, another 3 minutes.

3. Add the zucchini and cook for 2 minutes more. Add 5 cups water and ½ teaspoon salt. Bring to a boil, reduce the heat, and simmer for 15 minutes.

(*continued on next page*)

4. Add the turnips and the remaining leek, celery, and carrot. Simmer until the turnips are tender, 10 to 12 minutes.

5. Add the turnip greens and cook until wilted, about 2 minutes. Season with salt and pepper.

6. To serve, place two chicken pieces per person in large bowls and ladle the broth and vegetables on top.

Variations: Try this with your favorite Category 1 and 2 vegetables.

Just before serving, add 1 teaspoon minced fresh herbs such as oregano, thyme, or dill.

Each serving: 311 calories, 45 g protein, 19 g carbohydrates, 5 g fiber (net carbs: 14 g), 9 g sugar, 6 g fat (1 g saturated fat), 136 mg cholesterol, 524 mg sodium

Serving suggestion: Fiber #2 (+ Cheese Protein + ¼ Fat): Southwestern slaw with 2 to 2½ cups shredded cabbage, 3 tablespoons reduced-fat feta, 1 tablespoon each chopped cilantro and red onion, ¼ diced jalapeño, 2 teaspoons lime juice (more to taste), and ¼ teaspoon olive oil

Each serving, with suggestions: 435 calories, 52 g protein, 30 g carbohydrates, 10 g fiber (net carbs: 20 g), 14 g sugar, 10 g fat (2 g saturated fat), 146 mg cholesterol, 845 mg sodium

SPICY HERB-MARINATED CHICKEN AND VEGETABLE SKEWERS (MAKES 4 SERVINGS)

Thai red chili paste is available in the Asian food aisle of most supermarkets. For a smokier flavor, substitute adobo sauce from a can of chipotle chiles.

> 2 teaspoons olive or grapeseed oil
> 1 teaspoon Thai red chili paste
> 1 tablespoon lemon juice
> 1 teaspoon chopped fresh rosemary
> 1 teaspoon chopped fresh mint
> 1 teaspoon fresh thyme leaves
> Kosher salt
> 1¼ to 1½ pounds boneless, skinless chicken breast, cut into 1½-inch cubes
> 2 cups sliced yellow summer squash, cut 1 inch thick (2 medium squashes)
> 2 cups sliced zucchini, cut 1 inch thick (2 medium zucchini)
> ½ cup diced red bell pepper
> ½ cup diced green bell pepper
> Ground black pepper

1. In a medium bowl, mix together 1 teaspoon of the oil, the chili paste, lemon juice, rosemary, mint, thyme, and ¼ teaspoon salt. Add the chicken,

toss to coat, cover with plastic wrap, and refrigerate for 45 minutes to 1 hour.

2. Meanwhile, heat a grill to medium-high.

3. In a large bowl, toss the squash, zucchini, and red and green bell pepper with the remaining 1 teaspoon olive oil, ¼ teaspoon salt, and ¼ teaspoon black pepper. Thread the vegetables onto four metal skewers and grill 3 to 4 minutes. Flip and grill 3 to 4 minutes more, until just crisp-tender.

4. Meanwhile, thread the chicken onto four more skewers. Grill for 5 minutes. Flip the chicken skewers and cook another 6 to 8 minutes, until everything is cooked through.

5. Serve one vegetable skewer and one chicken skewer to each person.

Variation: For a Moroccan twist, instead of the rosemary, mint, and thyme, use ½ teaspoon ground cumin, ½ teaspoon ground coriander, and ½ teaspoon ground turmeric.

Each serving: 243 calories, 37 g protein, 6 g carbohydrates, 2 g fiber (net carbs: 4 g), 3 g sugar, 6 g fat (1 g saturated fat), 99 mg cholesterol, 433 mg sodium

Serving suggestion: Fiber #1: 1 cup grilled asparagus (7 or 8 medium spears); Fiber #2 (+ Cheese Protein + ½ Fat): 1½ cups grilled sliced eggplant, and spinach salad with 3 cups baby spinach, ¼ cup sliced red onion, ¾ ounce goat cheese, and 1½ teaspoons *Balsamic Vinaigrette*

Each serving, with suggestions: 436 calories, 50 g protein, 22 g carbohydrates, 11 g fiber (net carbs: 11 g), 9 g sugar, 16 g fat (6 g saturated fat), 121 mg cholesterol, 583 mg sodium

VEAL AND SPINACH MEATBALLS WITH TOMATO SAUCE
(MAKES 4 SERVINGS)

Frozen and fresh spinach both work well in this dish.

- ½ cup diced onion (1 small onion)
- 2 teaspoons olive or grapeseed oil
- 1½ teaspoons ground turmeric
- 2 tablespoons tomato paste
- 2 to 3 cups low-sodium chicken broth
- ½ teaspoon paprika
- ¼ teaspoon ground coriander
- ¼ teaspoon caraway seeds
- Kosher salt and ground black pepper
- 1 cup cooked spinach, squeezed dry and chopped (from 7 cups fresh spinach or one 10-ounce package frozen spinach)
- 1 egg white or 2 tablespoons pasteurized egg whites
- 1 pound ground lean veal, turkey breast, or grass-fed beef
- 3 tablespoons grated Parmesan cheese
- ¼ cup chopped fresh parsley

1. In a large, deep saucepan, cook the onion in the oil, stirring occasionally, until softened, 3 to 4 minutes. Add ½ teaspoon of the turmeric and the tomato paste, mixing well. Stir in 2 cups broth and simmer for 10 minutes.

2. Meanwhile, in a large bowl, mix together the paprika, the remaining 1 teaspoon turmeric, the coriander, caraway, ¼ teaspoon salt, and ¼ teaspoon pepper. Add the spinach and egg white, mixing well. Gently but thoroughly fold in the veal, being careful not to overmix. Form into 1½-inch balls.

3. Carefully lower the meatballs into the sauce and simmer, loosely covered, until the meatballs are cooked through and the sauce has reduced slightly, 25 to 30 minutes, adding more chicken broth if the sauce seems dry. Season with salt and pepper.

4. Serve sprinkled with the Parmesan and parsley.

Each serving: 270 calories, 33 g protein, 6 g carbohydrates, 2 g fiber (net carbs: 4 g), 2 g sugar, 12 g fat (4 g saturated fat), 120 mg cholesterol, 394 mg sodium

Serving suggestion: Fiber #1: 1½ cups steamed broccoli and cauliflower, mixed; Fiber #2 (+ ¾ Cheese Protein + ½ Fat): 1½ cups roasted diced eggplant; spring salad of 2 cups mixed baby greens with ½ ounce goat cheese and 2½ teaspoons *Basic Vinaigrette, herb variation*

Each serving, with suggestions: 437 calories, 43 g protein, 25 g carbohydrates, 11 g fiber (net carbs: 14 g), 9 g sugar, 20 g fat (8 g saturated fat), 135 mg cholesterol, 479 mg sodium

DINNER, PHASE 2

In this phase, you can substitute ½ cup cooked whole grains, such as multigrain pasta, brown rice, bulgur, and rye (see the chart in the Meal Plans in Chapter 10), for the quinoa in Phase 1 two nights a week. The recipes here are for those evenings (you can substitute other whole grains, but adjust the cooking time accordingly). You can continue to use the dinner recipes in Phase 1 or devise your own protein and vegetable combinations for the remainder of the week.

SNAPPER SOUP WITH CRACKED RYE (MAKES 4 SERVINGS)

Ask your fishmonger to scale and clean the fish and cut it into 3-inch serving pieces (keep the head, tail, and backbone for the broth).

    ½ cup diced onion (1 small onion)
    1 tablespoon olive or grapeseed oil
    4 garlic cloves, minced
    1½ teaspoons ground cumin
    1 teaspoon ground turmeric
    Generous pinch of cayenne pepper, or more to taste
    2 celery stalks, cut in half
    One 3½-pound whole yellowtail snapper, cleaned, scaled, and cut into
        3-inch chunks (head, bones, and tail reserved)
    Kosher salt
    1 cup cracked rye or whole rye berries (see *Note* below)
    Ground black pepper
    ¼ cup chopped parsley

1. In a medium pot, cook the onion in the oil, stirring occasionally, until softened, 3 to 4 minutes. Add the garlic, cumin, turmeric, and cayenne and cook for 30 seconds. Add 5 cups water; the celery; the fish head, tail, and backbone; and 1 teaspoon salt. Bring to a boil, reduce the heat to low, and simmer the broth for 15 minutes.

2. Remove the celery and fish bones with a slotted spoon. Add the rye and simmer until tender, 20 minutes to 1½ hours (see *Note*), adding more water if the soup appears dry.

3. Season the snapper with ¼ teaspoon salt, add to the soup, and simmer just until the fish flakes, 8 to 12 minutes.

4. Season the soup with salt and pepper and serve sprinkled with the parsley.

(*continued on next page*)

Variation: Small whole striped bass or pollock fillets are good alternatives to yellowtail snapper. If using fillets, ask your fish seller for some bones and a fish head; often, the seller will give them to you free.

Each serving: 348 calories, 45 g protein, 24 g carbohydrates, 8 g fiber (net carbs: 16 g), 12 g sugar, 7 g fat (1 g saturated fat), 0 mg cholesterol, 296 mg sodium

Serving suggestion: Fiber #2 (+ Cheese Protein + ¼ of your Fat): 1 cup garlic-roasted brussels sprouts with ¼ teaspoon olive oil and 3 tablespoons Parmesan

Each serving, with suggestions: 460 calories, 54 g protein, 33 g carbohydrates, 11 g fiber (net carbs: 22 g), 14 g sugar, 12 g fat (3 g saturated fat), 13 mg cholesterol, 547 mg sodium

Note: Whole rye berries are the healthiest choice, but you can use either cracked rye (20 minutes cooking time) or whole berries (1 to 1½ hours cooking time). Avoid rye flakes.

CIOPPINO WITH BROWN RICE (MAKES 4 SERVINGS)

This is a flexible variation on the San Francisco–style seafood stew, so use your favorite herbs and seafood combinations. For a quick weeknight pantry version, use a mix of frozen calamari and shrimp.

½ cup diced onion (1 small onion)
1 tablespoon olive or grapeseed oil
3 garlic cloves, minced
2 tablespoons tomato paste
One 8-ounce bottle clam juice, 1 cup low-sodium seafood broth, or 1 cup
    Shrimp or Fish Broth
½ cup dry white wine
2 teaspoons fresh thyme leaves or ½ teaspoon dried thyme
Generous pinch of cayenne pepper, or more to taste
1 dried bay leaf
¾ cup medium-grain brown rice (not quick-cooking)
Kosher salt
½ pound shrimp, peeled and deveined
½ pound mussels, clams, or calamari
½ pound white fish fillets (cod, halibut, sea bass, or other), cut into 2-inch pieces
Ground black pepper
¼ cup chopped parsley

1. In a medium pot, cook the onion in the oil, stirring occasionally, until softened, 3 to 4 minutes. Add the garlic and cook for 30 seconds. Stir in the tomato paste, mixing well. Add the clam juice, wine, thyme, cayenne, bay leaf, rice, ½ teaspoon salt, and 4 cups water. Bring to a boil, reduce the heat

to low, cover, and simmer until the rice is tender, about 45 minutes, adding more water if the rice appears dry.

2. Add the shrimp, mussels, and fish and cook until the fish flakes and the mussels open, 4 to 6 minutes (discard any mussels that do not open). Remove the bay leaf. Season with salt and pepper and serve sprinkled with the parsley.

Each serving: 352 calories, 32 g protein, 35 g carbohydrates, 2 g fiber (net carbs: 33 g), 2 g sugar, 7 g fat (1 g saturated fat), 126 mg cholesterol, 608 mg sodium

Serving suggestion: Fiber #2 (+ Cheese Protein + ¼ Fat): 2½ cups curly endive salad with radishes and cucumber, 3 tablespoons reduced-fat feta, and 2¼ teaspoons *Lemon Vinaigrette*; 1 cup grilled sliced eggplant

Each serving, with suggestions: 481 calories, 40 g protein, 45 g carbohydrates, 10 g fiber (net carbs: 35 g), 5 g sugar, 11 g fat (3 g saturated fat), 138 mg cholesterol, 956 mg sodium

STUFFED CABBAGE LEAVES (MAKES 4 SERVINGS)

This easy version of stuffed cabbage makes a fun family cooking project.

> 1 medium head green cabbage
> 2 teaspoons olive or grapeseed oil
> 2 tablespoons tomato paste
> 2 cups low-sodium chicken broth
> 1 teaspoon ground turmeric
> ½ cup minced onion (1 small onion)
> ½ cup chopped fresh parsley
> ½ teaspoon dried oregano leaves or ⅛ teaspoon ground oregano
> Generous teaspoon cayenne pepper, or more to taste
> 1½ cups cooked brown rice (½ cup raw rice simmered in 1 cup water for about 45 minutes)
> Kosher salt and freshly ground black pepper
> 1 pound ground lean veal, turkey breast, or grass-fed beef
> ¼ cup chopped fresh parsley

1. Bring a large pot of water to a boil. Add the cabbage and simmer for 5 minutes. Drain, rinse under cold running water, and set aside to cool.

2. When cool, separate the leaves and cut off the tough stem ends (try to keep the delicate leaves intact). Pat the leaves dry with paper towels.

3. Preheat the oven to 350°F.

(*continued on next page*)

4. Combine the oil, tomato paste, chicken broth, and ½ teaspoon of the turmeric in a medium saucepan, mixing well. Simmer for 10 minutes. Remove from the heat.

5. Meanwhile, in a large bowl, mix together the onion, parsley, oregano, the remaining ½ teaspoon turmeric, the cayenne, rice, ½ teaspoon salt, and ½ teaspoon pepper. Gently fold in the meat.

6. Lay out the leaves on your work surface, cupped upward. Spoon 2 tablespoons of the meat mixture into the center of a leaf. Fold both sides over the filling, toward the center, and roll up like an egg roll or burrito. Place the roll seam side down in a 9 by 13-inch baking pan. Repeat with the remaining meat mixture and cabbage, keeping the rolls in one layer, if possible.

7. Spoon the sauce on top of the cabbage rolls. Cover the pan with aluminum foil and bake for 45 minutes to 1 hour, or until the meat is cooked through. Season with salt and pepper and serve sprinkled with the parsley.

Each serving: 347 calories, 29 g protein, 32 g carbohydrates, 4 g fiber (net carbs: 28 g), 4 g sugar, 11 g fat (3 g saturated fat), 291 mg cholesterol, 144 mg sodium

Serving suggestion: Fiber #2 (+ Cheese Protein + Fat): 2 cups mustard greens cooked in ½ teaspoon olive oil; 1 cup diced cucumber with 3 tablespoons reduced-fat feta and 1 teaspoon chopped mint

Each serving, with suggestions: 486 calories, 38 g protein, 42 g carbohydrates, 8 g fiber (net carbs: 34 g), 8 g sugar, 16 g fat (5 g saturated fat), 437 mg cholesterol, 489 mg sodium

VEGETABLES

GRILLED VEGETABLES

Many of the Favorite Vegetables (see the chart in Chapter 10) are particularly good grilled. Brush them very lightly with oil before grilling them. Experiment by sprinkling them with different herbs, vinaigrettes, sauces, and cheeses at dinner. Make extra when you grill, and serve the leftover vegetables dressed with lemon juice, salsa, or other fat-free toppings for lunch.

MEDITERRANEAN SALAD

(MAKES 2 LUNCH SERVINGS, EACH 1 CUP CATEGORY 2 VEGETABLES)

This Turkish-inspired version of a Mediterranean salad is a great lunch side dish, as there is no added fat. It's a flexible recipe, so increase the amount of tomato according to your remaining lunch fruit allotment and adjust the lemon juice to taste.

> 2 cups diced cucumber (1 large cucumber)
> ½ cup diced tomato (1 small tomato)
> 3 tablespoons minced red or yellow onion
> 1 teaspoon capers, drained, rinsed, and coarsely chopped
> 1 tablespoon chopped fresh parsley
> 1 teaspoon chopped fresh mint
> 2 teaspoons lemon juice, plus more to taste
> Kosher salt and ground black pepper

Toss together the cucumber, tomato, onion, capers, parsley, mint, and lemon juice in a medium bowl. Season with salt, pepper, and more lemon juice, to taste. Serve immediately.

Variations: Add 4 or 5 thinly sliced radishes.
   Instead of mint, try dill or basil.
   Use 2 thinly sliced scallions (green onions) instead of the diced onion.

Each serving: 31 calories, 1 g protein, 7 g carbohydrates, 1 g fiber (net carbs: 6 g), 3 g sugar, 0 g fat (0 g saturated fat), 0 mg cholesterol, 48 mg sodium

SNACKS

KALE CHIPS (MAKES 4 DINNER OR AFTERNOON SNACK SERVINGS, EACH 1 CUP CATEGORY 1 VEGETABLES, ½ SERVING FAT)

This recipe may even convert the entire family to vegetable chips. The key is getting as much water as possible out of the leaves and baking them long enough so they get crisp but do not burn.

> 1 large bunch kale
> 2 teaspoons olive or grapeseed oil
> Kosher salt

(continued on next page)

1. Preheat the oven to 400°F.

2. Separate the kale bunch into individual leaves. Wash the kale well and shake off as much water as you can. Cut out the center ribs with a sharp knife. Tear the leaves into 2-inch pieces; you should have 4 to 5 cups. Place the kale on a dish towel, fold the towel over, and gently wring the towel to remove as much moisture as possible.

3. In a large bowl, toss the kale with the oil and ½ teaspoon salt. Scatter the kale in one layer on a large baking sheet. Bake for 5 minutes.

4. Remove from the oven and stir the kale with a silicone spatula to redistribute pieces at the edge toward the center, to ensure even browning. Return the kale to the oven and bake until the leaves are dark brown in spots but not blackened, stirring occasionally, 7 to 10 minutes (check the kale frequently during the last few minutes of baking to avoid burning).

5. Serve immediately, or let cool and store in a sealed container.

Variation: To make seasoned chips, mix the salt with ¼ teaspoon chili powder, onion powder, or garlic powder, or a mixture of your favorite spices.

Each serving: 53 calories, 2 g protein, 7 g carbohydrates, 1 g fiber (net carbs: 6 g), 0 g sugar, 3 g fat (0 g saturated fat), 0 mg cholesterol, 320 mg sodium

SAUCES AND BROTHS

FRESH TOMATO SALSA

(MAKES ABOUT 4 "FREE" CONDIMENT SERVINGS, ¼ CUP EACH)

Use this salsa on egg dishes, chicken, or fish. It is best the day it is made.

    1 cup diced tomato (1 large tomato)
    ½ small jalapeño, seeded and minced, or to taste
    2 tablespoons minced red onion
    1 garlic clove, minced
    2 tablespoons chopped fresh cilantro
    1 teaspoon lime juice, plus more to taste
    Kosher salt and ground black pepper

Mix together the tomato, jalapeño, onion, garlic, cilantro, and lime juice in a medium bowl. Season with salt, pepper, and more lime juice, to taste.

Each serving: 10 calories, 0 g protein, 2 g carbohydrates, 1 g fiber, 1 g sugar, 0 g fat (0 g saturated fat), 0 mg cholesterol, 41 mg sodium

SALSA VERDE

(MAKES 6 SERVINGS, ABOUT 2 TEASPOONS EACH—½ SERVING FAT)

Use this classic Mediterranean topping for grilled fish, chicken, or roasted vegetables.

> 1 garlic clove, coarsely chopped
> 1 tablespoon capers, drained and rinsed
> Kosher salt
> ¼ teaspoon Dijon mustard
> 3 tablespoons minced flat-leaf parsley
> 1 tablespoon minced fresh mint
> ¼ teaspoon grated lemon zest (only the colored part of the skin)
> 1 tablespoon lemon juice, plus more to taste
> 1 tablespoon olive or grapeseed oil
> Ground black pepper

Mash the garlic, capers, and a pinch of salt to a paste with a mortar and pestle. (Or finely chop the garlic and capers, place in a small bowl, and mash with the salt with the back of a spoon.) Stir in the mustard, parsley, mint, lemon zest, lemon juice, and oil. Season with more salt, pepper, and more lemon juice, to taste.

Variations: Mash 1 small anchovy fillet, drained and minced, with the capers.

Try different fresh herbs such as basil, chives, or oregano instead of the mint

Stir in 1 tablespoon minced shallot.

If you prefer a tangier sauce, add a splash of red wine vinegar.

Each serving: 23 calories, 0 g protein, 1 g carbohydrates, 0 g fiber, 0 g sugar, 2 g fat (0 g saturated fat), 0 mg cholesterol, 46 mg sodium (more if you add anchovy)

HOMEMADE TOMATO SAUCE (MAKES ABOUT 3 CUPS)

Use this sauce in the Phase 2 lunch pizza and lasagna recipes.

  1 cup diced onion (1 large onion)
  ¾ cup diced celery (about 3 stalks)
  ½ cup diced carrot (about 1 medium carrot)
  2 teaspoons olive or grapeseed oil
  3 tablespoons tomato paste
  2 teaspoons dried oregano leaves or 1 teaspoon ground oregano
  ⅛ teaspoon cayenne pepper
  1 dried bay leaf
  One 28-ounce can whole tomatoes or 2 pounds fresh tomatoes, peeled and diced
  Kosher salt and ground black pepper

In a medium saucepan, cook the onion, celery, and carrot in the oil, stirring occasionally, until the onion is softened, 4 to 5 minutes. Stir in the tomato paste, oregano, and cayenne and cook for 30 seconds. Add the bay leaf. Crush the canned tomatoes with your hands. Add the tomatoes, with their juices, to the other vegetables. Bring to a boil, reduce the heat to low, and simmer for 30 minutes, stirring occasionally, until sauce has thickened slightly. Season with salt and pepper. Remove the bay leaf before using.

SHRIMP OR FISH BROTH (MAKES ABOUT 2 SERVINGS, 1 CUP EACH—"FREE" CALORIES)

When you peel raw shrimp, save the shells and tails in a resealable plastic bag in the freezer to use for this quick broth. Or when you buy a whole fish from your fishmonger, ask for the head, tail, and backbone to make a fish version. Save the stalk from your morning fennel to use here. This broth freezes well.

  Shells and tails from 2 to 3 pounds raw shrimp, or heads, tails, and bones
    from 1 large or 2 small fish, gills and organs removed, rinsed well to
    remove blood
  ¼ cup dry white wine (optional)
  ½ onion, coarsely chopped
  6-inch piece fennel stalk, coarsely chopped
  1 carrot, peeled and coarsely chopped
  1 celery stalk, coarsely chopped
  1 dried bay leaf
  Generous pinch of cayenne pepper
  ¼ teaspoon kosher salt

In a medium pot, bring 2½ cups water to a boil. Add all the ingredients. Reduce the heat and simmer for 20 minutes, occasionally skimming away any foam that rises to the surface. Strain and cool. Store in the refrigerator and use within 3 days, or freeze in 1-cup containers.

Variation: Add a 2-inch piece of peeled gingerroot.

Each serving: 15 calories, 2 g protein, 0 g carbohydrates, 0 g fiber, 0 g sugar, 0 g fat (0 g saturated fat), 5 mg cholesterol, 200 mg sodium

SALAD DRESSINGS

Use these recipes as dinner accompaniments (at lunch, the recipes already include all of your fat), or build your own lunch (see "Create Your Own Phase 1 and 2 Menus" in Chapter 10) and save a portion of your fat serving to use on your salads and vegetables. The dressings are generous in vinegar to keep your fat calories down and to dress a large amount of greens, so they are meant to be used sparingly; you can adjust the amount of vinegar in each to your taste.

BASIC OR DIJON VINAIGRETTE
(MAKES 6 DINNER SERVINGS, 1½ TEASPOONS EACH—½ SERVING FAT)

The Dijon version is great when you're serving the dressing with grilled fish, grilled vegetables, and salads with tangy cheeses like feta.

> 2 tablespoons red wine vinegar or champagne vinegar
> 2 teaspoons minced shallot
> ¼ teaspoon minced garlic
> ½ teaspoon Dijon mustard (optional)
> 1 tablespoon olive or grapeseed oil
> Kosher salt and ground black pepper

Whisk together the vinegar, shallot, garlic, and mustard, if using, in a small bowl. Gradually whisk in the oil until blended. Season with salt and pepper to taste.

Variations: Add 2 teaspoons minced fresh parsley or chives.

For an Italian-style dressing, add ¼ teaspoon dried oregano leaves.

For an Asian twist, use rice vinegar instead of red wine vinegar and ginger instead of garlic.

Each serving: 22 calories, 0 g protein, 0 g carbohydrates, 0 g fiber, 0 g sugar, 2 g fat (0 g saturated fat), 0 mg cholesterol, 32 mg sodium

BALSAMIC VINAIGRETTE

(MAKES 6 DINNER SERVINGS, 1½ TEASPOONS EACH—½ SERVING FAT)

    2 tablespoons balsamic vinegar
    ½ teaspoon Dijon mustard
    ¼ teaspoon minced garlic
    1 tablespoon olive or grapeseed oil
    Kosher salt and ground black pepper

Whisk together the vinegar, mustard, and garlic in a small bowl. Gradually whisk in the oil until blended. Season with salt and pepper to taste.

Variation: To make a citrusy balsamic dressing, good with goat cheese–topped salads, add ½ teaspoon finely grated orange zest (the colored part only of the skin) instead of the garlic.

Each serving: 21 calories, 0 g protein, 0 g carbohydrates, 0 g fiber, 0 g sugar, 2 g fat (0 g saturated fat), 0 mg cholesterol, 32 mg sodium

LEMON VINAIGRETTE

(MAKES 6 DINNER SERVINGS, 2½ TEASPOONS EACH—½ SERVING FAT)

A light, tangy dressing for slaws, chilled steamed green beans, cucumbers, and other light vegetables.

    ¼ cup lemon juice, or more to taste
    2 teaspoons minced red onion
    2 teaspoons minced fresh parsley
    1 tablespoon olive or grapeseed oil
    Kosher salt and ground black pepper

Whisk together the lemon juice, onion, and parsley in a small bowl. Gradually whisk in the oil until blended. Season with salt and pepper to taste and more lemon juice, if desired.

Variation: For a Caesar dressing, add 2 anchovy fillets, drained and minced, and serve with 3 tablespoons grated Parmesan at dinner.

For a southwestern-style slaw, use lime juice instead of lemon and cilantro instead of parsley.

Each serving: 23 calories, 0 g protein, 1 g carbohydrates, 0 g fiber, 0 g sugar, 2 g fat (0 g saturated fat), 0 mg cholesterol, 28 mg sodium

BREADS

When working with quinoa flour, expect a sticky dough and resist the temptation to add more flour. (The flour will dry out more than wheat flour as it bakes.) The amount of quinoa flour needed will vary by brand, as some are very finely ground, others more coarsely. Adjust the amount of water by a few tablespoons as needed. Quinoa flour dough also requires a longer rising time than most yeast doughs.

PROTEIN BOOST DIET CRUSTY ROLLS (MAKES 14 ROLLS)

These satisfying rolls freeze well. To keep the bread light in texture, handle this dough as little as possible after the first rise—instead of shaping the dough into classic rounds, you slice it like biscotti and shape only the edges.

    1 envelope (2¼ teaspoons) active dry yeast
    1 cup quinoa flour, plus more for dusting
    ¾ cup whole wheat flour
    ½ cup semolina flour
    ⅓ cup flaxseed meal
    ⅓ cup wheat bran
    ⅓ cup whole chia seeds
    ¾ teaspoon kosher salt
    1 teaspoon olive or grapeseed oil, plus more for the bowl

1. Combine the yeast and 1¼ cups lukewarm water in the bowl of a stand mixer fitted with a paddle attachment. Mix well and allow to rest for 5 minutes.

2. In a medium bowl, whisk together 1 cup of the quinoa flour, the whole wheat and semolina flours, flaxseed meal, wheat bran, chia seeds, and salt. Add the oil to the dissolved yeast, then add half of the flour mixture. Mix on low speed for 15 seconds to incorporate the flours. Scrape down the sides of the bowl and the paddle and set aside for 5 minutes.

3. Add the remaining flour mixture and mix on medium-low speed until the dough comes together, scraping down the sides of the bowl and paddle as necessary; the dough will be sticky. Dust the work surface lightly with quinoa flour. Turn the dough out onto the work surface and let rest for 5 minutes.

4. Knead the dough for 5 minutes, adding up to 2 tablespoons quinoa flour if needed, until the dough holds together.

(*continued on next page*)

5. Lightly oil a large bowl. Transfer the dough to the bowl, cover loosely with plastic wrap, and set aside to rise until it has nearly doubled, about 1¼ hours.

6. Line a baking sheet with parchment paper.

7. Lightly press on the dough to deflate it. Cut the dough into two equal pieces. Shape one half into a 7 by 3-inch rectangle (it will look and feel like biscotti dough), handling the dough as little as possible. Score the dough into seven 1 by 3-inch pieces, then slice along the scores. Lay each piece on its side on the work surface. Gently pinch both ends lightly, then press them toward the center of the dough slightly to make a football shape. Place on the baking sheet several inches apart. Repeat with the other half of the dough. Loosely cover with plastic wrap and set aside to rise for 30 to 45 minutes or until slightly puffy; the rolls will not double in size.

8. While the rolls are rising, place a rack in the middle of the oven and pre-heat the oven to 400°F.

9. Remove the plastic wrap and bake the rolls for 10 minutes. Rotate the pan front to back and reduce the heat to 350°F. Bake until golden brown on the bottom (the rolls will be only lightly browned on top), about 20 minutes.

10. Cool on a wire rack. Store in a sealed container, or wrap each roll individually and freeze.

You can also mix the dough by hand: In Step 1, combine the yeast and water in a large bowl. In Step 2, stir in half the flour mixture with a wooden spoon. In Step 3, add the remaining flour mixture gradually, stirring with the wooden spoon, until all the flour has been added and no dry streaks remain. Continue with the rest of the recipe as written.

Each serving (1 roll): 136 calories, 5 g protein, 20 g carbohydrates, 5 g fiber, 0 g sugar, 4 g fat (0 g saturated fat), 0 mg cholesterol, 126 mg sodium

PROTEIN BOOST DIET QUINOA SANDWICH BREAD
(MAKES ONE 9-INCH LOAF, 14 SLICES)

This dough has a rich whole-grain flavor and texture rather than the light, airy texture of commercial sandwich breads made with processed flour, so it will not be as "tall" as many sandwich breads. If you knead the dough by hand, increase the amount of rising time by as much as 30 minutes to aerate the dough.

1 envelope (2¼ teaspoons) active dry yeast
1½ cups quinoa flour
1½ cups whole wheat flour
⅓ cup flaxseed meal
⅓ cup wheat bran
⅓ cup whole chia seeds
¾ teaspoon kosher salt
2 teaspoons olive or grapeseed oil
4 egg whites or ½ cup pasteurized egg whites
Cooking oil spray

1. Combine the yeast and 1 cup plus 2 tablespoons lukewarm water in the bowl of a stand mixer fitted with a paddle attachment. Mix well and allow to rest for 5 minutes.

2. In a medium bowl, mix together the quinoa and whole wheat flours, flaxseed meal, wheat bran, chia seeds, and salt. Stir the oil and egg whites into the dissolved yeast. Add half the flour mixture and mix on low speed for 15 seconds to incorporate the flours. Scrape down the sides of the bowl and the paddle and set aside for 5 minutes.

3. Add the remaining flour mixture and mix on medium-low until the dough comes together, scraping down the sides of the bowl and the paddle as necessary (the dough will be sticky). Replace the paddle attachment with the dough hook and knead on low speed for 6 minutes. Remove the bowl from the mixer, cover it loosely with plastic wrap, and set aside for the dough to rise until nearly doubled, about 1¼ hours.

4. Lightly coat a 9 by 5-inch loaf pan, preferably nonstick, with cooking oil spray. Gently deflate the dough and shape it into an oblong to fit the pan (it does not have to be perfectly smooth on top). Cover loosely with plastic wrap and set aside to rise until the dough almost reaches the top of the pan, 1¼ to 1½ hours.

5. After the loaf has been rising for 45 minutes, place a rack in the middle of the oven and preheat the oven to 350°F.

6. Remove the plastic wrap and bake the bread for 10 minutes. Remove from the oven and lightly tent the pan with aluminum foil. Return to the oven to bake until cooked through (180°F on an instant-read thermometer), 50 minutes to 1 hour. The loaf will be golden brown on the bottom but only light brown on top.

7. Cool completely on a wire rack before slicing. Store in a sealed container, or wrap well and freeze.

(*continued on next page*)

To mix by hand, follow the directions in the variation for *Protein Boost Diet Crusty Rolls*. To knead by hand, follow Steps 3 and 4, but knead the dough for 10 minutes, until it's smooth and elastic.

Each serving (1 slice): 160 calories, 6 g protein, 23 g carbohydrates, 6 g fiber (net carbs: 17 g), 0 g sugar, 5 g fat (0 g saturated fat), 0 mg cholesterol, 145 mg sodium

QUINOA PIZZA DOUGH OR FLATBREAD

(MAKES 3 PIZZAS, 2 SERVINGS EACH; OR 3 FLATBREADS, 4 SERVINGS EACH)

This pizza dough makes a hearty but thin crust that holds up well to toppings. It also makes a great flatbread to serve with soups and salads.

> 1 envelope (2¼ teaspoons) active dry yeast
> 1½ cups quinoa flour, plus more for dusting
> 1¼ cups whole wheat flour
> ½ cup wheat bran
> ¼ cup flaxseed meal
> Kosher salt
> 2 teaspoons olive or grapeseed oil, plus more for the bowl
> Olive oil, coarsely ground black pepper, and grated Parmesan cheese (optional), for topping flatbreads

1. Combine the yeast and 1¼ cups lukewarm water in the bowl of a stand mixer fitted with a paddle attachment. Mix well and allow to rest for 5 minutes.

2. In a medium bowl, combine the quinoa flour, whole wheat flour, wheat bran, flaxseed meal, and ¾ teaspoon salt. Add the oil to the dissolved yeast, then add half the flour mixture and mix on low speed for 15 seconds to incorporate the flours. Scrape down the sides of the bowl and the paddle and set aside for 5 minutes.

3. Add the remaining flour mixture and mix on medium-low until the dough comes together, scraping down the sides of the bowl and the paddle as necessary. Turn the dough out onto a work surface sprinkled lightly with quinoa flour and let rest for 5 minutes.

4. Dust the work surface very lightly with quinoa flour. Knead the dough for 5 minutes, until it is smooth and elastic.

5. Lightly oil a large bowl. Place the dough in the bowl, cover loosely with plastic wrap, and set aside to rise until almost doubled, about 1 hour (it will not rise as much as typical pizza dough).

6. Place a pizza stone in the bottom of the oven and preheat the oven to 450°F. (Alternatively, place a baking sheet upside down on the bottom rack in the oven.) Line a baking sheet with parchment paper.

7. To make pizza, follow the instructions for topping and baking the dough in the *Pizza* recipe.

8. To make flatbread, divide the dough into four pieces. Roll each into an 8 by 12-inch rectangle. Place two flatbreads on the parchment paper, an inch apart at least. Brush lightly with olive oil and sprinkle with salt, pepper, and 1 tablespoon Parmesan, if desired. Bake until golden brown on the bottom and around the edges, 8 to 10 minutes, watching closely during the last few minutes. Cool on a wire rack. Repeat with the remaining two flatbreads.

Variations: Top the flatbread with dried oregano or paprika.

Sprinkle the flatbread with fresh thyme leaves and minced garlic for the last 2 minutes of baking.

Each serving (flatbread): 145 calories, 5 g protein, 24 g carbohydrates, 4 g fiber (net carbs: 20 g), 1 g sugar, 3 g fat (0 g saturated fat), 0 mg cholesterol, 3 mg sodium

INDEX

resynchronizing of, 108
role in Protein Boost Diet of, 217
role in weight loss of, 5
sleep-hormone interactions and,
  97–121
See also cellular clock; circadian
  rhythm/clock
biotin, 183
birth control pills, 41, 62, 124, 126
bisphenol A (BPA), 38–39
Black Bean and Tuna Salad with
  Radicchio (recipe), 298–99
blood pressure
  antioxidants and, 180, 183
  circadian rhythms and, 98
  detoxification and, 167, 180, 187,
    188
  effects of too much weight on, 25
  estrogen-testosterone balance and,
    128, 131, 134
  evaluation of body fat and, 13
  fats and, 164
  fiber and, 158
  growth hormone and, 67
  herbs and spices and, 187
  Mediterranean diet and, 145
  metabolism role in weight gain and,
    13, 19, 24, 25
  protein/amino acids and, 150
  Protein Boost Diet and, 150, 158,
    164
  relaxation and, 86
  resveratrol and, 188
  sleep and, 116, 119
  stress and, 75, 77, 78, 86
  thyroid hormones and, 44, 50, 56
blood sugar
  antioxidants and, 179, 180, 181,
    183
  artificial sweeteners and, 160
  benefits of Protein Boost Diet and, 4,
    148, 150, 155, 156, 157, 160
  carbohydrates and, 4, 155, 156, 157,
    227
  cellular clock and, 104
  circadian rhythms and, 100, 101,
    105, 107
  cortisol and, 101
  detoxification and, 179, 180, 181,
    185, 187, 188
  drinks and, 185
  environmental toxins and, 38
  estrogen-testosterone balance and,
    134

exercise and, 243
fiber and, 157
fundamentals of Protein Boost Diet
  and, 217
glycemic load and, 155, 156, 157
growth hormone and, 67
herbs and spices and, 187
insulin and, 23, 24
Mediterranean diet and, 145
metabolism role in weight gain and,
  11, 17, 23, 24, 27
nighttime eating and, 107, 217
protein/amino acids and, 150
reservatrol and, 188
stress and, 35, 75, 81
tests concerning, 200
thyroid hormones and, 65
what to eat when and, 100, 217,
  227
See also glycemic load
blood tests, 1, 72, 73, 139, 140, 170,
  197–200
body mass
  antioxidants and, 180
  calcium and, 188–89
  chart for, 204–5
  detoxification and, 180, 188–89
  estrogen-testosterone balance and,
    132, 139
  exercise and, 284
  insulin and, 24
  measuring, 204–5
  metabolism role in weight gain and,
    12, 13–14, 24
  stress and, 86
  thyroid hormones and, 49
  toxic environment and, 38
  tracking progress and, 205–6
body rhythms. *See* biological clock;
  cellular clock; circadian rhythm/
  clock
body temperature, 1, 18, 20, 44, 45,
  65, 99, 104, 117, 120, 128–29,
  130, 164
bones, 58, 67, 126, 137, 188
bowel movements, 65, 93, 158. *See also*
  constipation
bracelet, 207, 209
brain
  antioxidants and, 177, 180, 181,
    183
  artificial sweeteners and, 160, 164
  circadian rhythm and, 98–103
  cognitive/thinking, 79, 80

brain (*cont.*)
  common impediments to weight loss
    and, 212, 213
  detoxification and, 177, 180,
    181,184
  dopamine and, 93, 94
  drinks and, 184
  emotional, 77, 79–80, 82, 241
  estrogen-testosterone balance and,
    124, 129, 131, 133, 136, 139
  exercise and, 91, 239
  fats and, 162, 164
  functions of, 90
  genetics and, 34
  growth hormone and, 70–72
  metabolism role in weight gain and,
    11, 14–15, 16, 17, 20, 23, 26–27
  probiotics and, 92, 93
  Protein Boost Diet and, 160, 162,
    164
  relaxation techniques and, 86, 241
  scheduled eating and, 220
  serotonin and, 90, 91, 97, 119, 124,
    129
  sleep and, 98–103, 109, 116, 119,
    120
  stress and, 26–27, 76, 77, 79–80,
    81–83, 86, 90, 91, 92, 93, 94
  thyroid hormones and, 1, 44, 45, 62,
    90
  tips for long-term success and, 207
  training the, 81–83, 94
  See also hypothalamus
breads, 203, 212, 215, 219, 329–33
breakfast
  circadian rhythms and, 100, 102,
    103, 106
  correct sequence of foods for, 221
  creating your own menus for, 236
  detoxification and, 168, 169
  ghrelin and, 102
  Meal Plans and, 226–27, 228–29,
    232–33, 236, 286–90, 291–92
  number of calories for, 236, 286,
    291
  recipes for, 286–92
  sample, 228–29
  scheduled eating and, 217, 220
  supplements for, 190
  what to eat for, 100, 106, 152, 153,
    154, 157, 158, 159, 161, 165, 216,
    217, 221, 226–27, 232–33, 236
breathing, 25, 85, 86, 88, 98, 112, 196,
  251. *See also* sleep apnea

buddies/partners, weight-loss, 208, 210,
  212

Caesar salad dressing (recipe variation),
  328
caffeine, 174, 184
calcium
  antioxidants and, 181, 190
  common impediments to weight loss
    and, 214
  detoxification and, 168, 181, 188–
    89, 190
  as favorite supplement, 190, 191
  functions of, 188–89
  milk and, 161
  Protein Boost Diet and, 161
  supplements and, 189, 190, 191
  thyroid hormones and, 57, 60–61,
    189–90
  vitamin D and, 189
  when to take, 190
calories
  burn rate of, 147, 149–52
  exercise and, 239, 240, 244, 283–84
  as factor determining weight, 14
  metabolism role in weight gain and,
    2, 3, 15, 19, 20, 27
  for Protein Boost Diet, 216, 217,
    236, 237
  severe restriction of, 15, 144, 166
  sleep and, 100, 105, 106
  stress and, 76
  thyroid hormones and, 44, 47
  See also specific meal or recipe
cancer, 25, 37, 73, 132, 133, 134, 157,
  160, 164, 165, 177, 179, 181, 182
capsaicin, 186
carbamazepine, 62
carbohydrates
  addiction to, 218
  antioxidants and, 177, 181
  blood sugar and, 4, 227
  and commercial low-carb diets, 144
  correct sequence of foods and, 221
  detoxification and, 171, 174, 177,
    181
  dopamine and, 94
  eating out and, 215
  energy and, 100
  estrogen-testosterone balance and, 127
  fats and, 162
  Favorite Foods and, 222
  functions of, 155–57
  glycemic load and, 155–56

curried lentil-veal ragout (recipe variation), 300
Curtsy Lunge (exercise), 280
Cushing's syndrome, 77–78
cycling, 88, 197, 248–49, 282–83
cytokines, 117

dairy products
  common impediments to weight loss and, 214
  detoxification and, 170
  fats and, 162–63
  as Favorite Foods, 225
  food sensitivities and, 170
  Meal Plans and, 226, 228–29, 232, 234–38
  Mediterranean diet and, 145
  organic, 202
  protein/amino acids and, 151, 153–54
  recipes and side dishes with, 288, 289, 290, 292, 305, 306, 307, 311, 312, 313, 315, 317
  role in Protein Boost Diet of, 151, 153–54, 162–63, 189
  shopping for, 202–3
  stocking the pantry with, 201
  when to eat, 228–29, 232, 234–38
danazol, 61–62
dancing, 282
Day 1 workout, 251, 252–56
Day 2 workout, 251, 257–61
Day 3 workout, 251, 262–66
Day 4 workout, 251, 267–71
Day 5 workout, 251, 272–73
Day 6 workout, 251, 274–77
Day 7 workout, 251, 278–81
dementia, 134, 145, 181
depression
  antioxidants and, 177, 180, 181, 182
  detoxification and, 177, 180, 181, 182
  dopamine and, 95
  effects of too much weight and, 25
  estrogen-testosterone balance and, 125, 129, 139
  exercise and, 89, 248
  fats and, 164
  genetics and, 35–36
  growth hormone and, 67, 69–70, 71
  hypothyroidism and, 32
  medications for, 42, 82

metabolism and, 30, 31, 32, 33
obesity and, 89
probiotics and, 93
protein/amino acids and, 151
Protein Boost Diet and, 151, 164
relaxation and, 85
serotonin and, 25, 89–91, 119
sleep and, 109, 111, 116, 119
stress and, 82, 85, 88, 89–91, 93, 95
thyroid hormones and, 1, 44, 52, 54, 57, 59
weight connection to, 89–91
deprivation diet. *See* restrictive/starvation diet
desserts. *See* sweets/desserts
Detox Smoothie, 6, 167–69, 201, 202, 213, 217, 228
detoxification, 166–91
  antioxidants and, 167, 168, 169, 174, 176–84, 185, 186, 187, 189
  benefits of Protein Boost Diet and, 6
  and body's detox defenses, 169
  calcium and, 168, 181, 188–89, 190
  Candida yeast and, 167, 171
  common impediments to weight loss and, 213–14
  cravings and, 218
  definition of, 166–67
  drinks and, 166, 174–76, 184–85
  fiber and, 6, 158
  food and, 166, 167, 169–70, 174–76
  gluten sensitivity and, 170–71
  heavy metals and, 173
  herbs/spices and, 176–84, 186–88
  Meal Plans and, 218
  mercury and, 173–74
  micronutrients and, 176–84, 189
  probiotics and, 171, 172–73
  resveratrol and, 188
  sleep and, 177, 185
  spices/herbs and, 176–84, 186–88
  sugar and, 6
  supplements and, 166, 173, 176–84, 190–91
  See also Detox Smoothie
DHEA (dehydroepiandrosterone), 122, 138–39
DHEA-S (dehydroepiandrosterone sulfate), 138–39, 199
diabetes
  antioxidants and, 179
  bariatric surgery and, 17
  benefits of Protein Boost Diet and, 156, 157

Emily (patient), 111–12
emotions, 10–11, 35, 62, 74, 111–12,
    124, 151, 179. *See also* mood;
    specific emotion
employee health programs, 250
energy
    antioxidants and, 177, 179, 183,
        184
    benefits of Protein Boost Diet and, 2
    carbohydrates and, 100, 155
    cellular clock and, 104
    circadian rhythms and, 100–101
    common impediments to weight loss
        and, 214
    detoxification and, 170, 176, 179,
        185, 186–88
    drinks and, 185
    estrogen-testosterone balance and,
        139
    exercise and, 239–40, 241, 243
    fats and, 165
    food sensitivities and, 170
    fructose and, 159
    fundamentals of Protein Boost Diet
        and, 217
    GABA and, 91, 92
    growth hormone and, 67
    herbs/spices and, 186–88
    hormone balance/imbalance and, 1
    metabolism role in weight gain and,
        3, 11, 18
    protein/amino acids and, 5, 143,
        217
    relaxation and, 86
    sleep and, 100–101, 104, 106, 109,
        112
    stress and, 78, 86, 87, 91, 92
    supplements and, 176
    thyroid hormones and, 1, 100–101
    timing of meals and, 100
    when you eat what and, 106
environment
    as factor influencing hormone
        balance and weight gain, 29,
        37–41
    genetics and, 33–37
    household, 33–34
    importance of, 5
    metabolism role in weight gain and,
        10–11
    sleep, 121
    stress/anxiety and, 34–37, 76
    toxins/obesogens in, 29, 37–41
    uterine, 34

epigallocatechin gallate (EGCG), 185
epinephrine, 183
Erik (patient), 116–17
estradiol, 126–27, 133, 135, 136, 138,
    199
estrogen
    balancing of testosterone, 122–40
    benefits of, 126–27
    detoxification and, 166
    functions of, 126–27
    growth hormone and, 67–68
    importance of, 127–28
    serotonin and, 90
    sleep and, 119
    thyroid hormones and, 62
    See also hormone replacement
        therapy; menopause; menstruation
exercise(s)
    antioxidants and, 177, 181
    for arms, 274–77
    for back of body, 262–66
    Backstroke, 273
    Close Hand Push-up, 275
    Cobra, 262, 273
    common impediments to weight loss
        and, 214
    for core muscles, 257–61, 272–73,
        278–81
    Crunches, 252, 272
    Curtsy Lunge, 280
    detoxification and, 177, 181, 186
    diary about, 208
    Dips, 277
    dopamine and, 95
    effects on appetite of, 241
    estrogen-testosterone balance and,
        132
    fats and, 165
    food intake and, 240
    Forward Lunge with Rotation, 267
    for front of body (including belly),
        252–56
    genetics and, 36
    goal of, 242
    in groups, 89, 284
    growth hormone and, 5, 67, 73
    herbs/spices and, 186
    importance of, 5, 239, 240
    insulin and, 5
    Kneeling Plank with Kicks, 279
    Leaning Toe Touches, 271
    Leg Raises, 253, 272
    for legs, 267–71, 272
    leptin and, 5

GABA (gamma-aminobutyric acid)
  antioxidants and, 183
  as favorite supplement, 191
  probiotics and, 93
  protein/amino acids and, 151
  role in Protein Boost Diet of, 147,
    151
  serotonin and, 90
  sleep and, 99, 102, 103, 120
  sources of, 92
  stress and, 91
  thyroid hormones and, 62, 64
gamma linoleic acid, 164
Garcinia cambogia, 186
garlic, 183, 187, 201, 226, 327, 328
gastrin, 151
gastrointestinal tract (GI)
  common impediments to weight loss
    and, 212–13
  detoxification and, 167, 170, 172–
    73, 187
  estrogen-testosterone balance and,
    126
  fiber and, 158
  food choices and, 26
  food sensitivities and, 170
  fructose and, 159
  herbs/spices and, 187
  metabolism role in weight gain and,
    26, 31
  probiotics and, 92–93
  protein/amino acids and, 149, 151
gender
  abdominal fat and, 127
  effects of too much weight and, 25
  growth hormone and, 68
  metabolism role in weight gain and,
    15
  sleep and, 118–19
  thyroid disorders and, 43
  See also women
genetically modified food, 175–76
genetics, 29, 33–37, 54, 106
GERD (gastroesophageal reflux
  disorder), 25
ghrelin
  breakfast and, 102
  circadian rhythm and, 98, 99, 102
  dinner and, 102
  fiber and, 158
  functions of, 2, 14, 16–17, 64, 102
  hormone triangle and, 14, 16–17, 18,
    19, 20
  lunch and, 102

Meal Plans and, 19
  metabolism role in weight gain and,
    10, 14, 16–17, 18, 19, 20, 26
  nighttime eating and, 107
  overview about, 16–17
  protein/amino acids and, 149
  scheduled eating and, 220
  sleep and, 98, 99, 102, 107, 112
  stress and, 26, 79
  thyroid hormones and, 2, 48, 64
ginger, 183, 187, 201, 211, 226, 327.
    See also specific recipe
ginger-soy marinated tofu (recipe
  variation), 287
glucocorticoids, 31–32, 41, 42, 61–62,
    124, 132, 133
glucose
  antioxidants and, 180, 181
  benefits of Protein Boost Diet and,
    148
  carbohydrates and, 155–56
  cellular clock and, 21–22, 104
  circadian clock and, 105
  detoxification and, 180, 181
  estrogen-testosterone balance and,
    123
  fats and, 164
  glycemic load and, 155–56
  growth hormone and, 66
  insulin and, 21–22, 23, 25
  Mediterranean diet and, 145
  metabolism role in weight gain in,
    21–22, 23, 24, 25, 35
  protein and, 148
  shopping and, 203
  sleep-weight connection and, 104,
    105
  stress and, 35
  tests concerning, 199, 200
  when you eat what and, 106
  See also blood sugar; sugar
glutamine, 154
glutathione, 178, 179, 183. *See also*
  L-glutathione
gluten, 153, 155, 170–71, 172, 199,
    203, 219
gluteus: exercises for, 278–81
glycemic load
  benefits of Protein Boost Diet and, 6
  carbohydrates and, 155–56, 157
  circadian rhythms and, 99, 100,
    101–2, 103, 106
  estrogen-testosterone balance and,
    123–24

legumes/lentils (*cont.*)
  recipes with, 288, 293, 294, 295,
    299, 300, 301–2, 308–10
  role in Protein Boost Diet of, 145,
    150, 152, 153, 154, 156, 157, 158,
    172
  shopping and, 202
  starch and, 157
  stress and, 92
  when to eat, 217, 221, 227, 228–35,
    237–38, 293
Lemon Vinaigrette (recipe), 321, 328
Lemony Roast Salmon or Snapper
  (recipe), 314–15
Lentil-Veal Ragout (recipe), 300–301
leptin
  antioxidants and, 176, 178, 179
  benefits of Protein Boost Diet and,
    6, 148
  calcium and, 189
  carbohydrates and, 156
  cellular clock and, 104
  circadian rhythm and, 98, 99
  detoxification and, 166, 176, 178,
    179, 187, 189
  efficiency/inefficiency of, 16, 18, 19,
    24, 45, 47–48, 49, 97, 99, 100,
    117, 122, 127, 148, 156, 178
  environmental toxins and, 37
  estrogen-testosterone balance and,
    123, 127, 132
  exercise and, 5
  fats and, 162, 164
  functions of, 2, 5, 9, 10, 14, 18, 45,
    47–48, 50, 76, 101
  fundamentals of Protein Boost Diet
    and, 217
  glycemic load and, 156
  growth hormone and, 63
  herbs/spices and, 187
  hormone triangle and, 14–16, 17, 18,
    19, 20
  insulin and, 23
  metabolism role in weight gain and,
    9, 10, 14–16, 17, 18, 19, 20, 23,
    24, 26
  nighttime eating and, 107
  overview about, 14–16
  paradox of, 15
  protein/amino acids and, 6, 112, 143,
    150, 151, 217, 227
  relaxation and, 85
  resistance to, 16, 19, 23, 24, 48, 65, 85,
    112, 123, 127, 147, 162, 164, 176

  role in Protein Boost Diet of, 146
  sensitivity to, 6, 65, 187
  sex hormones and, 122
  sleep and, 97, 98, 99, 100, 101, 104,
    107, 110, 112, 117, 196
  stress and, 26, 76, 79, 85
  supplements and, 176
  thyroid hormones and, 2, 45, 47–48,
    49, 50, 58, 63, 65, 66
  timing of meals and, 100
  too much, 50, 147
Leslie (patient), 113–14
leucine, 150
levothyroxine, 57, 58, 59, 62, 63
L-glutathione, 179, 181, 183, 190
LH (luteinizing hormone), 123, 199
lifestyle
  common impediments to weight loss
    and, 212
  hormone-replacement therapy and,
    134
  need for change in, 27, 210
  Protein Boost Diet as, 214
  sedentary, 12, 29, 30, 240, 241
  thyroid hormones and, 49
light/dark cycles. *See* biological clock;
  circadian rhythm/clock
lithium, 40, 42, 54, 55
liver
  antioxidants and, 179, 180, 181, 183
  carbohydrates and, 156
  cellular clock and, 104
  common impediments to weight loss
    and, 214
  detoxification and, 167, 168, 169,
    174, 179, 180, 181, 183, 185
  drinks and, 185
  effects of too much weight and, 25
  estrogen-testosterone balance and,
    126, 128
  exercise and, 243
  fats and, 164
  growth hormone and, 66
  insulin and, 22
  nighttime eating and, 107
  protein/amino acids and, 150
  tests concerning, 198
  timing of meals and, 107
  toxic environment and, 37
L-theanine, 88, 184, 191
L-tyrosine, 95
Lucy (patient), 129
lunch
  circadian rhythms and, 100, 102, 106

supplements and, 189
thyroid hormones and, 101
timing of meals and, 100
toxic environment and, 37, 38
Monica (patient), 69–70
monosodium glutamate, 213
monounsaturated fat, 6, 63, 145, 163
mood
  antioxidants and, 180, 181, 182, 183
  benefits of Protein Boost Diet and, 2,
    6, 147, 164
  detoxification and, 170, 171, 180,
    181, 182, 184
  dopamine and, 95
  drinks and, 184
  estrogen-testosterone balance and,
    124, 129, 130, 140
  exercise and, 239, 241, 248
  fats and, 6, 164
  food sensitivities and, 170
  growth hormone and, 43, 67
  hormone balance/imbalance and, 1
  medications for, 42
  menopause and, 129, 130
  metabolism role in weight gain and,
    18, 33
  probiotics and, 93
  protein/amino acids and, 143, 151,
    152
  relaxation and, 85
  serotonin and, 90, 91
  sleep and, 110, 117
  stress and, 74, 76, 82, 83, 85, 87, 90,
    91, 93, 95
  thyroid hormones and, 43, 44, 45,
    62, 90, 129, 130
  See also emotions
Moroccan-spiced soup (recipe
    variation), 299
Moroccan-style chicken and vegetable
    skewers (recipe variation), 317
motivation
  benefits of Protein Boost Diet and,
    147
  buddies/partners and, 210
  dopamine and, 93
  estrogen-testosterone balance and,
    129, 139
  hormone balance/imbalance and, 1,
    46, 71
  stress and, 74, 80, 81, 85
  tips for long-term success and, 207,
    209

multivitamins, 61, 190
muscles/joints
  antioxidants and, 179, 180, 182
  benefits of Protein Boost Diet and,
    148
  BMI and, 14
  calcium and, 188
  carbohydrates and, 156
  cellular clock and, 104
  detoxification and, 179, 180, 182, 188
  estrogen-testosterone balance and,
    126, 132
  exercise and, 240, 241, 242, 243,
    245–46, 251, 252
  fats and, 162, 165
  growth hormone and, 67, 73, 126
  hormone balance/imbalance and, 1
  insulin and, 22
  protein/amino acids and, 150, 151,
    154
  relaxation and, 87
  sleep and, 104, 118, 119
  stress and, 78, 87
  thyroid hormones and, 44, 58, 62, 65
mustard-glazed salmon (recipe
    variation), 314
myokines, 240

National Cholesterol Education
    Program, 161
National Dairy Council, 161
National Heart, Lung, and Blood
    Institute (NHLBI), 13
Nature-Throid, 60
neuropeptide Y, 118, 127
neurotransmitters, 91, 124–25, 152,
    166, 180, 181, 183. *See also
    specific neurotransmitter*
niacin, 61–62, 179, 180, 183
Niçoise Salad (recipe), 297–98
night sweats, 125–26, 131
nighttime eating, 30, 107–8, 196, 217,
    227
noradrenaline, 10, 62, 64, 75, 77, 80,
    90, 99, 113, 152, 166, 242
norepinephrine, 181
Northeastern University: exercise study
    at, 89
nuclei accumbens, 80
nutmeg, 201, 211, 226, 307
nuts/seeds
  antioxidants and, 183
  carbohydrates and, 156

nuts/seeds *(cont.)*
    detoxification and, 183
    dopamine and, 95
    environmental toxins and, 39
    fats and, 161, 162, 164
    as Favorite Foods, 225, 226
    fiber and, 157
    food sensitivities and, 169
    GABA and, 92
    herbs/spices and, 187, 201, 226
    Meal Plans and, 228–29, 231, 232,
        233, 234, 235, 237–38
    Mediterranean diet and, 145
    protein/amino acids and, 151, 152
    recipes with, 286, 290
    serotonin and, 91
    shopping for, 202
    stocking the pantry and, 201
    thyroid treatment and, 57
    when to eat, 211, 228–29, 231, 232,
        233, 234, 235, 237–38, 286
    See also type of nut or seed

obesity/overweight
    antioxidants and, 178, 179, 182
    calcium and, 189
    carbohydrates and, 156
    causes of, 49–50
    cellular clock and, 104
    characteristics of, 12–14
    circadian rhythm and, 98, 105
    depression and, 89, 90–91
    detoxification and, 170, 175, 178,
        179, 182, 189
    disadvantages of, 11–12
    dopamine and, 94
    environmental toxins and, 37
    estrogen-testosterone balance and,
        123, 125, 127, 136
    evaluation of, 12–14
    exercise and, 243, 249–50
    fiber and, 157
    food sensitivities and, 170
    genetics and, 33–34
    glycemic load and, 156
    growth hormone and, 68–69
    health effects of, 25
    metabolism role in weight gain and,
        11–14, 19
    nighttime eating and, 107
    prevalence of, 11–12
    protein/amino acids and, 150
    serotonin and, 90–91

sleep and, 98, 104, 105, 106, 107,
        109, 110–11, 118
    socializing and, 90
    stress and, 80, 89, 90–91, 94
    thyroid hormones and, 48, 49–50
    what you eat and, 106
    zinc as treatment for, 182
obesogens, 29, 31, 37–41, 174
oils
    antioxidants and, 183
    to avoid, 203
    cookware and, 201
    detoxification and, 183
    eating out and, 215
    fats and, 161, 162, 164–65, 311
    as Favorite Food, 226
    hydrogenated, 203
    Meal Plans and, 228–38
    Mediterranean diet and, 145
    recipes with, 286–89, 291–304,
        306–9, 311–32
    for relaxation, 89
    role in Protein Boost Diet of, 165
    shopping and, 203
    stocking the pantry with, 201
    in toxic environment, 40
    when to eat, 228–35, 237–38, 286,
        287, 311
    See also salad dressings; *specific
        recipe*
oligofructose, 172
omega-3 fatty acids, 91, 163, 164, 173,
        174, 191, 197
omega-6 fatty acids, 164–65
optimism: feelings of, 147, 209
oral contraceptives, 171
organic food, 39, 201–2
orlistat, 177
osteoarthritis, 25, 128
osteoporosis, 126, 188
overweight. *See* obesity/overweight
oxidative stress
    antioxidants and, 6, 177–78, 179,
        181, 183
    benefits of Protein Boost Diet and, 6
    detoxification and, 167, 168, 177–
        78, 179, 181, 184, 185, 187
    drinks and, 184, 185
    health effects of too much weight
        and, 25
    herbs/spices and, 187
    metabolism role in weight gain and,
        24, 36

milk and, 161
PRO diet and, 145
protein/amino acids and, 152
role in Protein Boost Diet of, 165
shopping and, 203
sources of, 163
total daily amount of, 217
as type of fat, 162, 163
when to eat, 227
See also specific recipe
sauces and broths
eating out and, 215
recipes for, 324–27
schedules
for meals, 4, 5, 24, 105–7, 108, 195–96, 217, 220–21
for sleep, 108–9, 120–21
for successful launch of diet, 195–97
seafood. *See* fish/seafood
Seafood Ceviche (recipe), 311–12
Sean (patient), 71–72
sedentary lifestyle, 12, 29, 30, 240, 241
selenium, 19, 54, 63, 157, 178, 182, 183, 190, 200
serotonin
antioxidants and, 182, 183
benefits of Protein Boost Diet and, 147, 148
brain and, 90, 91, 97, 119, 124, 129
depression/mood and, 25, 89–91, 147
detoxification and, 166, 182
in diet pills, 177
estrogen-testosterone balance and, 124, 129
fats and, 164
genetics and, 34
health effects of too much weight and, 25
protein/amino acids and, 148, 150, 151, 155
relaxation and, 87
sleep and, 97, 110, 119
stress and, 80, 87, 89–91
thyroid hormones and, 62, 64
sertraline, 91
setbacks, 208–9, 210
sex drive, 71, 74, 90, 109, 116, 130, 137, 138, 139
sex hormones
circadian rhythm and, 98
environmental toxins and, 40–41
growth hormone and, 69, 122
insulin and, 122

leptin and, 15, 122
Meal Plans and, 19
metabolism role in weight gain and, 15, 19, 32
sleep and, 97, 98
thyroid hormones and, 128–30
See also specific hormone
SHBG, 199
shopping, 196, 201–3, 209
Shrimp or Fish Broth (recipe), 326–27
Shrimp Quinoa Risotto (recipe), 303
Side Lunges (exercise), 260
Side Plank (exercise), 258
Side Step-Ups (exercise), 261
skin
antioxidants and, 181, 183
detoxification and, 169, 181
dry, 1, 32, 44, 71, 125, 128, 130
estrogen-testosterone balance and, 125, 130
growth hormone and, 71
hypothyroidism and, 32
thyroid hormones and, 1, 44, 128, 130
skipping meals, 30, 212, 214
sleep
amount of, 196
antioxidants and, 177
bedtime and, 120–21
benefits of Protein Boost Diet and, 6, 147, 156
brain and, 98–103, 109, 116, 119, 120
carbohydrates and, 112, 156
cellular clock and, 103–4, 105–7
circadian rhythm/clock and, 98–103, 104, 105–7, 108, 120
common impediments to weight loss and, 214
cortisol and, 101–3, 104, 107, 110, 113, 117
detoxification and, 177, 185
diary about, 208
disturbances, 109–14
environment for, 121
estrogen-testosterone balance and, 119, 125, 129, 130–31, 140
exercise and, 120
fragmentation, 109, 114–15
GABA and, 91
ghrelin and, 98, 99, 102, 107, 112
glycemic load and, 227
growth hormone and, 6, 63, 67, 73, 98, 101, 102, 110, 113, 114, 118, 196

ABOUT THE AUTHOR

Ridha Arem, MD, is a world-renowned endocrinologist and director of the Texas Thyroid Institute. He has served as clinical professor of medicine at Baylor College of Medicine for many years and was also chief of endocrinology and metabolism at Ben Taub General Hospital in Houston. He was the founder and editor in chief of *Clinical Thyroidology*, an official publication of the American Thyroid Association, and is the author of the groundbreaking bestseller *The Thyroid Solution*.

www.AremWellness.com
www.TexasThyroidInstitute.com